HMO——
RATE SETTING
& FINANCIAL
STRATEGY

HMO
RATE SETTING
& FINANCIAL
STRATEGY

Charles William Wrightson, Jr.

Health Administration Press Perspectives
Ann Arbor, Michigan   1990

95   94   93   92   91   5   4   3   2   1

Library of Congress Cataloging-in-Publication Data

Wrightson, Charles William.
    HMO rate setting and financial strategy / Charles William Wrightson, Jr.
    p.   cm.
    ISBN 0-910701-49-0
    1. Health maintenance organizations—United States—Rates.
2. Health maintenance organizations—United States—Finance. I. Title.
RA413.5.U5W75   1990   362.1'0425—dc20   89-20072 CIP

Health Administration Press
A division of the Foundation of the
   American College of Healthcare Executives
1021 East Huron Street
Ann Arbor, Michigan 48104–9990
(313) 764-1380

Table of Contents

Foreword by Gino A. Nalli xiii

Preface xvii

Acknowledgments xxi

Part I   The Current Competitive Environment

Chapter 1   Introduction and Background **3**

1.1   Introduction 3
1.2   The Debate over Premium Rate Setting 5
1.3   The Health Maintenance Organization Amendments
      of 1988 6
1.4   National Health Policy in the 1980s 6
1.5   Increased Competition in Health
      Care Markets 11
1.6   Outline 15

Chapter 2   History of HMOs **25**

2.1   Introduction 25
2.2   Prepaid Group Practice Plans 26
2.3   The Health Maintenance Organization Act
      of 1973 27
2.4   Development of the HMO Industry:
      1973–1988 31

Chapter 3   Key Features of the HMO Concept **45**

3.1   Introduction 45
3.2   Differences between HMOs and Other Forms
      of Health Insurance 49
3.3   HMO Cost-Containment Methods 51

3.4　HMO Risk-Sharing Models 58

Chapter 4　**The Debate between HMOs and Employers** ... **69**

4.1　Introduction 69
4.2　Key Issues of Concern to Employers 70
4.3　Premium Rate Setting: The HMO Perspective 81
4.4　The Health Maintenance Organization Amendments
　　　of 1988 88
4.5　Summary 101

Part II　HMO Rate Setting

Chapter 5　**Rating and Underwriting** **113**

5.1　Introduction to Rating 114
5.2　Underwriting for Group Health Insurance................ 123
5.3　The Statistical Nature of the
　　　Underwriting Process 128
5.4　Marketing, Underwriting, and Rating 134
5.5　HMO Underwriting Methods 137

Chapter 6　**Community Rating** **143**

6.1　Introduction 143
6.2　Federal Legislation and Regulations 144
6.3　Community-Rating Methods 147
6.4　Community Rating by Class 174

Chapter 7　**Alternative Rating Methods** **195**

7.1　Introduction 195
7.2　Adjusted Community Rating 199
7.3　Kaiser Permanente's Adjusted
　　　Community-Rating System 206
7.4　Experience Rating 213
7.5　Group-Specific Rating 218
7.6　Rating and Data Analysis Strategies 232

Chapter 8　**Selection Bias and Premium Rate Setting** **245**

8.1　Introduction 245
8.2　What Is Selection Bias? 247
8.3　HMOs and ''Skimming'' 252
　　Appendix　Selection Bias: An Overview 258

Part III HMO Competitive Strategy

Chapter 9   Issues, Trends, and Goals Affecting HMO Competitive Strategy **295**

9.1   Introduction 295
9.2   Current Issues Affecting HMO
        Competitive Strategy 297
9.3   Forecast of Trends 299
9.4   Immediate Goals for HMOs 300
9.5   Financial Strategies 307
9.6   Other HMO Competitive Strategy Issues 313
9.7   Conclusion 324

Epilogue 333

Glossary of HMO Actuarial Terminology 341

Index 345

About the Author 354

List of Figures

5-1 Distribution of Actual-to-Expected Costs by Size of Group:
50 Members 130

5-2 Distribution of Actual-to-Expected Costs by Size of Group:
100 Members 131

5-3 Distribution of Actual-to-Expected Costs by Size of Group:
500 Members 132

5-4 Distribution of Actual-to-Expected Costs by Size of Group:
1,000 Members 133

5-5 Distribution of Actual-to-Expected Costs by Size of Group:
2,500 Members 134

5-6 Distribution of Actual-to-Expected Costs by Size of Group:
5,000 Members 135

6-1 Overview of Premium Rate–Setting Practices 151

List of Tables

2-1   Selected HMO Organizations from 1900 to 1970 28
2-2   Growth of HMO Industry.. 31
2-3   1980 HMO Membership 33
2-4   HMO Plan Characteristics, January 1988............................... 35
2-5   HMO Enrollment Growth (Number of Members Added) and
Growth Rate for Calendar Years 1981 to 1987 36
2-6   30 Largest Plans Ranked by Enrollment, January 1988............... 37
2-7   HMO Membership Growth by Model Type,
June 1980 to January 1988 38
2-8   HMOs and Enrollment by State Headquarters, January 1988 40
2-9   Number of TEFRA Risk HMOs and Enrollees, June 1985
to December 1986.. 41
2-10   Number of Risk HMOs by Model Type, June 1985 to
December 1986 42
2-11   Kaiser Permanente Medical Care Program Total Enrollment,
by Region.. 42
2-12   Kaiser Permanente Medical Care Program
Community Rate Increases for 1985 to 1989 43
6-1   Types of Premium Rate Structures.. 149
6-2   Operating Budget for Staff-Model and Group-Model HMOs 156
6-3   Development of Medical Service Capitation Cost
(Based on Fee-for-Service Charge Method) 160
6-4   Determination of Total HMO Capitation Rate
(Including Medical Services Costs, Adjustments,
Administration, and Other Loadings).. 163
6-5   Community Rating by Class: Example 1 180
6-6   Community Rating by Class: Example 2 183
6-7   Baseline Data for Community Rating by Class Using
Age/Sex Factors: Example 3 186

6-8   Derivation of Medical Service Cost for Ajax Box Company
Using Community Rating by Class: Example 3 188

6-9   Derivation of Premium Rate for Three-Tier Contracts
Using Community Rating by Class: Example 3 189

7-1   Example of Adjusted Community Rating 202

List of Exhibits

3-1 HMO Cost-Containment Methods 52

3-2 Summary of GAO Report on Physician Incentive Payments
by Prepaid Health Plans 64

6-1 Derivation of Community Rate Increase Factor 158

6-2 Flexible Forms of Community Rating: Two-Tier
Rate Structure, Standard PMPM Revenue Requirement 166

6-3 Flexible Forms of Community Rating: Three-Tier
Rate Structure, Standard PMPM Revenue Requirement 167

6-4 Flexible Forms of Community Rating: Recomposition of
Premiums to Match In-Force Rates 171

6-5 Flexible Forms of Community Rating: The Effect
of Different Contract Mixes 172

6-6 Flexible Forms of Community Rating: The Effect
of Different Assumptions for Contract Mixes, Contract Sizes,
and In-Force Rates 173

Foreword

HMO Rate Setting and Financial Strategy will serve as a needed and valuable resource. It is an excellent technical handbook on rate setting, and it is more than that. It discusses the art of rate setting as well, and places it within the HMO industry's historical context and within a framework of competitive strategy. It is this multidimensional perspective that makes the book such a useful reference.

I served as president of a large and successful regional HMO for nearly ten years. From that perspective I know the rate-setting process is the HMO's ultimate bottom line. How good are the HMO's utilization review programs? How do its premiums compare competitively? How administratively efficient is its operation?

More recently, I am a consultant for large corporations and other purchasers of care. From this perspective my observation is that purchasers are increasingly squeezed by their commitment to provide employees good health coverage and by the relentless rise in costs, from which cost-containment promises have provided little relief.

Cost-containment efforts have followed two basic strategies. Cost shifting to the patient/consumer was the first strategy. If a patient were responsible for more of his health care bill through increased deductibles, copayments, or other out-of-pocket expenses, the reasoning went, he would be a more prudent consumer. While a reasonable approach for primary care services, cost sharing offers limited potential for saving when medical needs are catastrophic or when a patient needs sophisticated technological interventions.

The second strategy was based on the designation of an independent third party to oversee the appropriateness and necessity of a patient-physician interface. Preadmission certification and second surgical opinions are examples of this cost-containment approach. While these programs achieved some initial savings, providers altered practice patterns to minimize oversight, so long-term and recurrent savings are more difficult to assess.

Given these experiences, major purchasers are increasingly looking to managed care as the most viable cost-containment strategy. By formally integrating the financing and delivery of health services, a managed care network puts the provider in a position of clinical as well as financial responsibility. The managed care industry, which HMOs spawned in the 1970s, has evolved into a plethora of related acronyms in the 1980s— PPOs, EPOs, DRGs, and others—as purchasers of health care experiment with different models of managed care. As more and more major purchasers establish managed care perspectives within their health benefits programs, HMOs should enjoy significant recognition and opportunity for their experience and accomplishments in this environment.

HMOs, however, are not without their detractors. HMOs have been criticized as failing to deliver on the promises of effective and cost-efficient health care. Indeed, it is sometimes argued that the marketing and pricing strategies of HMOs have accelerated increases in an employers' medical plan costs.

Lack of understanding as to how HMO premiums are established has exacerbated purchaser skepticism with HMOs. Until recently, HMOs have contributed to this skepticism by responding inadequately to legitimate questions with regard to pricing practices. If HMOs are to recover the high ground in the managed care industry, they will need to communicate better with institutional purchasers. It is in this regard that *HMO Rate Setting and Financial Strategy* makes a significant contribution.

For those in the HMO industry, this book will certainly serve as a convenient reference. The book's technical discussion will not lose the nonfinancial manager—the medical director, the marketing executive; Wrightson's is an understandable presentation of rate-setting methodologies. Beyond this, however, the book sensitizes the HMO manager to the critical issue of the effect of rate setting on major corporate purchasers. In the chapters entitled "The Debate between HMOs and Employers" and "Selection Bias and Premium Rate Setting," Wrightson acknowledges the controversy and objectively reviews what is and is not known about the complicated effect of HMOs on employers' overall costs. These discussions serve as a valuable aid to HMO management in both setting prices and presenting prices to the marketplace.

Finally, this book will serve as a welcomed guide to benefit managers and other executives responsible for purchasing their company's medical benefits. Corporations are recognizing a need to buy health care more proactively in terms of benefits, administration, and cost. As corporate purchasers sharpen their buying acumen, and as well-run HMOs are recognized as potential solutions to a company's health care cost challenge, the need for appropriate resources to assist the corporate purchaser is clear. This book is such a resource.

Gino A. Nalli
The Wyatt Company

Preface

During the past 15 years, the health maintenance organization (HMO) industry has become a significant provider of medical services and a major source of health insurance coverage in the United States. Today, more than one of every seven employees (and their families) belongs to an HMO. One of every 20 elderly persons eligible for Medicare receives health care through an HMO.

An HMO provides comprehensive medical services to its enrolled members for a fixed, prepaid fee or premium. In addition to ensuring access to medical services, HMOs emphasize continuity of care and "health maintenance" services such as well-baby care, physicals, immunizations, and other preventative health services. Because revenues are fixed and paid in advance, cost containment is a high priority. Thus, HMOs have incentives to provide high-quality services in an efficient and effective manner, while preserving access and continuity of care.

The threat of rising medical costs has been a significant public policy issue for several decades. As early as 1929, the Committee on the Costs of Medical Care, a blue-ribbon panel, published a landmark report on this topic. In the following decades, health insurance coverage expanded substantially in the United States as regional Blue Cross and Blue Shield plans developed. After World War II, private insurance companies entered the health insurance marketplace and, by the 1970s, they rivaled the market share held by Blue Cross. In the late 1970s, the health care cost-containment debate intensified, and "pro-competition" proposals came to the forefront of national health policy discussions.

The cost of health care for employers is their share of the premiums paid to HMOs and other carriers such as Blue Cross plans, private insurance companies, preferred provider organizations (PPOs), third-party administrators (TPAs), and other medical providers or insurers. Many larger employers now "self-insure" their health plans and directly pay the claims for services used by their employees (and associated administrative expenses) rather than insurance premiums.

Today, health care cost containment is a major goal for employers and other purchasers of health care coverage. For the past two decades, medical care costs have consistently outpaced other measures of inflation such as the consumer price index. In 1988, many employers experienced increases in indemnity plan premiums that exceeded 30 percent.

In recent years, there has been an ongoing, at times rancorous, debate between employers and HMOs over the methods used to determine premiums charged to employers. The debate has centered on issues such as equity (whether HMO methods of setting premiums are fair to employers), cost savings (whether employers actually save money by offering HMOs), and selection bias (whether HMOs receive favorable selection and profit by enrolling healthier, lower-cost enrollees).

The majority of HMOs have obtained a certification from the federal government, referred to as federal "qualification." To be federally qualified, HMOs must follow regulations governing permissible rating methods. Since 1973, being federally qualified has meant that an HMO has had to use community rating for the employers that it serves.

On 24 October 1988, President Reagan signed into law a bill (Pub. L. No. 100–517) that dramatically changed the premium-rating requirements for federally qualified HMOs. This legislation, the Health Maintenance Organization Amendments of 1988, allows much greater rating flexibility for HMOs and appears to respond to many concerns raised by employers. However, the debate continues between HMOs and employers over premium rate–setting practices. A major objective of this book is to explore the dimensions of this debate.

HMO premium rate setting is a complex and multifaceted topic. The situation faced by HMOs that compete in multiple-choice open enrollments for members of an employment group is especially complex, involving an interplay of rate differentials, provider availability, benefit packages, and cost-sharing differentials. Yet few published studies provide comprehensive data on premium rates charged by HMOs and indemnity plans in employer-sponsored, multiple-option health benefits programs. The other objectives of this book are (1) to examine alternative rate-setting methodologies available to HMOs, (2) to analyze the key issues that are at the heart of the current debate over premium rate setting by HMOs, (3) to present data for analysis of a range of issues related to premium rate setting in multiple-option health benefits programs sponsored by employers, and (4) to assess competitive strategies that can be used by HMOs.

Evaluation of the following issues is central to assessing the impact of increased competition in health care markets:

1. What alternative methods can be used by HMOs for premium rate setting? How does community rating differ from experience rating in setting health insurance premium rates?

2. What is the relationship between indemnity and HMO premiums? There has been very little published information on the overall level and distribution of HMO and indemnity premium rates, especially with respect to employer-sponsored, multiple-option health benefits programs. Do HMOs "shadow price" or set rates based on "what the market will bear," as has been suggested by some employers and health benefits consultants? Do HMOs that profess to be "community rated" actually use community-rating methods in setting employer premiums?

3. What strategies are HMOs using to respond to the increasingly competitive health care environment faced by many plans? How can financial and other strategies be used to improve the competitive position of the plan?

4. Other key issues surrounding HMO rate setting include the following: (a) how to reconcile the historical use of community-rating methods by HMOs with employers' strong objection to the cross-subsidies that are necessarily a part of community rating, (b) with respect to major philosophical differences between HMOs and employers, how to reconcile the desires of most major employers for experience rating, self-insurance, or "paying what my employees actually cost" with a principal tenet of HMO philosophy—prepayment, and (c) the many difficult technical issues that create confusion and hamper resolution of problems related to the HMO/employer relationship need to be addressed, including selection effects and selection bias in multiple-option health benefits plans, the "regression to the mean" phenomenon, and whether HMOs actually produce "cost savings" from the employer perspective.

The key issues surrounding the topic of HMO premium rate setting are explored in this book. In addition, the theory underlying rating for group health insurance products is examined, the methods that HMOs use to set premium rates are described and explained, and potential alternative methods are discussed.

Part I (Chapters 1–4) provides a description of the current competitive environment faced by HMOs and background information concerning HMO operations and the status of the HMO industry. Special attention is paid to the relationship between employers and HMOs. Although HMOs continue to receive a great deal of support from employers, a number of concerns continue to be raised about different aspects of the HMO/employer relationship.

Part II (Chapters 5–8) describes rate-setting methods used by HMOs and also contains technical information related to underwriting procedures for health insurance and the effect of selection bias on premium rate setting.

Part III is devoted to HMO financial strategy and current trends that will likely have an effect on the financial performance of the HMO industry in the future.

Acknowledgments

The motivation for this book was provided by the need for a comprehensive source of information that would be useful to HMO personnel, employee health benefit managers, and others interested in financial issues related to the "managed care" segment of the health care system. However, the book would not have been possible without the encouragement and support of several groups. The members of the HMO industry with whom I have worked in the past provided the inspiration and encouragement for this effort. Actuarial Research Corporation (ARC) provided the support and technical resources to undertake the project.

Several persons made significant contributions to the book. Ann Evans of Kaiser Foundation Health Plan provided substantial assistance for the description of Kaiser's adjusted community-rating system in Chapter 7. Portions of Chapters 7 and 9 were developed jointly with Gordon Trapnell, F.S.A., of ARC and were presented at the 1988 Group Health Institute in Chicago. Karen Wintringham, of Health Insurance Plan of Greater New York, and John Wilkin, F.S.A., of ARC, carefully reviewed two drafts of virtually every chapter, and their suggestions greatly improved the content of the book. Jim Genuardi, of ARC, provided valuable technical assistance throughout the preparation of the manuscript.

In addition, a number of persons were kind enough to review draft versions of the manuscript:

- Richard Anderson, Kaiser Foundation Health Plan
- David Baker, CIGNA Healthplan of Arizona
- Bruce Bradley, Rhode Island Group Health Association
- Robert Crane, Kaiser Foundation Health Plan
- Peter Fox, Lewin/ICF

- Brent Greenwood, Towers, Perrin, Forster & Crosby
- George Halvorson, Group Health, Inc.
- Dwaine Hartline, Bay State Health Care
- Mark Joffe, Group Health Association of America
- Jim Mays, ARC
- Nelda McCall, SRI International
- David McKusick, ARC
- Denise Mount, Rhode Island Group Health Association
- Gino Nalli, The Wyatt Company
- Mary O'Hara, Physicians Health Plan of Minnesota
- Harry Sutton, Towers, Perrin, Forster & Crosby
- Deborah Szmuszkovicz, Rhode Island Group Health Association
- Gordon Trapnell, ARC
- Margaret Wrightson, Georgetown University
- Carole Zimbrolt, Physicians Health Plan of Minnesota

The book benefited greatly from their comments and suggestions.

Part I

The Current
Competitive
Environment

Chapter 1

Introduction and Background

Never has the parable of the three blind men feeling the elephant been more apt than in the case of the American health care industry and its participants today. The pace of change is simply breathtaking to all of us in the trenches who are watching it happen to us and trying to discern its future directions. Not a week goes by that we do not read of some new business combination, acquisition, or product development. We have indeed been like the three blind men—representing in this case the insurer, provider, and health maintenance organization (HMO) sectors—all feeling a fast moving elephant in the hope of determining what it is and where it's going.

Robert Patricelli, "Musings of a Blind Man: Reflections on the Health Care Industry"

1.1 Introduction

Since passage of the Health Maintenance Organization (HMO) Act of 1973, the HMO industry has grown from a few major plans serving selected geographic areas to a highly developed, nationwide industry. There has been rapid growth in both the number of plans and total HMO membership over the past 15 years. In 1970, there were 33 plans serving 3 million members. By 1980, there were 236 HMOs serving 9 million members, and, as of January 1988, these figures had increased to over 650 HMOs serving 30 million members, or about 12 percent of the U.S. population. The HMO industry is an established part of the U.S. health care delivery system.

HMOs are considered important health care actors in the following national health policy issues:

- *Cost containment through competition in health markets.* HMOs offer a means for controlling health care costs by increasing competition in health markets and by implementing effective "managed care" techniques. HMOs are playing an increasingly important role in employer-sponsored health care programs, especially multiple-option health benefits programs. HMOs represent the primary alternative to traditional health insurance and fee-for-service medicine.[1]

- *Medicare.* In 1982, the Tax Equity and Fiscal Responsibility Act (TEFRA) permitted HMOs to contract with Medicare on a risk basis. This program has grown rapidly as HMOs have signed up to participate in the Medicare risk program. (The growth has slowed recently, primarily due to HMO concerns over payment adequacy and rating-related factors.)

- *Medicaid.* Since 1981, there has been a trend toward prepaid capitation financing in state Medicaid programs. Prepaid health plans and HMOs have played major roles in these programs.

HMOs are involved in both the delivery and the financing of health services to their enrolled membership population. Thus, HMOs can be viewed as a subset of two distinct industries: (1) the health care industry, as related to the organization, production, and delivery of medical services; and (2) the health insurance industry, as related to the financing and underwriting of HMO benefit packages sold to employers and other purchasers.

Historically, the primary emphasis in most HMOs has been devoted to the development of an effective health care delivery system and implementation of the functional components required for operation of the HMO, including medical/operations, marketing, finance, planning, management information systems (MIS), provider relations, member relations, utilization review, and quality assurance. In many cases, little emphasis has been given to the traditional functions associated with group health insurance operations such as underwriting and actuarial functions, development of detailed pricing guidelines or rate manuals, in-depth analysis of claims experience and expense allocations, traditional insurance accounting principles, and negotiation of premium payment and settlement formulas with large and medium-sized clients (contract holders).

Because HMOs have placed so much emphasis on their delivery system, they have often overlooked the insurance aspect of their business (i.e., that they are making financial guarantees based on the payment of a premium). Since their guarantees involve the delivery of medical services, they represent a significant amount of financial risk.

This general pattern is changing, however, as more plans are now forced to pay attention to the insurance aspects of their business. This is a result of many factors, including heightened competition, diversification of HMO product lines, pressures exerted by major employer clients, decreased levels of HMO profitability, and recognition of the need for increased financial sophistication in a highly competitive environment.

1.2 The Debate over Premium Rate Setting

As recently as the early 1980s, HMOs were advocated by most knowledgeable sources and experts as being effective in helping employers to contain health care costs, while offering employees alternative choices for obtaining quality health care services. Since then, however, many employers have developed mixed feelings concerning HMOs. Some employers are firmly convinced that offering HMOs in their health benefits programs actually increases the overall health care costs they pay, and they would like to see evidence of the quality of HMO services. On the other hand, there are other employers who are firmly convinced that HMOs have actually produced cost savings in total outlays for health benefits and increased employee satisfaction.

Many HMO representatives believe they have been unfairly criticized. Most HMO personnel agree that they have operated in good faith in their relationships with employers, according to their standard operating procedures and within the limits of both federal and state requirements. They also believe that they have developed effective cost-containment mechanisms and strong managed care components in their plans. Thus, they are firmly convinced that they are cost-effective—that for a given population, HMOs will produce lower total costs than either standard fee-for-service medical practice or a preferred provider organization (PPO)—and that they provide high-quality health care services to their enrolled membership.

At the present time, there is considerable disagreement over many aspects of the HMO/employer relationship. A distinct "employer perspective" and a distinct "HMO perspective" have developed. Chapter 4 includes an examination of the HMO/employer relationship and the issues that are being debated. Particular attention is devoted to one of the most difficult issues: HMO premium rate–setting practices.

1.3   The Health Maintenance Organization Amendments of 1988

Congress has enacted legislation to add flexibility to the premium rate–setting methods permissible to federally qualified HMOs. The Health Maintenance Organization Amendments of 1988 (Pub.L.No. 100–517) were signed into law by President Reagan on 24 October 1988. The proposed amendments allow HMOs the option to set rates based on "adjusted community-rating" methods. These methods permit federally qualified HMOs to determine premium rates for an employer group based on the anticipated revenue requirements for that group. Thus, the HMO can base the rates on the prior cost and utilization experience of the group. However, the rating must be done in a prospective manner.

The adjusted community-rating option specifically disallows "experience rating as practiced by indemnity carriers." This is meant to prohibit retroactive refunds or dividends for good experience based on the actual utilization or cost experience of a group (i.e., retroactive payments are not permitted if an employer's health costs are less than the premiums paid for a contract period). However, it does permit HMOs to practice a modified form of experience rating where rates are set prospectively for individual employers based on the HMO's projected revenue requirements for that group. Therefore, it is permissible to take into account the group's historical or projected utilization, intensity, and cost experience in setting future premium rates for that group.

This legislation has the potential to significantly influence the current debate over HMO premium rate–setting practices. In particular, it will permit federally qualified HMOs to determine rates on a group-specific basis. Thus, the legislation eliminates a major constraint for HMOs to respond effectively to employers' desires for premium rates that reflect the actual costs generated by their employees who are enrolled in HMOs.

1.4   National Health Policy in the 1980s

The Health Care Financing Administration (HCFA) estimates that U.S. health expenditures will exceed $1.5 trillion and consume 15 percent of the gross national product (GNP) by the year 2000.[2] For comparison purposes, national health expenditures were $27 billion in 1960 (5 percent of the GNP), $132 billion in 1975 (9 percent of the GNP), and $500 billion in 1987 (11 percent of the GNP).[3] Although most observers agree that health costs must be contained, there is a lack of consensus—indeed, there are major disagreements—over the content and focus of cost-containment efforts.

During the past decade, there has been a fundamental shift in national health policy.[4] Most policies under serious consideration by the federal government or private employers favored competitive approaches rather than the regulatory approaches that filled the national policy agenda in the 1970s.[5] However, except for the legislation described below, incremental year-to-year changes and budget-cutting proposals continued to play important roles in shaping major health programs like Medicare and Medicaid.

Policy proposals of the 1980s have ranged from new reimbursement methods for major providers to changes in the tax treatment of employer-sponsored health insurance to the promotion of HMOs and alternative delivery systems (coupled with increased consumer choice). A particular focus was the introduction of financial incentives to encourage cost-conscious choices and to discourage overutilization of health services. In the past few years, the focus has shifted to promotion of managed care systems with the accompanying requirements for utilization review and control.

Federal Initiatives

A detailed review of all major health legislation proposed by the Reagan administration is beyond the scope of this book.[6] However, several initiatives have had a major impact on the HMO industry and on the relationship between employers and HMOs:

1. *Medicare risk contracts.* The Tax Equity and Fiscal Responsibility Act of 1982 permits HMOs and competitive medical plans (CMPs) to participate on a risk basis as contractors with the Medicare program. The regulations implementing this provision of the law were published in January 1985 and, soon thereafter, many HMOs applied to become contractors. To participate, an HMO must either be federally qualified or be certified as a CMP. Risk contractors must provide all Medicare-covered services and may provide additional services (and require a supplemental premium paid directly by enrollees). HMOs are paid by the Medicare program on a capitation basis according to the Adjusted Average Per Capita Cost (AAPCC), which is calculated annually by the Office of the Actuary in HCFA. The HMO reimbursement

rate differs based on the characteristics (age, sex, institutional status, welfare status, and county of residence) of each Medicare enrollee.

2. *Prospective payment system.* In 1983, a new method of paying hospitals for Medicare patients was introduced. The prospective payment system (PPS) established per-case reimbursement amounts based on diagnosis-related groups (DRGs). Formerly, hospitals were reimbursed on the basis of incurred costs. The change from cost reimbursement to a prospectively determined fixed fee per admission has had a significant impact on the hospital industry. In general, there has been a substantial reduction in hospital length of stay, which has been attributed to the introduction of DRGs.[7]

3. *Medicare Catastrophic Act.* In July 1988, Congress enacted the most sweeping expansion of Medicare since its creation in 1965. The focus of this legislation was to protect Medicare beneficiaries from catastrophic health care expenses. Major features of the bill included: unlimited, free hospital care after payment of the annual Part A deductible ($560 in 1989); a limit on out-of-pocket costs for Part B physician and outpatient services of $1370 in 1990, rising to $1900 in 1993; an increase from 100 days to 150 days per year of care in skilled nursing facilities (SNFs), removal of the three-day prior hospitalization requirement, and significant reduction in SNF cost sharing; removal of the 210-day limit on hospice care; a new prescription drug benefit, whereby Medicare would pay 50 percent of outpatient drug bills that exceed $600 (indexed) in 1991 (rising to 80 percent reimbursement in 1993); new benefits for breast cancer screening exams and respite care; and more generous treatment of income permitted to spouses of persons who spend down for Medicaid. The additional benefits are financed by an additional Part B monthly premium of $4 in 1989 (rising to $10.20 in 1993) and an added, income-related premium based on a percentage of annual income tax liability for each Medicare beneficiary over specified threshold amounts (up to a maximum of $800 per person or $1600 per couple in 1989, rising to a maximum of $1050 per person or $2100 per couple in 1993). In 1989, there were several proposals to repeal or amend the Medicare Catastrophic Act, primarily in response to complaints concerning the income-related premium. The Medicare Catastrophic

act was repealed in November 1989. A limited number of provisions of the Act (primarily those affecting the Medicaid program) were maintained.

4. *COBRA requirements.* A number of additional requirements related to health insurance coverage were placed on employers as a result of the Consolidated Omnibus Budget Reconciliation Act of 1985 (COBRA) that was passed in April 1986. COBRA requires that employers extend an option for continuation of coverage to workers and their dependents who might otherwise lose health care coverage due to layoffs or terminations. Spouses who would lose coverage due to divorce, separation, or death of the subscriber are also covered by COBRA. In particular, eligible workers, spouses, and dependents are allowed to continue coverage in the employer's group health plan for up to 18 months if coverage is lost due to a layoff and up to 36 months if coverage is lost due to divorce, separation, or death.

5. *Tax Reform Act of 1986.* In a revision to Section 89 of the Internal Revenue Code, the Tax Reform Act of 1986 specified rules that an employer's welfare benefit plans (i.e., life, health, disability, pension, and so on) must pass in order to be considered nondiscriminatory by the Internal Revenue Service. The purpose of these provisions is to ensure that tax-exempt fringe benefit plans do not excessively favor the officers of the firm and other highly compensated employees. The new Section 89 rules, which went into effect 1 January 1989, impose new taxes on an employer's highly compensated employees if the company's welfare plans do not pass nondiscrimination tests. Section 89 requires employers to conduct a series of tests to determine whether a sufficient percentage of their employees who are not highly compensated are covered or eligible to participate in welfare plans such as group health and life insurance programs. If a company fails the nondiscrimination tests, its highly compensated employees will be taxed on all or a portion of their benefits. To comply with Section 89 requirements, it is anticipated that employers will face a large administrative burden, including substantial data collection and reporting requirements. Implementation of the Section 89 requirements was delayed in 1989, and there were proposals for Congress to modify or rescind them. In November 1989, the Section 89 requirements of the Tax Reform Act of 1986 were repealed.

6. *SOBRA changes for Medicare risk contractors.* The Sixth Omnibus Budget Reconciliation Act (SOBRA) contained the following changes for HMOs that participate as Medicare risk contractors: (a) repeal of the "2 for 1" conversion requirement for HMOs that had Medicare cost contracts prior to the risk contract, (b) restrictions on issuance of new waivers to plans with less than 50 percent non-Medicare and non-Medicaid enrollees, (c) other requirements concerning prompt payment of claims, use of reserve funds, provision of explanation of enrollee rights, disclosure of financial transaction information, and permitting Medicare enrollees to disenroll from HMOs and CMPs at any local social security office, (d) prohibition of HMOs and CMPs under risk contracts from making incentive payments to physicians to encourage reduced or limited services to Medicare and Medicaid beneficiaries, and (e) required studies regarding HMO quality of care, refinements to the AAPCC and Adjusted Community Rate (ACR), and the impact of HMO physician incentive payments.

In addition to these pieces of legislation, a variety of other legislative proposals were enacted in the past decade, including numerous changes to the Medicare and Medicaid programs.

Congressional Proposals

In addition to the legislative proposals that were passed and implemented, a number of other major pieces of legislation have not passed. These proposals, however, are important indicators of the direction of national health policy and the types of issues that are being seriously considered.

1. *Tax cap proposals.* Employees do not pay taxes on payments made by employers for group health insurance (i.e., employer-paid health insurance premiums are excluded from employees' wages subject to income and social security taxes). There have been several bills introduced in Congress that have advocated changing the treatment of tax-favored group health benefits. Some of these bills proposed placing an upper limit on the amount of employer payments that would be exempt from taxes. It is felt that the open-ended tax subsidy for the purchase of employer-sponsored health insurance significantly reduces the incentives for cost-conscious choices regarding alternative

health plans. A cap on the tax subsidy would encourage employers to offer workers a choice of health plans and also force employees to be more sensitive to costs since they would be required to pay more for high-cost plans.[8]

2. *Medicare voucher proposals.* To encourage consumer choice and cost containment in the Medicare program, there have been several bills introduced in Congress for Medicare voucher proposals. Under these bills, Medicare beneficiaries would be given vouchers that they could use to purchase health insurance coverage in lieu of the standard Medicare coverage. The objectives of these proposals are to stimulate competition and the development of alternative health plans for Medicare eligibles. In this way, an expanded set of choices would be made available to program eligibles, and costs would be contained through market competition.[9]

3. *Mandated employer-sponsored health insurance proposals.* These proposals attempt to expand health insurance coverage to persons who are currently uninsured by mandating that employers provide coverage for all of their eligible employees. One bill, sponsored by Senator Kennedy and Representative Waxman, was the subject of congressional hearings, and a modified version was reported by the Senate committee. Under this bill, employers would be required to cover all workers who work more than 17.5 hours per week. A minimum set of benefits (i.e., covered services, cost-sharing limits, required employer contributions) is also set by the legislation.

1.5   Increased Competition in Health Care Markets

During the 1980s, there has been an increasing reliance on market forces to contain health costs. In the previous section, a variety of legislative and national health policy issues were discussed. Although these activities produced major changes in federal health programs, perhaps even greater changes have occurred in the private sector.

In the past decade, private sector initiatives aimed at cost containment have proliferated, including the restructuring of employer-sponsored health programs to take advantage of the market power of organized purchasers of health services.[10] Other market approaches focused on consumers, with expanded choice of alternative plans and increased cost sharing to enhance sensitivity to costs. Specific market-based strategies have included (1) growing numbers of alternative delivery systems and rapidly growing enrollment in HMOs and PPOs, (2) increasing price competition among health plans, (3) greater cost sharing in employer-sponsored health programs, (4) improving consumer awareness and knowledge in choice of health plans and health care services, (5) raising the capacities of employers and other third-party payers to be "prudent buyers" of health care services, and (6) increasing individual and institutional consideration of health care costs and the cost effectiveness of alternative options when decisions are made regarding health care choices.[11]

In addition to these attempts to "unleash competitive forces" in health insurance and services, there has been a fundamental restructuring of the private health insurance marketplace in the 1980s. The combination of these actions has profoundly changed the environment for HMOs. Just as the growth of the HMO industry has coincided with efforts to make health care markets more competitive, now HMOs must adjust to the altered landscape when making strategic decisions to ensure future growth and profitability.

Changes in the Health Insurance Marketplace

In 1988, virtually every urban and suburban area of the United States had more health care providers and organized health plans than in the previous decade. This has led to an atmosphere of significantly heightened competitive activity in the health care marketplace. Frech and Ginsburg[12] discuss the changes that have taken place in the market for health insurance:

> In the 10 years [from 1977 to 1987] the health insurance market has become more competitive and cost-containment efforts have increased markedly. [p. 280]
>
> In the past decade the insurance market has changed dramatically. Most large employers are now self-insured. Although many employers use commercial insurers and Blue Cross/Blue Shield plans as administrators, insurers must compete with third-party administrators (TPAs) for employer business. Employers have also taken a more active interest in the benefit structure and administration of their plans. In addition, preferred provider organizations (PPOs) have begun to transform the nature of fee-for-service health insurance, and health maintenance organizations (HMOs) have become a more significant part of the health insurance market. [p. 281]
>
> Increased use of self-insurance increases the competitiveness of the

insurance market in several ways. First, as employers gain more control over their plans, cost-containment initiatives are likely to be incorporated more rapidly. Their ability to pursue a benefit structure with cost sharing is facilitated, since the Blues advantage based on exemption from premium taxes is eliminated. Second, self-insurance has opened the insurance market to an additional type of competitor, the TPA. While the insurance market does not have high entry barriers, we believe that the entry of a new type of competitor is providing an additional spur to competition and innovation. [p. 284]

The health care financing system is still in transition. Most agree that the system of 1987 is only a preliminary response to the powerful forces of change. [p. 289]

Growth of HMOs

Health maintenance organizations are part of an alternative health care delivery system that is unlike traditional fee-for-service medical practice. Because of their cost-containment and managed care characteristics, HMOs have been touted by competition advocates as important agents for changing the health care industry in ways that will control expenditures for health care services.

> The growth of HMOs between 1977 and 1987 has been nothing short of spectacular. HMOs increased their market share from 2.5 percent in 1977 to 11.5 percent in 1987, with the most rapid growth occurring in the latter half of the period. This growth has increased the competitiveness of the health insurance market in several ways. First, the growth of HMOs means that additional competitors have entered the market. These new competitors are particularly valuable for competition because many of them come from backgrounds other than traditional health insurance and because they have introduced a different product into the market. Second, these new competitors have been able to reduce the advantage of hospital and physician discounts that some Blue plans have. Because of their ability to channel patients to providers with whom they contract, even HMOs with relatively small market shares have been able to negotiate substantial discounts, often larger than those allowed the Blue plans.[13]

There have been interaction effects between the growth of the HMO industry and changes in the private health insurance industry. Most Blue Cross plans have started HMOs and, in some cases, statewide networks of plans. Many of the larger insurance companies (Prudential, CIGNA, AETNA, Metropolitan, Travelers) have also entered the HMO market, either through acquisitions or start-ups. In general, private health insurers are well versed in the required marketing, underwriting, data systems, claims processing, and actuarial functions, and they bring these skills and capabilities, plus considerable capital resources, to their sponsored HMOs. New areas of HMO operation for insurers include more extensive provider relations, clinic operations (for staff-model plans), and other aspects of delivering health services.

In addition, most observers believe that HMOs have had a stimulative effect on competitive response from private insurers. In this way, HMOs may have contributed to recent attempts by insurers to develop PPOs and managed care indemnity plans.

HMOs have experienced rapid growth over the past 15 years. Both the number of plans and total HMO membership have increased significantly since passage of the HMO Act of 1973. From a relatively modest start (33 plans serving 3 million members in 1970), the HMO industry has become a significant provider of medical services and a major source of health insurance coverage in the United States. By 1980, there were 236 HMOs serving 9 million members and, by the beginning of 1988, these figures had increased to 650 HMOs serving 30 million members.

Thus, the growth of HMOs and HMO enrollment has coincided with efforts to make health care markets more competitive and to contain health care costs. In most areas, HMOs have felt pressure from increased competition. In particular, HMOs face greater numbers of competitors, and price competition has become stronger in many areas. Other problems experienced by many HMOs include decreased profitability, slower enrollment growth, and increased difficulty in maintaining the competitive position of the plan. Recent trends affecting HMOs are discussed in more detail in Chapter 2.

Summary

Virtually every urban and suburban area of the United States has more health care providers than they had in the 1970s, with more competition among them. Yet competition has engendered new types of problems, prompting a second round of reform proposals and refinements aimed at more effectively managing health markets with increased levels of competition. Luft discusses the issue of biased selection and puts forth ways to handle the problem of selection bias in health care markets.[14] Enthoven calls for a ''managed competition'' approach:

> The essence of managed competition is the use of the available tools to structure cost-conscious consumer choice among health plans in the pursuit of equity and efficiency in health care financing and delivery. The market

in a system of managed competition should be viewed not as merely two-sided but as three-cornered, including consumers, health plans, and sponsors. Health plans integrate the financing and provision of care. The goal of managed competition is to reconcile equity and efficiency, at least to a reasonable degree.[15]

From now until the year 2000, it is likely that major changes will continue to occur in the U.S. health care system. Whether or not the current focus on pro-competitive proposals will continue is debatable. In the extreme, some observers believe that pressures on purchasers and providers of health services will become so intense that eventually a broad-scale national health insurance plan will be enacted with universal coverage and government controls. In any event, a number of extremely difficult problems must be addressed in the next decade, including (1) rapidly rising health care costs and the need for cost containment, (2) extending access to health services to the 37 million uninsured persons in the United States and others with inadequate health insurance, (3) effective management of medical technology, and (4) rationing of health services.[16]

Looking ahead, the problems facing policymakers are difficult. The current health system in the United States is characterized by decentralization, individual choice, pluralistic centers of power (with much control in the hands of physicians), and high levels of third-party payment. Reforming the current system to one that emphasizes rational use of technology, equitable access, managed care, cost containment, and mild (but effective) forms of rationing will doubtless prove to be a formidable challenge.

1.6   Outline

This book is organized in three parts. The remainder of Part I delineates and discusses the current status of the HMO industry. Chapter 2 provides a brief review of the history of HMOs and the development of the HMO industry. The emphasis is on the early history of HMOs, including traditional HMO principles and philosophy. It also focuses on the period from 1973 to 1988, addressing (1) the changes that occurred in the HMO industry during this period, (2) the external factors that had a major impact on HMOs, and (3) how the industry evolved from a newly formed, fledgling industry into a nationwide force.

Chapter 3 describes the key features of HMOs and discusses how they differ from other types of health care organizations. Unique characteristics of HMOs such as risk-sharing arrangements, utilization control mechanisms, and cost-containment techniques are also described.

Chapter 4 focuses on the debate between employers and HMOs over premium rate–setting practices. It discusses recent developments that have had (or are likely to have) a major impact on HMOs. The competitive environment for HMOs has changed significantly over the past few years, and the influence of recent developments on the operations, financial results, and competitive position of HMOs can already be seen.

Part II turns to the topic of alternative rate-setting methods for HMOs. Chapter 5 presents an introduction to rating and underwriting for group health insurance. Chapter 6 describes community-rating methods. Chapter 7 discusses other rate-setting methods that can be used by HMOs. The impact of selection bias for premium rate-setting is described in Chapter 8.

Part III focuses on HMO competitive strategy. At the present time, many plans are maintaining the basic approach and strategy that has been successful for them in the past. However, given the dynamic, increasingly competitive environment, other HMOs are employing a variety of different strategies in attempts to respond to competitive pressures and to improve the competitive positions of their plans for the future. In Chapter 9, emphasis will be placed on the types of competitive strategies—both general and financial—that are being used, and on the advantages, disadvantages, and potential implementation problems associated with each strategy.

Notes

1. Regardless of the competitive impact of HMOs, many observers believe that the importance of HMOs is derived from their effective management and allocation of health resources.
2. R. H. Arnett et al., "Projections of Health Care Spending to 1990," *Health Care Financing Review* 7, no. 3 (1986): 1; and M. L. Berk, A. C. Monheit, and M. M. Hagen, "How the U.S. Spent Its Health Care Dollar: 1929–1980," *Health Affairs* 7, no. 4(Fall 1988): 46–60; Division of National Cost Estimates, HCFA, "National Health Expenditures, 1986–2000," *Health Care Financing Review* 8, no. 4 (1987): 1–36.
3. K. R. Levit and M. S. Freeland, "National Health Care Spending," *Health Affairs* 7, no. 5 (1988): 124–36; R. M. Gibson, "National Health Expenditures, 1979," *Health Care Financing Review* 2, no. 1 (1980): 1; and

   D. Shalowitz, "Health Care Spending Tops $500 Billion," *Business Insurance* 22, no. 49 (1988).
4. For a review of competition literature in the early 1980s, see: A. Enthoven, *Health Plan: The Only Practical Solution to the Soaring Cost of Health Care* (Reading, MA: Addison-Wesley, 1980); M. Olson, *A New Approach to the Economics of Health Care* (Washington, DC: American Enterprise Institute, 1981); C. C. Havighurst, *Deregulating the Health Care Industry* (Cambridge, MA: Ballinger, 1982); J. A. Meyer, ed., *Market Reforms in Health Care: Current Issues, New Directions, Strategic Decisions* (Washington, DC: American Enterprise Institute, 1983); W. McClure, "Implementing a Competitive Medical Care System through Public Policy," *Journal of Health Politics, Policy and Law* 7, no. 1(1982): 2–44; J. Christianson and W. McClure, "Competition in the Delivery of Medical Care," *New England Journal of Medicine* 301, no. 15(1979): 815.
5. Examples include the National Health Planning and Resources Development Act (Pub.L.No. 93–641, 1974); certificate of need programs; state-run hospital rate-setting commissions; the Carter administration's Hospital Cost Containment Act of 1977 (H.R. 6575, 95th Congress, 1977), reintroduced as S. 570, 96th Congress, 1979; and the Carter administration's National Health Insurance Act (H.R. 5400, 96th Congress, 1979).
6. For a broad review of the Reagan administration's record, see J. L. Palmer and I. V. Sawhill, *The Reagan Experiment* (Washington, DC: Urban Institute Press, 1982).
7. See J. Feder, J. Hadley, and S. Zuckerman, "How Did Medicare's Prospective Payment System Affect Hospitals?" *New England Journal of Medicine* 317, no. 14(1987): 867–73.
8. For examples of proposed legislation that advocated "tax caps," see National Health Care Reform Act (H.R. 850, introduced by Representatives Richard Gephardt and David Stockman, 97th Congress, 1981); S. 433 (introduced by Senator David Durenberger, 97th Congress, 1981); S. 139 (introduced by Senator Richard Schweiker, 97th Congress, 1981). See also P. Ginsburg, "Altering the Tax Treatment of Employment-Based Health Plans," *Milbank Memorial Fund Quarterly* 59 (Spring 1981): 233.
9. See, for example, the Medicare Voucher Act of 1986 (S. 1985, introduced by Senator David Durenberger on behalf of the Department of Health and Human Services, 99th Congress, 1985); the Voluntary Medicare Option Act (introduced by Representatives Willis Gradison and Richard Gephardt, 97th Congress, 1981). See also P. Ginsburg, "Medicare Vouchers and the Procompetition Strategy," *Health Affairs* 1, no. 1(1981): 39.
10. P. D. Fox, W. B. Goldbeck, and J. J. Spies, *Health Care Cost Management: Private Sector Initiatives* (Ann Arbor, MI: Health Administration Press, 1984); S. Sullivan, *Managing Health Care Costs: Private Sector Initiatives* (Washington, DC: American Enterprise Institute, 1984); G. Halvorson, *How to Control Your Company's Health Costs* (Englewood Cliffs, NJ: Prentice-Hall, 1988).

11. See W. Greenberg, "Introduction to Special Issue on Competition in the Health Care Sector: Ten Years Later," *Journal of Health Politics, Policy and Law* 13, no. 2(1988): 223–26; J. H. Hibbard and E. C. Weeks, "Consumers in a Competition-Based Cost Containment Environment," *Journal of Public Health Policy* 9, no. 2(1988): 233–49; C. C. Havighurst, "The Changing Locus of Decision Making in the Health Care Sector," in *Health Policy in Transition: A Decade of Health Politics, Policy and Law*, ed. Lawrence D. Brown (Durham, NC: Duke University Press, 1987); S. H. Altman, and M. A. Rodwin, "Halfway Competitive Markets and Ineffective Regulation: The American Health Care System," *Journal of Health Politics, Policy and Law* 13, no. 2(1988): 323–40.
12. H. E. Frech, III and Paul B. Ginsburg, "Competition Among Health Insurers, Revisited," *Journal of Health Politics, Policy and Law*, 13, no. 2(1988): 279–92.
13. Frech and Ginsburg, "Competition Among Insurers," 283.
14. H. S. Luft, "Compensating for Biased Selection in Health Insurance," *Milbank Memorial Fund Quarterly* 64, no. 4(1986): 566.
15. A. Enthoven, "Managed Competition of Alternative Delivery Systems," *Journal of Health Politics, Policy and Law* 13, no. 2(1988): 307.
16. Other relevant problems include AIDS, the aging of the population, and increasing demands for long-term care services. Some observers believe that advanced technology and medical breakthroughs, more than anything else, are the driving forces behind medical care cost increases. See V. R. Fuchs, "The 'Competition Revolution' in Health Care," *Health Affairs* 7 no. 2(1988): 5–24; W. B. Schwartz, "The Inevitable Failure of Current Cost-Containment Strategies," *Journal of the American Medical Association* 257, no. 2(1987): 220; and R. J. Samuelson, "Why Medical Costs Keep Soaring," *Washington Post*, 30 November 1988. Of course, part of the cost equation depends on the "relative" use of available technology. For example, if cost-containment efforts are unsuccessful, we will undoubtably be forced to adopt, either explicitly or implicitly, some method of rationing health services (on the basis of age, ability to pay, cost of the service, waiting time in queue, or other means).

Suggested Readings

Altman, Stuart H., and Rodwin, Marc A. "Halfway Competitive Markets and Ineffective Regulation: The American Health Care System." *Journal of Health Politics, Policy and Law* 13, no. 2(1988): 323.
Enthoven, Alain C. *Health Plan: The Only Practical Solution to the Soaring Cost of Medical Care*. Reading, MA: Addison-Wesley, 1980.
Fox, Peter D.; Goldbeck, Willis B.; and Spies, Jacob J. *Health Care Cost Management: Private Sector Initiatives*. Ann Arbor, MI: Health Administration Press, 1984.

Frech, H. E., III, and Ginsburg, Paul B. "Competition among Health Insurers, Revisited." *Journal of Health Politics, Policy and Law* 13, no. 2(1988): 279.

Havighurst, Clark C. *Deregulating the Health Care Industry: Planning for Competition.* Cambridge, MA: Ballinger, 1982.

Helms, R. B., and Hackbarth, G. M. "The Reagan Approach Calls for Subtle Support: Government Urges Private Sector ADS Initiatives." *Business and Health* 1, no. 3(1984): 11.

Manning, Willard G.; Newhouse, Joseph P.; Duan, Naihua; Keeler, Emmett B.; Leibowitz, Arleen; and Marquis, M. Susan. "Health Insurance and the Demand for Medical Care: Evidence from a Randomized Experiment." *American Economic Review* 77, no. 3(1987): 251.

McClure, Walter. "Implementing a Competitive Medical Care System through Public Policy." *Journal of Health Politics, Policy and Law* 7, no. 1(1982): 2.

Melhado, Evan M.; Feinberg, Walter; and Swartz, Harold M., eds. *Money, Power, and Health Care.* Ann Arbor, MI: Health Administration Press, 1988.

Schwartz, W. "The Inevitable Failure of Current Cost-Containment Strategies." *Journal of the American Medical Association* 257, no. 2(1987): 220.

Additional Readings

HMOs and National Health Policy:
Competition and Cost Containment

Arnett, Ross H., III; McKusick, David R.; Sonnefeld, Sally T.; and Cowell, Carol S. "Projections of Health Care Spending to 1990." *Health Care Financing Review* 7, no. 3(1986): 1.

Bishop, Christine E. "Competition in the Market for Nursing Home Care." *Journal of Health Politics, Policy and Law* 13, no. 2(1988): 341.

Blumberg, Mark S. "Inter-Area Variations in Age-Adjusted Health Status." *Medical Care* 25, no. 4(1987): 340.

Boland, Peter. "Trends in Second-Generation PPOs." *Health Affairs* 6, no. 4(1987): 75.

Brown, Lawrence D. "Afterword." *Journal of Health Politics, Policy and Law* 13, no. 2(1988): 361.

_____. "Competition and Health Cost Containment: Cautions and Conjectures." *Milbank Memorial Fund Quarterly/Health and Society* 59, no. 2(1981): 145.

_____. "Introduction to a Decade of Transition." In *Health Policy in Transition: A Decade of Health Politics, Policy and Law,* edited by Lawrence D. Brown. Durham, NC: Duke University Press, 1987.

_____. *Politics and Health Care Organizations: HMOs as Federal Policy.* Washington, DC: Brookings Institution, 1983.

————, ed. *Health Policy in Transition: A Decade of Health Politics, Policy and Law.* Durham, NC: Duke University Press, 1987.

Christianson, Jon B. "The Impact of HMOs: Evidence and Research Issues." *Journal of Health Politics, Policy and Law* 5, no. 2(1980): 354.

Davies, Allyson Ross; Ware, John E., Jr.; Brook, Robert H.; Peterson, Jane R.; and Newhouse, Joseph P. "Consumer Acceptance of Prepaid and Fee-For-Service Medical Care: Results from a Randomized Controlled Trial." *Health Services Research* 21, no. 3(1986): 429.

de Lissovoy, Gregory; Rice, Thomas; Gabel, Jon; and Gelcer, Heidi. "Preferred Provider Organizations One Year Later." *Inquiry* 24, no. 2 (1987): 127.

Ellwood, Paul M., Jr.; Anderson, Nancy N.; Billings, James E.; Carlson, Rick J.; Hoagberg, Earl J.; and McClure, Walter. "Health Maintenance Strategy." *Medical Care* 9, no. 3(1971): 291.

Enthoven, Alain C. "Competition of Alternative Delivery Systems." In *Competition in the Health Care Sector: Past, Present, and Future,* edited by Warren Greenberg. Germantown, MD: Aspen Systems, 1978.

————. "Consumer-Choice Health Plan." *New England Journal of Medicine* 298, no. 12(1978): 650.

————. "Managed Competition in Health Care and the Unfinished Agenda." *Health Care Financing Review,* 1986 Annual Supplement: 101–119.

————. "Managed Competition of Alternative Delivery Systems." *Journal of Health Politics, Policy and Law* 13, no. 2(1988): 305.

————. "Theory and Practice of Managed Competition in Health Care Finance." Paper presented as one of the Professor F. de Vries lectures, North Holland.

Evans, Robert G. "Finding the Levers, Finding the Courage: Lessons from Cost Containment in North America." In *Health Policy in Transition: A Decade of Health Politics, Policy and Law,* edited by Lawrence D. Brown. Durham, NC: Duke University Press, 1987.

Feldman, Roger. "Health Insurance in the United States: Is Market Failure Avoidable?" *Journal of Risk and Insurance* 54, no. 2(1987): 298.

Feldman, Roger, and Sloan, Frank. "Competition among Physicians, Revisited." *Journal of Health Politics, Policy and Law* 13, no. 2(1988): 239.

Frank, Richard G., and Welch, W. P. "The Competitive Effects of HMOs: A Review of the Evidence." *Inquiry* 22, no. 2(1985): 148.

Frech, H. E., III. "The Long-Lost Free Market in Health Care: Government and Professional Regulation of Medical Care." In *A New Approach to the Economics of Health Care,* edited by Mancur Olson. Washington, DC: American Enterprise Institute, 1981.

Frech, H. E., III, and Ginsburg, Paul B. "Competition among Health Insurers." In *Competition in the Health Care Sector: Past, Present, and Future,* edited by Warren Greenberg. Germantown, MD: Aspen Systems, 1978.

Gabel, Jon, and Ermann, Dan. "Preferred Provider Organizations: Performance, Problems, and Promise." *Health Affairs* 4, no. 1(1985): 24.

Ginsburg, Paul B. "The Grand Illusion of Competition in Health Care." *Journal of the American Medical Association* 249, no. 14(1983): 1857.

_____. "Medicare Vouchers and the Procompetition Strategy." *Health Affairs* 1, no. 1(1981): 39.

_____. "Procompetition in Health Care: Policy or Fantasy." *Milbank Memorial Fund Quarterly/Health and Society* 60, no. 3(1982): 386.

Ginzberg, Eli. "Competition and Cost Containment." *New England Journal of Medicine* 303, no. 19(1980) 1112.

Goldberg, Lawrence G. "The Competitive Response of Blue Cross to the Health Maintenance Organization." *Economic Inquiry* (January 1980): 55–68.

_____. "The Determinants of HMO Enrollment and Growth." *Health Services Research* 16, no. 4(1981): 421–38.

Goldberg, Lawrence G., and Greenberg, Warren. "The Emergence of Physician-Sponsored Health Insurance: A Historical Perspective." In *Competition in the Health Care Sector: Past, Present, and Future,* edited by Warren Greenberg. Germantown, MD: Aspen Systems, 1978.

_____. "Health Insurance without Provider Influence: The Limits of Cost Containment." *Journal of Health Politics, Policy and Law* 13, no. 2(1988): 293.

Greenberg, Warren. "Introduction." *Journal of Health Politics, Policy and Law* 13, no. 2(1988): 223.

_____. *National Health Issues: A Perspective on Cost Containment.* Nutley, NJ: Hoffman-La Roche, 1981.

Havighurst, Clark C. "The Changing Locus of Decision Making in the Health Care Sector." In *Health Policy in Transition: A Decade of Health Politics, Policy and Law,* edited by Lawrence D. Brown. Durham, NC: Duke University Press, 1987.

_____. "Controlling Health Care Costs: Strengthening the Private Sector's Hand." *Journal of Health Politics, Policy and Law* 1(1977): 471.

_____. "The Role of Competition in Cost Containment." In *Competition in the Health Care Sector: Past, Present, and Future,* edited by Warren Greenberg. Germantown, MD: Aspen Systems, 1978.

Iglehart, John K. "Competition and the Pursuit of Quality: A Conversation with Walter McClure." *Health Affairs* 7, no. 1(1988): 79.

Jensen, Gail; Morrissey, Michael; and Marcus, John. "Cost Sharing and the Changing Pattern of Employer-Sponsored Health Benefits." *Milbank Memorial Fund Quarterly/Health and Society* 65, no. 4(1987): 521–50.

Joskow, P. L. "Reimbursement Policy, Cost Containment and Non-Price Competition." *Journal of Health Economics* 2, no. 2(1983): 167.

Lave, J. R. "Competitive Bidding and Public Insurance Programs."*Journal of Health Economics* 3, no. 2(1984): 195.

Luft, Harold S. "Competition and Regulation." *Medical Care* 23, no. 5(1985): 383.

————. "Trends in Medical Care Costs: Do HMOs Lower the Rate of Growth?" *Medical Care* 18, no. 1(1980): 1.

Manning, Willard G.; Leibowitz, Arleen; Goldberg, George A.; Rogers, William H.; and Newhouse, Joseph P. "A Controlled Trial of the Effect of a Prepaid Group Practice on Use of Services." *New England Journal of Medicine* 310, no. 23(1984): 1505.

McClure, Walter. "On Broadening the Definition of and Removing Regulatory Barriers to a Competitive Health Care System." *Journal of Health Politics, Policy and Law* 3, no. 3(1978): 303.

McMahon, Walter W. "The New Competition in Health Care: Implications for the Future." In *Money, Power, and Health Care,* edited by Evan M. Melhado, Walter Feinberg, and Harold M. Swartz. Ann Arbor, MI: Health Administration Press, 1988.

Melhado, Evan M. "Competition Versus Regulation in American Health Policy." In *Money, Power, and Health Care,* edited by Evan M. Melhado, Walter Feinberg, and Harold M. Swartz. Ann Arbor, MI: Health Administration Press, 1988.

Melhado, Evan M.; Feinberg, Walter; and Swartz, Harold M. "Introduction." In *Money, Power, and Health Care,* edited by Evan M. Melhado, Walter Feinberg, and Harold M. Swartz. Ann Arbor, MI: Health Administration Press, 1988.

Meyer, Jack A., ed. *Market Reforms in Health Care: Current Issues, New Directions, Strategic Decisions.* Washington, DC: American Enterprise Institute, 1983.

————, ed. *Incentives vs. Controls in Health Policy: Broadening the Debate.* Washington, DC: American Enterprise Institute, 1985.

Mitchell, Samuel A., and Virts, John R. "Health Care Cost Containment: What is Too Much?" *Health Affairs* 5, no. 4(1986): 112.

Newhouse, Joseph P. "The Structure of Health Insurance and the Erosion of Competition in the Medical Marketplace." In *Competition in the Health Care Sector: Past, Present, and Future,* edited by Warren Greenberg. Germantown, MD: Aspen Systems, 1978.

————. "Has the Erosion of the Medical Marketplace Ended?" *Journal of Health Politics, Policy and Law* 13, no. 2(1988): 263.

————. "Is Competition the Answer?" *Journal of Health Economics* 1, no. 1(1982): 109.

Newhouse, Joseph P.; Schwartz, William B.; Williams, Albert P.; and Witsberger, Christina. "Are Fee-For-Service Costs Increasing Faster than HMO Costs?" *Medical Care* 23, no. 8(1985): 960.

Nexon, D. "The Politics of Congressional Health Policy in the Second Half of the 1980s." *Medical Care Review* 44, no. 1(1987): 65.

Olson, Mancur, ed. *A New Approach to the Economics of Health Care.* Washington, DC: American Enterprise Institute, 1981.

O'Rourke, Thomas W. "Consumer Sovereignty in a Competitive Market: Fact or Fiction." In *Money, Power, and Health Care,* edited by Evan M. Melhado, Walter Feinberg, and Harold M. Swartz. Ann Arbor, MI: Health Administration Press, 1988.

Pauly, M. "Is Medical Care Different?" In *Competition in the Health Care Sector: Past, Present, and Future,* edited by Warren Greenberg. Germantown, MD: Aspen Systems, 1978.

Pauly, Mark V. "Is Medical Care Different? Old Questions, New Answers." *Journal of Health Politics, Policy and Law* 13, no. 2(1988): 227.

Pauly, Mark V., and Langwell, Kathryn. "Research on Competition in the Financing and Delivery of Health Services: Future Research Needs." In *Research on Competition in the Financing and Delivery of Health Services,* edited by Louis F. Rossiter. DHHS Pub. No. (PHS) 83–3328–2. Washington, DC: U.S. Government Printing Office, 1983.

―――. "Research on Competition in the Market for Health Services: Problems and Prospects." *Inquiry* 20, no. 2(1983): 142.

Sapolsky, Harvey; Altman, Drew; Greener, Richard; and Moore, Judith D. "Corporate Attitudes toward Health Care Costs." *Milbank Memorial Fund Quarterly* 59, no. 2(1981): 561.

Vignola, Margo L. *Health Maintenance Organizations Confronting Tighter Markets.* New York, NY: Salomon Brothers, 1987.

HMOs and National Health Policy: The Demand for Medical Care

Chernick, Howard A.; Holmer, Martin R.; and Weinberg, Daniel H. "Tax Policy toward Health Insurance and the Demand for Medical Services." *Journal of Health Economics* 6, no. 1(1987): 1.

Holmer, Martin. "Tax Policy and the Demand for Health Insurance." *Journal of Health Economics* 3, no. 3(1984): 203.

HMOs and National Health Policy: HMOs in the Medicaid and Medicare Programs

Freund, Deborah A. "Competitive Health Plans and Alternative Payment Arrangements for Physicians in the United States: Public Sector Examples." *Health Policy* 7, no. 2(1987): 163.

Freund, Deborah A., and Neuschler, Edward. "Overview of Medicaid Capitation and Case-Management Initiatives." *Health Care Financing Review,* 1986 Annual Supplement: 21–30.

Ginsburg, Paul B. "Medicare Vouchers and the Procompetition Strategy." *Health Affairs* 1, no. 1(1981): 39.

Ginsburg, Paul B., and Hackbarth, Glenn M. "Alternative Delivery Systems and Medicare." *Health Affairs* 5, no. 1(1986): 6.

Langwell, Kathryn M., and Hadley, James P. "Capitation and the Medicare Program: History, Issues, and Evidence." *Health Care Financing Review,* 1986 Annual Supplement: 9–20.

Chapter 2

History of HMOs

Given all these developments, a slower rate of HMO growth is understandable and a signal that the HMO industry is entering a new era. The new era will be one of more efficient and effective management of a soundly established competitive healthcare marketplace. Market growth will be secondary to developing or refining systems and strategies that can produce managed care—care that can undergo analysis for appropriateness in the rendition, effectiveness of outcome, and reasonableness in price. Practitioners skilled at producing high quality healthcare, while making frugal practice decisions, will give new meaning to the term "preferred providers." HMO managers will devise methods for identifying and contracting with such providers, initiating a shift away from the current popularity of "free choice," open-ended HMO offerings. In this new era, the individual consumer's influence will lessen while employer/payer power will be made manifest.

The InterStudy Edge, 1988

2.1 Introduction

This chapter provides an overview of the history of health maintenance organizations. After a brief review of the prepaid group practice movement, the distinguishing characteristics of HMOs are described, and the development of the HMO industry is discussed.

The term "health maintenance organization" was coined in 1970 by Paul Ellwood and others during policy sessions that focused on ways for the federal government to encourage the prepaid group practice form of health care delivery.[1] In February 1971, President Nixon unveiled a detailed proposal for HMO development that was the centerpiece of a major address to Congress on national health policy.[2]

After three years of legislative struggles over general philosophical approaches and specific provisions of the legislation, President Nixon signed the Health Maintenance Organization Act of 1973 into law on 29

December 1973.[3] This law, Public Law 93–222, provided the framework for development of the nascent HMO industry.

The HMO concept, however, was built upon a long history of prepaid group practice (PGP) dating back to the 1920s and 1930s. The next section provides a brief review of the predecessors to modern HMOs. In fact, many of these PGP plans, formed approximately 50 years ago, still exist today. They provided the foundation for the HMO industry of today and still constitute a substantial share of the total HMO enrolled membership population.

2.2   Prepaid Group Practice Plans

Rapidly rising medical costs have been a significant public policy issue since the 1920s. In an attempt to shed light on this issue, a blue-ribbon panel was established in 1927 to study the American health system, in general, and health care costs, in particular. In 1932, this panel (known as the Committee on the Costs of Medical Care) issued a comprehensive report that made the following recommendations:

> Medical service, both preventive and therapeutic, should be furnished largely by organized groups of physicians and other associated personnel in order to maintain high standards and to develop or preserve a personal relationship between patient and physician.
>
> The cost of medical care should be placed on a group prepayment basis—by insurance and/or taxation. An individual fee basis should be continued for those who prefer the present method.
>
> Organized groups of consumers [should] unite in paying into a common fund agreed annual sums, in weekly or monthly installments, and in arranging with organized groups of medical practitioners working as private group clinics, hospital medical staffs, or community medical centers, to furnish them and their families with virtually complete medical services. By "organized groups of consumers" the Committee means industrial, fraternal, educational or other reasonably cohesive groups.[4]

Although many prepaid clinics had been developed in the early 1900s and existed prior to 1930, the report by the Committee on the Costs of Medical Care greatly strengthened and legitimized the concept of prepaid group practice. The conclusions of the report, however, were strongly criticized by the American Medical Association, and organized medicine continued to fight the PGP form of health care delivery through the 1970s and 1980s.

In the 1960s, another blue-ribbon panel, the National Advisory

Commission on Health Manpower, again endorsed prepaid group practice as a superior system for cost-effective health care delivery, compared to fee-for-service medicine by individual practitioners. The report published by the commission in 1967 contained a detailed review of the Kaiser Permanente program as a model for this type of health care delivery system.[5]

Table 2-1 is a listing of many of the early prepaid group practice plans.[6] Most of the plans were built around clinics or medical groups that offered "prepaid medical care" to subscribers. A few of the plans, however, were organized around individual physicians in private practice (e.g., the Foundation for Medical Care of San Joaquin County, Stockton, California). These plans were the forerunners of the individual practice association (IPA) HMOs.

2.3 The Health Maintenance Organization Act of 1973

The HMO Act of 1973 (Pub. L. No. 93–222) was signed into law by President Nixon on 29 December 1973. The HMO Act resulted from three years of intense legislative activity that involved many actors, including the Group Health Association of America (GHAA), existing prepaid group practice plans, the political lobbies of interested parties (the American Medical Association, the American Hospital Association), administration representatives, and many members of the House and Senate. The act established a broad base of support for HMO development efforts. The major objective of the law was to focus attention on the HMO concept and to stimulate the interest of consumers and providers in making health care delivery available through HMO plans. In addition, assistance was provided to a limited number of demonstration projects.

The HMO Act of 1973 prescribed a broad set of requirements that an HMO must meet in order to become a federally qualified plan. To meet the requirements, an HMO has to successfully complete a rigorous qualification review process. By becoming federally qualified, the plan receives the federal government's "seal of approval" and is permitted to mandate employers under the "dual-choice" provision, along with the other benefits of the law. The act covered several specific requirements:

- Requirements for the contractual relationship between medical providers with the plan

Table 2-1: Selected HMO Organizations from 1900 to 1970

Plan	Date of Establishment	Sponsor
Western Clinic, Tacoma, WA	1906, 1910[a]	Medical partnership
Bridge Clinics in Oregon and Washington	1911	Individual practitioner
Palo Alto Medical Clinic, Palo Alto, CA	1929, 1947[a]	Medical partnership
Ross-Loos Clinic, Los Angeles, CA	1929	Medical partnership
Community Hospital Association, Elk City, OK	1929	Cooperative
Group Health Cooperative of Puget Sound (1947), Seattle, WA (formerly Medical Securities Clinic)	1935	Cooperative (originally a medical partnership)
Group Health Association, Washington, DC	1937	Cooperative
Physicians Association of Clackamus County, Gladstone, OR	1938	Medical partnership
Kaiser Foundation Health Plan, Oakland, CA and Portland, OR	1942	Industry
Community Health Center, Two Harbors, MN	1944	Union cooperative
Labor Health Institute, St. Louis, MO	1945	Teamsters Union
Miners' Clinics—9 group practice plans in PA, OH, and WV	1946	United Mine Workers Union
Health Insurance Plan of Greater New York, NY	1947	City, physicians, and community
Foundation for Medical Care of San Joaquin County, Stockton, CA	1954	Medical society
Community Health Association of Detroit, MI	1956	United Auto Workers Union
Group Health Plan of St. Paul, MN	1957	Indemnity insurance company

Continued

Table 2-1: Continued

Plan	Date of Establishment	Sponsor
Columbia Medical Plan, Columbia, MD	1969	Connecticut General Life Insurance, Johns Hopkins University, and the Rouse Company
Harvard Community Health Plan, Boston, MA	1969	University
Kaiser Foundation Health Plan, Denver, CO	1969	Industry, community

Source: Adapted from R. G. Shouldice and K. H. Shouldice, *Medical Group Practice and Health Maintenance Organizations* (Arlington, VA: Information Resources Press, 1978), 28–29.

ªThe second figure is the date the prepayment plan was first offered.

- Designation of mandatory and optional health services
- Requirements for community rating
- Permissible cost-sharing features
- Allowable organizational forms
- Requirements for quality assurance programs
- Consumer participation and health education requirements
- Requirements for financial solvency and fiscal soundness

In addition, the act required employers to make equal contributions to HMOs that were no less than the contributions they made to the other health plans they offered. The act also provided for a dual-choice mandate through which HMOs could ensure that they were offered by employers who had 25 or more employees living in the HMO's service area. Thus, the law attempted to give HMOs increased market access in areas where employers were reluctant to offer HMOs as part of their health benefits program.

Since passage in 1973, the HMO Act has been amended six times (in 1976, 1978, 1979, 1981, 1986, and 1988). The amendments have served to modify particularly rigid portions of the law, and they have also responded to changes in the health care environment that have affected HMOs.

Originally, HMOs were classified into three basic categories: staff-model plans, group-model plans, and IPAs. Staff-model plans have most, if not all, of their physician providers on staff, and their basic form of compensation is salaries. Bonuses based on the financial performance of the plan may be an important component of physician compensation. Staff physicians practice in medical clinics that are owned and operated by the HMO. Some staff-model plans own their own hospitals. Most plans, however, use community hospitals.

In group-model plans, there is a contractual relationship between the health plan and the multispecialty group that provides primary care and specialist physician services. Some of these medical groups are 100 percent dedicated to the HMO (like Kaiser's Permanente Medical Groups), and others have fee-for-service practices that are not connected to the HMO. Under the law, group-model plans, by definition, must provide a specified percentage of their services to HMO members. Physician reimbursement for services provided to HMO enrollees is usually based on a capitation rate that is negotiated between the HMO and medical group. Profit-sharing is typically an important element of compensation. Since both bonuses and profit sharing tend to reward the physicians for their individual and collective performance, there are important similarities between staff-model and group-model HMOs.

Although HMOs share many of the characteristics of the traditional prepaid group practice plans, the HMO Act attempted to broaden the types of plans that could be included under the HMO umbrella. A major policy decision was made to include the IPA-model plans as HMOs (i.e., the medical foundation plans like San Joaquin, plans sponsored by the local medical societies, and other plans based on individual practitioners rather than organized medical groups).

The three categories of group, staff, and IPA were applicable for HMO classification purposes until the early 1980s. In 1981, a fourth category, direct contract model, was added to the HMO Act. HMOs could contract directly with physicians under this model.

During the past five years, a new category of "network-model" HMOs has been established as many plans have attempted to broaden their appeal and organizational structure by expanding to additional physician groups in their communities.[7] In addition, there has been a blurring of organizational forms for HMOs, as many "hybrid" plans have developed, incorporating features of PPOs, "open-ended" HMOs, and joint ventures with insurance companies to permit "triple options" and alternative premium payment methods such as mini-premium and administrative services only (ASO) plans. In some cases, federally qualified HMOs have started separate nonqualified plans in order to escape from the restrictions of the HMO Act on these new forms of organization and practice.

Table 2-2: Growth of HMO Industry

Month/Year	No. of Plans	HMO Enrollment (in millions)
1970	33	3.0
6/74	142	5.3
6/75	178	5.7
6/76	175	6.0
6/77	165	6.3
6/78	198	7.3
6/79	215	8.2
6/80	236	9.1
6/81	243	10.3
12/81	254	10.5
6/82	265	10.8
12/82	272	11.6
6/83	280	12.5
12/83	293	13.7
6/84	306	15.1
12/84	337	16.7
6/85	393	18.9
12/85	480	21.1
6/86	595	23.7
12/86	626	25.8
6/87	640	28.6
12/87	650	29.3
1/88	653	30.3

Source: InterStudy, *HMO Census* (various years).

2.4 Development of the HMO Industry: 1973–1988

After passage of the HMO Act in 1973, many new HMOs were started with funds from the federal grant and loan program (some plans participated as part of demonstration projects prior to 1973). Many plans received grants for feasibility assessment and preoperational start-up costs, and many plans received federal loans to assist during the initial years of plan operation. Table 2-2 shows the growth in the number of plans and HMO membership from 1970 to 1987.

From 1970 to 1980, although the number of HMOs increased from 33 to 236 plans, HMO membership growth increased from only 3 million to 9 million members (less than 4 percent of the U.S. population), substantially below the initial projections of HMO membership growth for this period. This result has been attributed to several factors. Basically,

HMOs are complicated organizations to start, and it takes substantial amounts of time and resources to develop the organization and build membership. In addition, in some parts of the country (e.g., the Southeast and many parts of the Southwest), providers were strongly opposed to the HMO concept and actively blocked or discouraged HMO development.

However, on the West Coast and in many areas of the Northeast and Midwest, the HMO industry got a strong start during this period, and numerous new HMOs flourished. By 1980, many major cities had several operational HMOs that were showing strong growth and achieving significant market share. Among those cities were Minneapolis-St. Paul; Boston; Rochester, New York; Washington, DC; Portland, Oregon; and many cities in California.

Many of the newly formed HMOs, however, experienced slow enrollment growth. As of June 1980, the traditional prepaid group practice plans that had existed before 1973 still had the largest share of the total HMO membership population. For example, in 1980 the 15 largest HMOs had 63.6 percent of the total number of HMO members, and all of these plans started prior to 1973. The total membership for the 15 largest HMOs in 1980 is displayed in Table 2-3.

During the early 1980s, the HMO movement blossomed into a full-fledged industry. Several factors facilitated this development. First, HMOs became accepted on Wall Street and in the major financial markets. This opened new avenues of access to capital for many plans and encouraged the growth of multiplan organizations. Expansion of established HMOs into new markets became commonplace. Second, after years of diffusing at a relatively slow rate, the HMO concept had become more familiar to consumers and membership growth increased rapidly. By the end of 1984, there were 337 established HMOs with 16.7 million members. Third, in areas of the country where providers had resisted the HMO movement, barriers began to break down, primarily due to provider concern about (1) competing against new staff-model and group-model HMOs, (2) maintaining patient loads as the supply of physicians increased, and (3) being left out or bypassed as new IPAs were developed. In these areas, it was more common for IPAs, controlled by providers, to develop. Fourth, HMO premium rates, which initially were significantly higher than indemnity rates in most parts of the country (resulting in part from the recapturing of HMO start-up costs), were now generally more competitive as HMOs increased their rates more slowly than indemnity plans from 1973 to 1980. In many areas, by 1980, HMO premiums were the same as or even lower than indemnity premiums.[8]

Table 2-3: 1980 HMO Membership

Plan	1980 Enrollment	Year Started	Type of HMO
1. Kaiser—Northern California	1,672,154	1945	Group
2. Kaiser—Southern California	1,565,634	1945	Group
3. Health Insurance Plan (NY)	774,475	1948	Group
4. Group Health Cooperative of Puget Sound	283,625	1947	Staff
5. Kaiser—Oregon	233,600	1947	Group
6. Ross-Loos Health Plan (CA)	190,601	1929	IPA
7. Wisconsin Physician Service	162,606	1970	IPA
8. Group Health Plan (St. Paul)	144,061	1957	Staff
9. INA Health Plan of California	125,809	1966	Staff
10. Kaiser—Cleveland, OH	122,151	1964	Group
11. Kaiser—Hawaii	116,022	1958	Group
12. Kaiser—Denver, CO	113,256	1969	Group
13. Group Health Association, Washington, DC	110,941	1937	Staff
14. Harvard Community Health Plan, Boston, MA	92,384	1969	Staff
15. Health Alliance Plan, Detroit, MI	82,659	1960	Group
Total: Top 15	5,789,978		
Total: All HMOs	9,099,858		
Top 15 as % of Total: 63.6%			

This fact, combined with the comprehensive services and reduced cost sharing offered by HMOs, greatly increased the appeal of HMOs to consumers.

During the past few years, several trends have had an effect on HMOs. First, competition in health care markets has increased substantially since 1980. HMOs have been a major part of this trend, but other new types of plans (i.e., PPOs, open-ended HMOs, managed care indemnity, triple options, and point-of-service multi-option plans) have also developed

Second, employers have become more sophisticated purchasers of health care services. This has resulted in increased interaction between HMOs and employers regarding a host of issues including rating, quality of care, and data on utilization and costs of services delivered by HMOs.

Third, although HMO enrollment growth has been strong, many established HMOs have suffered financial losses during the past few years. Many attribute this to "underpricing," but other factors, such as increased competition and changes in the risk level of the enrolled membership population, must also be considered.

Fourth, a majority of the new HMOs have been organized as for-profit companies rather than nonprofit organizations, a reversal of the historic trend in the industry. Several established HMOs have changed from nonprofit to for-profit status. In some cases, newly converted plans have held initial public stock offerings to raise capital. Although Wall Street was bullish on HMOs in the early and mid-1980s, the depressed and erratic earnings of most publicly held HMOs have created a negative environment for HMOs on Wall Street and in financial circles. This has adversely affected the ability of many HMOs to obtain access to needed capital and financial resources. The most notable case was Maxicare, which was unsuccessful in its attempt to create a national HMO chain through mergers and acquisitions of other HMO organizations.

Fifth, it appears that, in some geographic areas, the HMO industry has reached a point of maturation, saturation, or both. Some cities now have more HMOs than they can sustain. Nevertheless, many established HMOs now cover most large and medium-sized cities in the United States, and the HMO industry is acknowledged as a strong competitor to Blue Cross plans and private insurance carriers.

There have been forecasts of an industry shakeout and consolidation within the next decade, and it has already occurred in several areas. In general, however, the HMO industry has become an established part of the U.S. health care delivery system. Although significant changes are expected to continue, including the development of "hybrid" plans,[9] it appears that HMOs will continue to play an important role in an increasingly competitive health care marketplace.

Plan Characteristics

Table 2-4 lists characteristics of HMOs and the distribution of HMO enrollment as of January 1988. According to the *InterStudy Edge,* 653 HMOs existed in January 1988, and these plans had a total enrollment of 30,313,198 members.[10] This was the first month that HMO enrollment had exceeded 30 million members.

However, although the number of plans and total HMO enrollment continued to increase, the rapid growth experienced by HMOs had slowed significantly in 1987. The number of new HMO members for the year ending December 1987 was lower than the two preceding years, and the rate of growth decreased from 22.3 percent in 1986 to 13.6 percent in 1987 (see Table 2-5).

Table 2-4: HMO Plan Characteristics, January 1988

Characteristic	Enrollment: Total as of January 1988	Percent of Total Enrollment	No. of Plans: Total as of January 1988	Percent of Plans
Size of Plan:				
1– 4,999	240,912	0.8%	123	18.8%
5,000–14,999	1,584,653	5.2	171	26.2
15,000–24,999	1,770,474	5.8	92	14.1
25,000–49,999	3,862,503	12.7	109	16.7
50,000–99,999	6,545,320	21.6	92	14.1
100,000 or More	16,309,336	53.8	66	10.1
Age of Plan:				
< 1 Year	131,813	0.4	45	6.9
1–2 Years	3,622,723	12.0	262	40.1
3–5 Years	4,832,373	15.9	139	21.3
6–9 Years	6,492,716	21.4	90	13.8
10 or More	15,233,573	50.3	117	17.9
Model Type:				
Staff	3,772,842	12.4	69	10.6
Group	7,864,587	25.9	69	10.6
Network	5,975,817	19.7	100	15.3
IPA	12,699,952	41.9	415	63.6
Federal Qualification:				
Qualified	24,211,917	79.9	341	52.2
Not Qualified	6,101,281	20.1	312	47.8
Profit Status:				
For-Profit	14,272,049	47.1	433	66.3
Not-For-Profit	16,041,149	52.9	220	33.7
All Plans:	30,313,198	100.0%	653	100.0%

Source: InterStudy, *The InterStudy Edge Supplement: A Special Report of HMO Growth and Enrollment as of January 1988* (Excelsior, MN: InterStudy, 1988), 10.

The modal category for plan size was 5,000 to 14,999 members (26.2 percent of all plans), but HMOs were distributed fairly evenly throughout the size categories (see Table 2-4). In terms of membership, however, large HMOs of 100,000 or more members had 53.8 percent of the total HMO membership, even though they accounted for only 10.1 percent of the total number of plans. Thus, most HMO members are concentrated in the largest plans. As of January 1988, these plans had a total of 11,774,974 members, approximately 39 percent of total HMO membership (see Table 2-6).

Table 2-5: HMO Enrollment Growth (Number of Members Added) and Growth Rate for Calendar Years 1981 to 1987

Year	HMO Enrollment[a] (in millions)	No. of HMO Members Added (in millions)	Annual Rate of HMO Enrollment Growth[b]
1981	10.5	0.8	8.2
1982	11.6	1.1	10.5
1983	13.7	2.0	18.1
1984	16.7	3.1	21.9
1985	21.1	4.3	26.3
1986	25.8	4.7	22.3
1987	29.3	3.5	13.6

Source: InterStudy, *The InterStudy Edge: Quarterly Report of HMO Growth and Enrollment as of December 31, 1987* (Excelsior, MN: InterStudy, 1988), 4.
[a]Enrollment at end of year (December).
[b]December-to-December comparison.

Seven of the top ten plans were staff or group models, and seven plans were started before 1970. The ten largest HMOs accounted for 7,664,806 members or approximately 25 percent of the total HMO membership. The greatest number of HMOs (40.1 percent) were either one or two years old. However, these plans accounted for only 12.0 percent of HMO members. The oldest plans (ten years or more) had 50.3 percent of the total HMO membership enrolled in their plans.

Originally, staff-model and group-model HMOs were the predominant types of plan. Since 1980, however, IPA-model HMOs have had the fastest growth, in terms of both the number of plans and the number of HMO members. In June 1980, there were 97 IPAs serving 1.7 million members. By January 1988, there were 415 IPAs serving 12.7 million members, a membership increase of over 600 percent in less than eight years (see Table 2-7).

There have also been strong trends with respect to federal qualification and profit status. In the 1970s, most HMOs were nonprofit organizations and most plans were federally qualified. During the early 1980s, there was a significant shift toward for-profit enterprises, and many plans decided to forgo the federal qualification process. In recent years, new HMOs have tended to be for-profit and not to be federally qualified. Although the majority of HMO members continue to belong to federally qualified and nonprofit plans, the trends are in the opposite directions.

The greatest concentration of HMOs and HMO membership has

Table 2-6: 30 Largest Plans Ranked by Enrollment, January 1988

Plan Name	HMO Members	Combined HMO and Open-Ended Members	Model Type	Plan Age	Profit Status[a]
1. Kaiser Fdn. Hlth. Pl./No. CA	2,101,655		Group	42	NP
2. Kaiser Fdn. Hlth. Pl./So. CA	1,873,256		Group	42	NP
3. Health Ins. Plan of Grtr. NY	889,900	898,200	Group	40	NP
4. Health Net (CA)	508,148		Network	8	NP
5. HMO of Pennsylvania	490,665		IPA	11	P
6. CIGNA Healthplans of CA	442,554		Staff	58	P
7. Maxicare—So. CA	357,850		IPA	15	P
8. Harvard Comm. Hlth. Pl. (MA)	350,046		Network	18	NP
9. Grp. Hlth. Coop. Puget Sound (WA)	332,168		Staff	41	NP
10. Kaiser Fdn. Hlth. Pl./NW (OR)	318,564		Group	42	NP
11. HMO Illinois	296,624		Network	10	P
12. HMO of New Jersey	272,161		IPA	4	P
13. MedCenters Hlth. Pl.—Partners National Health Plan (MN)	271,148	298,875	Network	15	NP
14. Health Alliance Plan of MI	255,054		Network	27	NP
15. Bay State Health Care (MA)	227,383		IPA	8	NP
16. PacifiCare of California	220,276		Network	9	P
17. Blue Choice (NY)	206,203		IPA	3	NP
18. Foundation Health Plan (CA)	199,674		IPA	10	P
19. Blue Care Network of S.E. MI	197,724		IPA	6	NP
20. CIGNA Healthplan of AZ-Phoenix	194,730		Staff	15	P
21. Kaiser Fdn. Hlth. Pl./Mid-Atlantic (DC)	190,814		Group	15	NP
22. FHP, Inc./California	183,465		Staff	27	P
23. Kaiser Fdn. Hlth. Pl./CO	180,459		Group	18	NP

Continued

Table 2-6: Continued

Plan Name	HMO Members	Combined HMO and Open-Ended Members	Model Type	Plan Age	Profit Status[a]
24. Health Options (FL)	179,816	185,907	IPA	7	P
25. Group Health, Inc. (MN)	177,627	222,520	Network	30	NP
26. Kaiser Fdn. Hlth. Pl./OH	177,181		Group	23	NP
27. Maxicare Indiana, Inc.	173,979		IPA	9	P
28. TakeCare Corporation (CA)	170,000		Network	9	NP
29. SHARE Health Plan (MN)	168,100		Network	13	NP
30. Comprecare Colorado	167,750		IPA	13	P
Total	11,774,974				

Source: InterStudy, *The InterStudy Edge Supplement: A Special Report of HMO Growth and Enrollment of January 1988* (Excelsior, MN: InterStudy, 1988), 12.

Notes: Table 2-3 reflects only enrollment of individual HMOs. This membership does not accurately reflect a national firm's presence in the industry. The ranking is based on pure HMO membership only, not on combined HMO and open-ended HMO membership. If open-ended membership were included, the list would differ. Physicians Health Plan of Minnesota, for example, would rank 7th with combined membership of 386,000.

[a]P = profit; NP = nonprofit.

Table 2-7: HMO Membership Growth by Model Type, June 1980 to January 1988

Model Type	No. of Plans, June 1980	No. of Plans, January 1988	Percent Increase
Staff	63	69	9.5
Group	76	69	−9.2
Network	—[a]	100	—
IPA	97	415	327.8
Total	236	653	176.7

Source: InterStudy, *HMO Census* (various years).

[a]Network-model HMOs were not identified as a separate model type in 1980.

been in California (see Table 2-8). As of June 1980, California had 32 plans and 4 million members; the next closest states had 16 plans (Wisconsin) and 1 million members (New York). By January 1988, however, HMO enrollment growth had spread to all areas of the United States. Although California was still the leading state with 51 plans and 7.5 million members, there were many states with sizable HMO enrollments. Five states had more than 30 HMOs (Florida, Illinois, New York, Ohio, and Texas), and nine states had over 1 million HMO members (Florida, Illinois, Massachusetts, Michigan, New York, Ohio, Pennsylvania, Texas, and Wisconsin).

The number of Medicare eligibles enrolled in HMOs with risk contracts has also grown substantially (see Table 2-9). Although HMOs only began the risk contracts for Medicare (under the Tax Equity and Fiscal Responsibility Act) in 1985, the number of enrollees exceeded 1 million for the first time in 1987. Recent growth has been slowed as many HMOs have reconsidered the financial impacts of the risk contracts. Several demonstration projects and studies are under way to examine the reimbursement procedures and other aspects of the risk contracts between HMOs and the Health Care Financing Administration. The highest concentration of HMOs with risk contracts has been among the IPA models (see Table 2-10).

Although overall industry trends are useful for indicating the general direction of the industry, it should be noted that individual HMOs may have quite different characteristics from the pattern of the industry as a whole. As in most other industries, there are HMOs that are experiencing rapid growth, average growth, and no growth. Similarly, with respect to financial results, some plans are strong performers, while others are average or weak performers.

The largest HMO, Kaiser Permanente, has demonstrated above-average performance for a sustained period of time (consistent growth and financial strength for more than 30 years). With respect to enrollment growth, Kaiser had experienced its largest increase in membership in its history between December 1986 and December 1987. In the next year, 1988, this record growth was doubled, with an increase of over 490,000 members. The rate of increase varied among the different Kaiser regions (see Table 2-11). With respect to financial performance, Kaiser has maintained its strong financial position throughout the 1980s. In the process, the company has been able to control premium rate increases (see Table 2-12).

Table 2-8: HMOs and Enrollment by State Headquarters,
              January 1988

State	No. of Plans	HMO Enrollment	Combined HMO and Open-ended Enrollment[a]
Alabama	9	136,710	
Arizona	19	566,620	
Arkansas	6	43,580	
California	51	7,510,074	7,510,427
Colorado	21	600,352	602,250
Connecticut	12	544,687	545,010
Delaware	7	121,668	121,915
Dist. of Columbia	3	363,274	
Florida	40	1,177,227	1,215,910
Georgia	12	313,629	314,310
Guam	3	55,042	
Hawaii	5	219,643	
Idaho	2	10,508	10,759
Illinois	34	1,611,774	1,613,051
Indiana	13	488,688	
Iowa	11	241,830	
Kansas	14	202,118	202,259
Kentucky	7	210,859	
Louisiana	10	289,114	290,940
Maine	3	10,995	
Maryland	12	595,569	595,603
Massachusetts	19	1,237,722	
Michigan	22	1,454,170	
Minnesota	11	873,782	1,226,019
Missouri	17	515,428	517,546
Montana	1	936	
Nebraska	5	74,161	77,462
Nevada	4	131,339	
New Hampshire	3	124,205	
New Jersey	16	768,857	
New Mexico	5	175,259	
New York	34	2,219,650	2,234,100
North Carolina	11	369,459	
North Dakota	5	65,771	
Ohio	43	1,261,649	1,263,358
Oklahoma	10	169,302	
Oregon	11	536,700	537,000
Pennsylvania	24	1,036,010	

Continued

Table 2-8: Continued

State	No. of Plans	HMO Enrollment	Combined HMO and Open-ended Enrollment[a]
Rhode Island	3	185,557	
South Carolina	6	147,251	
South Dakota	1	18,322	
Tennessee	10	238,467	249,014
Texas	36	1,126,467	1,143,232
Utah	7	228,326	
Vermont	1	14,092	
Virginia	13	400,478	
Washington	11	493,782	
West Virginia	1	51,188	
Wisconsin	28	1,077,930	1,081,129
Wyoming	1	2,977	
All Plans	653	30,313,198	30,763,538

Source: InterStudy, *The InterStudy Edge Supplement: A Special Report of HMO Growth and Enrollment as of January 1988* (Excelsior, MN: InterStudy, 1988), 7.

[a]Twenty states headquartered 40 HMOs which reported open-ended membership in addition to pure HMO enrollment. The combined HMO and open-ended membership is reflected in this column. Open-ended membership of 450,340 added to pure membership of 30,313,198 equals a combined HMO and open-ended enrollment of 30,763,538.

Table 2-9: Number of TEFRA Risk HMOs and Enrollees, June 1985 to December 1986

Month/Year	Risk HMOs	Risk Enrollees
6/85	25	262,098
12/85	67	499,673
6/86	111	727,758
12/86	121	945,135
4/89	133	1,061,582

Source: InterStudy, *1986 December Update of Medicare Enrollment in HMOs* (Excelsior, MN: InterStudy, 1987), 9; Health Care Financing Administration, Office of Prepaid Health Care, "Monthly Report on TEFRA HMO/CMP Contracts," 1 April 1989.

Table 2-10: Number of Risk HMOs by Model Type,
June 1985 to December 1986

Model Type	6/85 No. of HMOs	6/85 Percent of Total	12/85 No. of HMOs	12/85 Percent of Total	6/86 No. of HMOs	6/86 Percent of Total	12/86 No. of HMOs	12/86 Percent of Total
Group	2	8%	11	16%	14	13%	17	14%
IPA	11	44	26	39	54	49	58	48
Network	6	24	17	25	26	23	28	23
Staff	6	24	13	19	17	15	18	15
Total	25	100%	67	99%	111	100%	121	100%

Source: InterStudy, *1986 December Update of Medicare Enrollment in HMOs* (Excelsior, MN: InterStudy, 1987), 17.

Table 2-11: Kaiser Permanente Medical Care Program
Total Enrollment, by Region

Region	December 1987	December 1988[a]	Absolute Increase	Percent Increase
Northern California	2,086,516	2,215,123	128,607	6.16%
Southern California	1,855,862	1,967,329	111,467	6.01
Northwest	310,819	339,493	28,674	9.23
Hawaii	147,067	162,060	14,993	10.19
Ohio	173,287	192,598	19,311	11.14
Colorado	173,101	195,190	22,089	12.76
Mid-Atlantic States	175,417	225,452	50,035	28.52
Texas	51,330	69,895	18,565	36.17
Northeast	92,498	100,599	8,101	8.76
North Carolina	56,140	78,670	22,530	40.13
Kansas City	14,266	20,538	6,272	43.96
Georgia	9,206	71,127	61,921	672.62
Total/Percent Change	5,145,509	5,638,074	492,565	9.57%

Source: "Kaiser Permanente Program Statistics," distributed at Kaiser Permanente Conference, New York, NY, 24 January 1989.
[a]Preliminary estimate as of January 1989.

Table 2-12: Kaiser Permanente Medical Care Program
Community Rate Increases for 1985 to 1989

	Percent Increase by Year[a]					Five-Year Average Increase
Region	1985	1986	1987	1988	1989	
Northern California	9.8%	5.7%	5.5%	6.4%	12.9%	8.0%
Southern California	7.8	5.9	3.6	4.9	9.6	6.3
Northwest	6.9	2.0	0.0	2.9	12.2	4.7
Hawaii	9.8	6.5	3.8	3.7	10.0	6.7
Ohio	4.5	0.0	0.0	6.9	13.0	4.8
Colorado	4.7	3.5	0.0	0.0	5.7	2.8
Mid-Atlantic States	4.2	0.0	0.0	3.8	7.3	3.0
Texas	9.4	4.5	0.0	2.0	9.8	5.1
Northeast[b]	8.5	2.3	1.1	9.2	20.6	8.1
North Carolina	—	6.9	3.9	9.7	20.3	10.0
Kansas City	—	4.3	0.0	4.9	8.6	4.4
Georgia	—	5.7	−7.0	4.5	10.8	3.3
Weighted Average Increase	11.1%	5.2%	3.6%	5.0%	8.2%	6.6%

Source: "Kaiser Permanente Program Statistics," distributed at Kaiser Permanente Conference, New York, NY, 24 January 1989.

[a]For a region the community rate increase is a weighted average of increases in basic rates for groups, which may vary because of differences in benefits, differences in contract renewal dates, and differences in rate structures.

[b]The increases for the Northeast region are weighted averages of the increases for the Hartford, Stamford, New York, and Massachusetts subregions.

Notes

1. P. M. Ellwood et al., "Health Maintenance Strategy," *Medical Care* 9, no. 3(1971): 291.
2. Richard M. Nixon, *Health Message from the President of the United States: Relative to Building a National Health Strategy,* 18 February 1971, 92nd Congress (Washington, DC: U.S. Government Printing Office, 1971).
3. For an excellent discussion of the legislative activities and political environment that attended the development of the HMO Act of 1973, see Chapter 5 in L. D. Brown, *Politics and Health Care Organization: HMOs as Federal Policy* (Washington, DC: Brookings Institution, 1983).
4. Committee on the Costs of Medical Care, *Medical Care for the American People* (Chicago: University of Chicago Press, 1932).
5. P. S. Bing, *Report of the National Advisory Commission on Health Manpower,* vol. 1 and 2 (Washington, DC: U.S. Government Printing Office, 1967).

6. For a review of the early prepaid group practice plans, see R. G. Shouldice and K. H. Shouldice, *Medical Group Practice and Health Maintenance Organizations* (Arlington, VA: Information Resources Press, 1978); and William A. MacColl, *Group Practice and Prepayment of Medical Care* (Washington, DC: Public Affairs Press, 1966).

7. Although network models are not a separately identified category under the HMO Act, they are counted regularly by InterStudy and other organizations that study HMOs.

8. However, there are significant variations in premiums for health coverage both across different geographic areas and also between different employers in the same area for the same form of indemnity coverage. In some areas, average HMO premiums were higher in 1980 than average indemnity premiums, while they were lower in other areas. In some cases, significant differences existed between premiums for different HMOs, with some plans in the same area above average indemnity premiums while other plans were below.

9. See P. Fox, and M. Anderson, "Hybrid HMOs, PPOs: The New Focus," *Business and Health* 3, no. 4(1986): 20–27; P. Boland, ed., *The New Healthcare Market: A Guide to PPOs for Purchasers, Payors and Providers* (Homewood, IL: Dow Jones-Irwin, 1985).

10. InterStudy, *The InterStudy Edge, Supplement: A Special Report on HMO Growth and Enrollment as of January 1988* (Excelsior, MN: InterStudy, 1988), 10.

Suggested Readings

Brown, L. D. *Politics and Health Care Organization: HMOs as Federal Policy.* Washington, DC: Brookings Institution, 1983.

Fox, Peter D. "The Future of HMOs," *Compensation and Benefit Management* 5, no. 2(1989): 101–106.

Gruber, Lynn R.; Shadle, Maureen; and Polich, Cynthia L. "From Movement to Industry: The Growth of HMOs," *Health Affairs* 7, no. 3(1988): 197–208.

Luft, Harold S. *Health Maintenance Organizations: Dimensions of Performance.* New York: John Wiley and Sons, 1981.

MacColl, William A. *Group Practice and Prepayment of Medical Care.* Washington, DC: Public Affairs Press, 1966.

Starr, Paul. *The Social Transformation of American Medicine.* New York: Basic Books, 1982.

Welch, W. P. "The Elasticity of Demand for Health Maintenance Organizations." *Journal of Human Resources* 21, no. 2(1986): 252.

Wilner, Susan. "Health Promotion and Disease Prevention in HMOs." *Health Affairs* 5, no. 1(1986): 122.

Chapter 3

Key Features of the HMO Concept

Anyone involved in delivering or insuring health care services knows that there is a massive restructuring underway in the industry. Less well understood, but fundamentally important, is the way in which the financial risk for health care has been migrating among the parties involved. Without a vision of where risk should be in the system, the managed care revolution is like a traveler without a plan—not knowing where you are going, and (assuming that) any road will get you there.

Robert Patricelli, "Financial Risk Takes a Modern Odyssey through Health Care"

3.1   Introduction

What then are the key features of an HMO that distinguish it from other forms of health care delivery and financing? First, it might be useful to review the characteristics of the traditional prepaid group practice concept. The principal PGP characteristics are related to the medical, financial, and organizational features of PGP plans. The medical considerations focus on the multispecialty medical group practice to ensure access, availability, continuity, and quality of medical care. The financial considerations include the insurance function (e.g., for spreading risks and costs among enrollees) and the prepayment feature (all enrollees pay a predetermined and fixed periodic payment), which are directly linked to the cost-containment goals of the plan. The organizational considerations focus on an organized health plan, built around an established medical group, providing administrative, planning, and management services (e.g., for the financing and delivery of health services to the enrolled membership population).[1]

The Kaiser Permanente program has often been described as embodying the characteristics of the PGP concept.[2] For example, Saward cited the key features as (1) prepayment, usually by monthly dues, (2) multispecialty group practice, (3) integrated medical facilities, including both hospitals and medical clinics, (4) voluntary enrollment by consumers, based on the choice of two or more health plan options, (5) payment of physicians and hospitals on the basis of fixed fees (per time period) or capitation for each enrollee, regardless of the amount of care provided, and (6) coverage of the full spectrum of comprehensive health services, including preventive services.[3] Alternatively, Williams discussed the Kaiser Permanente program characteristics and objectives from the perspectives of the various consumer, provider, and purchaser groups that are affected by the program.[4] From the user's (consumer's) viewpoint, the following features of the program are important:

1. *Community service.* The program accepts the responsibility for medical services for every member of a defined population, recognizing such services as the contractual right of that member.

2. *Comprehensive coverage.* The program provides comprehensive coverage of clinic, hospital, home, and other services, and will adjust prepaid benefits to suit special requirements of a consumer group.

3. *One identified point of entry for both primary and specialized care.* Plan medical offices and hospitals provide members with outpatient care by appointment during the day, plus inpatient care as needed, and urgent ambulatory care day or night.

4. *Continuity of service.* The patient may choose a doctor from the staff available for primary care and may be referred to other specialists as necessary. The patient's medical record is maintained as a single unit available to any staff member on the case.

5. *Shared financial risk through per capita prepayment.* Kaiser Health Plan dues, paid monthly and paid wholly or partially by employers or from union-negotiated health and welfare funds, can also be paid by individual members. The medical care costs of those receiving services are spread over the entire enrollment. Prepayment through dues lends itself to continuity of service, as well as to stability and predictability of income from a management viewpoint.

The following features are significant from the viewpoint of the physician (provider):

1. *Group practice.* An integrated group of well-trained and well-supervised physicians, including qualified specialists and general practitioners, is organized by departments and works as a team with nurses and other allied health professions.

2. *Hospital-based practice.* A professional staff provides outpatient and inpatient services in a Kaiser Foundation Hospital and all of its attached or adjacent Permanente Medical Group Offices, except in areas where patient load and geographic distribution of members requires the operation of satellite clinics affiliated with the regional hospital.

3. *Elimination of the "money question."* The group practitioner, paid a reasonably good income out of capitation revenue, can provide whatever services each patient needs without concern about whether the family can afford it and without being influenced by the opportunity for a fee for a service.

Finally, from the business (purchaser's) point of view, the program offers the following important features:

1. *Distribution of authority and responsibility.* The Kaiser Permanente program operates in the spirit of a joint venture of the medical profession and professional management, organized separately but committed to working together in a contractual marriage of clinical responsibility and fiscal accountability.

2. *"Making it pay."* As a completely private enterprise, the Kaiser Permanente program is under direct pressure to make revenue and expenditures balance. Its predetermination of income and predictable costs, with no place to pass the buck, give it full incentive to operate the program as efficiently and economically as possible while meeting service commitments to members.

3. *Capital development.* The program, out of member revenues, supports service operations and covers depreciation reserves. It is designed to produce a modest surplus of income over outgo, and thereby generates sufficient capital borrowing power to provide for renewal and expansion of facilities. Capitation income, being relatively stable and predictable, lends itself to planning the rational development of resources.

4. *Free enterprise.* Kaiser Permanente's program policy gives all subscribers, upon joining or upon periodic renewal of contract, the opportunity to choose from two or more alternative health plans. This policy insures that enrollment will be voluntary.

5. *Regional autonomy.* Each Kaiser Permanente medical group, health plan, and hospital is organized as part of a region having fiscal autonomy and considerable independence of action, while maintaining a high degree of conformity from region to region in principles and patterns of operation. Each region has central control of purchasing and supplies, budgeting, cost accounting, rate setting, facilities planning, and capital management for all facilities within the region.

How do HMOs differ from these basic PGP concepts? As discussed in Chapter 2, some plans were started as prepaid group practices before 1973 when the term "HMO" was initiated. Also, most of the staff-model and group-model plans follow PGP concepts, so many HMOs incorporate many of the characteristics of the traditional prepaid group practice plans. The primary differences relate to the broad scope of the HMO concept, which includes a wider variety of organizational forms. However, in some ways, the specific requirements that have been legislated or promulgated in federal regulations for HMOs are more confining in terms of acceptable organizational characteristics, especially regarding federally qualified HMOs. As a result of the HMO Act of 1973, the term "HMO" has come to include all prepaid health plans. In particular, both prepaid group practice plans and individual practice association plans are included. Federal qualification requires a specific set of organizational and health care delivery system requirements for HMOs.

The issue of the key distinguishing characteristics of HMOs has been addressed by several authors. For example, Luft discussed the following key features of the HMO concept:

1. The HMO assumes a contractual responsibility to provide or assure the delivery of a stated range of health services. This includes at least ambulatory care and inpatient hospital services. This implies that the member has the legal right to expect necessary treatment from the HMO.

2. The HMO serves a population defined by enrollment in the plan. The existence of a *defined population* means that an HMO can know, at any point in time, to whom it is obligated to provide services, and it can estimate its demand for services. This is critical for planning purposes.

3. Subscriber enrollment is voluntary, which means that potential enrollees must have a choice among alternative health care pro-

viders. Voluntary enrollment implies that the HMO is competing against other providers for members and thus has an incentive to meet member demands for services.

4. The consumer pays a fixed annual or monthly payment that is independent of the use of services. Thus, the HMO does not gain substantial revenue by providing more services. This does not exclude the possibility for some minor charges related to utilization.

5. The HMO assumes at least part of the financial risk or gain in the provision of services. This implies that the HMO, which provides or assures the delivery of services, also has a financial incentive to reduce the excessive use of health services.[5]

In addition, it was originally believed that health maintenance (with emphasis on preventive services and early diagnosis and treatment) should be a critical component of the HMO concept. The HMO has a financial incentive to provide services of a preventive nature in order to avoid larger expenditures in the future (although the cost efficiency of preventive services has been questioned by some). The belief that health maintenance should be a critical component of the HMO concept is still held by many observers.

Further, providers in the HMO system operate within a fixed budget and are responsible for delivering appropriate services to a defined population that is enrolled in the plan. Thus, the HMO concept has an inherent set of financial incentives that makes it appealing for controlling costs. In principle, dealing with fixed revenues forces HMO providers to make trade-offs (cost-efficient choices) between alternative methods of treatment and delivering care. The HMO concept also incorporates the goals of accessibility, continuity, and quality of the health care services delivered to enrolled members. The removal of financial barriers when receiving care helps to focus attention on the goal of HMOs to contain costs (through reduced inpatient utilization and more appropriate use of services) and to increase access to health services at the same time.

3.2 Differences between HMOs and Other Forms of Health Insurance

HMOs compete against a variety of other forms of health coverage: Blue Cross plans, private insurance carriers, preferred provider organizations, self-insured health plans, third-party administrators (TPAs), and so on. In this section, we review the differences between HMOs and other forms of health insurance.

The different ways that Americans obtain financial protection against costs they incur for health services can be divided into three primary categories: indemnity insurance plans, service benefit plans, and direct service delivery plans. Plans that provide indemnity benefits reimburse or "indemnify" the subscriber for medical expenses that are incurred. Service benefit plans guarantee to purchase the services (except perhaps for a fixed copayment) in return for "prepayment" through premiums. These plans usually require patients to go to participating providers and usually pay the physician or hospital directly. HMOs are part of the third category, direct service delivery plans, in which health services are provided directly to the subscriber by the organization that receives the premiums.

Indemnity plans for health insurance were initiated by private insurance companies, and indemnity insurance grew rapidly after World War II.[6] The early Blue Cross plans, which started in the 1930s, were the original service benefit plans.[7] As discussed earlier, many prepaid group practice plans (the forerunners of present-day HMOs) also started in the 1920s and 1930s as the first direct service plans.

Each type of health plan uses different methods to attempt to control plan costs. Indemnity plans attempt to control their potential liabilities through reimbursement policies that provide incentives for the subscriber to limit services. These incentives may include exclusion of discretionary or noncovered services; requirements for cost sharing by the subscriber through deductibles, coinsurance, or copayments; and the establishment of fixed, or maximum, reimbursement schedules for designated services. With a plan that provides service benefits, an eligible person receives care directly from a participating medical provider (hospital or physician), and the provider makes a claim for reimbursement from the service benefit plan. Cost control under a service benefit plan is dependent on the relationship between the plan and providers, including agreements that the providers will accept the plan's payments as reimbursement for services rendered.

As discussed earlier, HMOs and other direct service plans provide health care services directly to members. The methods used by HMOs to contain costs are described in Section 3.3. Most HMOs try to use their direct and close relationship with providers as a major component of their cost-containment program.

Over time, insurance companies, the Blue Cross plans, and HMOs have all made numerous changes in the types of health plans they offer to consumers, blurring the distinctions and traditional boundaries between them. For example, Blue Cross plans have gravitated away from pure service benefit plans (with "first-dollar" coverage of inpatient hospital and other services) and now offer plans with indemnity insurance features. In addition, many insurance companies now offer hybrid plans that contain a number of managed care features similar to HMOs. To further blur the boundaries, many Blue Cross plans and insurance companies own HMOs that they offer to employers along with their other health plans.

3.3   HMO Cost-Containment Methods

There are a number of methods used by HMOs to control health services utilization and to contain health care costs.[8] The different types of cost-containment mechanisms have been grouped into two categories: factors related to plan operation and direct cost-containment measures (see Exhibit 3-1). HMO risk-sharing models and related issues are discussed in the next section.

Cost-Containment Methods Related to Plan Operation

The first step toward cost containment involves basic aspects of plan operations, including benefit package design, underwriting and eligibility determination, provider selection, health care delivery methods and practice patterns, quality-of-care review and cost-effectiveness review, and financial data analysis capabilities. Careful definition of covered services, use of optional copayments or other cost sharing, and limitations on services all reduce the unnecessary use of services. Development of the provider network requires particular attention and detailed consideration. Careful selection of major providers (such as primary care practitioners, specialists, hospitals, clinical laboratories, and pharmacies) can produce a low-cost, high-quality network of providers (e.g., physicians who deliver high-quality services with practice patterns that result in lower than average costs (per member per month) through lower utilization, less intense services, and care delivered in lower-cost settings). The most cost-effective methods of health care delivery are chosen based on the evaluation of alternatives for physician organization (salaried versus indi-

Exhibit 3-1: HMO Cost-Containment Methods

I. **Factors Related to Overall Plan Operation**
   A. Benefit package design: definition of covered services, optional copays or other costsharing or limitations on services (mandated vs. optional)
   B. Providers
      1. Careful selection of provider network: MDs (PCPs and specialists), hospitals, labs, pharmacies
      2. Use of physician extenders, PAs, NPs
      3. Use of other low-cost providers
   C. Health care delivery methods and practice patterns
      1. Physician care: salaried vs. group practice vs. FFS; use of physician extenders (PAs, NPs); referral procedures
      2. Hospitalization patterns: extent of use of alternative settings (e.g., outpatient surgery)
      3. Gatekeepers, case management, managed care
      4. Role of medical director
      5. Ancillary services: lab, radiology, pharmacy, dental
   D. Financial data requirements, analysis, and rate making
      1. MIS requirements and capabilities
      2. IBNR monitoring
      3. Premium rate setting
      4. Plan solvency
      5. Plan profitability
      6. Other financial analysis issues

II. **Direct Cost-Containment Methods**
   E. Provider reimbursement methods and contractual arrangements
      1. Reimbursement procedures
      2. Limitations or specifications for acceptable practice patterns
   F. Utilization control mechanisms
      1. Inpatient
         a. Prospective: prior authorization, screening, or certification; second opinion surgery
         b. Concurrent review: length of stay, discharge planning
         c. Retrospective: utilization review
      2. Physician
         a. PCPs: Profiling, analysis of practice patterns to identify outliers, potential inappropriate patterns, and high-cost practitioners
         b. Analysis of specialist utilization and referral patterns
         c. Analysis of gatekeepers to identify and correct problems in system, procedures, or individual providers
      3. Ancillary services
      4. Role of medical director

Continued

Exhibit 3-1: Continued

G. Claims analysis, utilization review, and enforcement
  1. Denial of noncovered services, or procedures to limit future occurrence of noncovered services
  2. Patient education: inappropriate ER use, and so on
  3. Provider education
  4. Provider sanctions: denial of claims, drop, and so on
H. Third-party recoveries (enhancements to revenue, or offsets to expenses)
  1. Coordination of benefits/third-party liability
  2. Medicare
     a. Part A
     b. Part B
  3. Reinsurance
  4. Other revenue recovery methods
     a. Capitation revenue (enrollment errors)
     b. Copays or other cost sharing
     c. Denied services (recovery from providers or enrollees)
  5. Key issues
     a. Data requirements
     b. Secondary priority for new plan
     c. Potential benefits vs. actual costs (organizational, administrative, personnel)

---

vidual practitioners versus contract with a multispecialty group practice), gatekeeper requirements and referral protocols, policies for hospitalization (versus the use of alternative settings, such as for outpatient surgery), policies for the use of ancillary services, and the definition of the role of the medical director in setting and enforcing practice patterns.

The financial data analysis capabilities of a plan can be used in cost-containment efforts. These capabilities can be greatly enhanced through a well-designed management information system (MIS) that permits analysis of detailed financial, utilization, and demographic data. The plan should be able to make detailed financial analyses and have rate-making capabilites that are based on the historical experience of the plan and that give adequate feedback to management on the source of its gains and loses.

If any of these capacities is missing or inadequate, the plan will be likely to encounter difficulties in following through on cost-containment initiatives. For example, computerized data systems for enrollment, utilization, and financial data are necessary for understanding the financial condition of the plan (including estimation of required reserves) and the effectiveness of current utilization control mechanisms.

Accurate estimation of liabilities for incurred but unpaid medical claims, and establishment of adequate reserves for these liabilities, are critical to maintaining plan solvency. The cash float, the time lag between receipt of capitation revenues and payments for medical services incurred, makes it possible for the financial status of an HMO to appear acceptable but then to deteriorate very quickly. Because monthly revenues are received in advance and payments for services incurred during the month may be paid with a lag of one to three months or longer, a plan may experience substantial positive cash flow. However, unless adequate provision has been made for the total claims that have been incurred, including those that are incurred but not reported (IBNR), plan liabilities will be understated and the financial condition of the plan will appear more favorable than it actually is. Estimating the IBNR liability is especially difficult for a new health plan with unknown bill flow patterns, data systems that may be under development, and new administrative procedures that may change over time. Further, the growth in the number of members of new plans tends to conceal the problem of unpaid liabilities because the current claims paid always reflect a smaller enrollment.

Financial analysis and rate-making capabilities are also important components. The long-term solvency of a prepaid health plan will depend, in part, on its ability to analyze its prior financial experience and to set premium rates in an appropriate manner. Rate setting requires accurate projections of health services utilization rates, medical service costs, and administrative expenses. Plans without good data systems and experienced financial personnel will be limited in their ability to prepare accurate cost estimates.

Direct Cost-Containment Measures

The second category of HMO cost-containment mechanisms comprises direct techniques that can be used by plans to help reduce or contain health care costs. Alternative forms of these methods can be found in Exhibit 3-1. The objective of these methods may be (1) to reduce the frequency of medical services and claims, (2) to reduce the expenditure (reimbursement) for services rendered, or (3) to change the point of service to less costly locations or procedures. The direct cost-containment measures focus primarily on specific cost-related activities. Four types of these methods are identified in Exhibit 3-1: (1) provider reimbursement methods, (2) utilization control mechanisms, (3) utilization and quality review techniques, and (4) third-party recoveries. The first category indicates how much is paid out by the plan to providers. The second and third categories focus on the methods and techniques that HMOs employ to produce what is commonly termed "managed care." The fourth category involves all of the procedures that HMOs can use to minimize costs by maximizing what can be legitimately collected from other sources of revenue (i.e., recoveries from reinsurance, coordination of benefits, and third-party liability).

Because reimbursement of major providers (physicians and hospitals) is the largest expenditure category for HMOs, the procedures and contractual arrangements governing provider reimbursement comprise a major area of potential cost containment for most HMOs. Many plans have been successful in negotiating favorable contract terms with hospitals, physician groups, pharmacies, laboratories, mental health providers, and other providers. These arrangements have included discounts (sometimes substantial percentages) from normal billed charges; capitation reimbursement (fixed payment rate per enrollee); per diem hospital rates (fixed payments per day of hospital care provided); reimbursement according to fixed, or maximum, fee schedules (usually significantly below the area's prevailing charge levels); and other provider payment methods or innovative reimbursement mechanisms that offer advantages to the HMO.

In many cases, provider contracts include provisions for risk sharing whereby providers are at risk for part of their compensation from the plan. These arrangements vary widely, and providers can share in bonuses or incentive payments, if utilization targets or financial goals are met, and they can be at risk for losing potential compensation, if adverse financial experience is encountered. Risk-sharing models are discussed in more detail in the next section.

The second category focuses on methods used by HMOs to control utilization of health services by enrolled members. In general, HMOs have gained an excellent reputation for their ability to control health services utilization. Originally, most plans focused on inpatient utilization as the source of the greatest cost savings. Methods used by HMOs to control inpatient utilization included the following:

- Programs aimed at confirming that a hospital admission was medically necessary (prior authorization, second opinion surgery)

- Programs aimed at reducing length of stay (concurrent review, setting expected length of stays, review and evaluation of patients while in the hospital, discharge planning)

- Programs aimed at identifying new and accepted treatment alternatives for high-cost inpatient procedures (drug therapy versus heart bypass surgery for ischemic heart disease)

- Programs aimed at substituting care in a less costly setting (outpatient surgery)

- Programs aimed at providing comprehensive case management services for patients with high-cost, complicated or chronic illnesses or conditions (neonatal; AIDS; head, neck, or spinal cord injuries)

- Programs aimed at identifying physicians with patterns of unnecessarily high use of inpatient services (utilization review)

Most plans have progressed to considering all forms of health services utilization (i.e., outpatient services, ancillary services, and prescription drugs) as potential targets of utilization control programs.

The third category of direct cost-containment methods involves retrospective review and analysis of claims and practice patterns and follow-up programs based on the results of the analysis. As the capabilities of HMO data systems have developed and expanded, more detailed analyses of claims data and physician practice patterns have been possible.

For closed-panel plans with physicians whose patients are nearly all HMO members (primarily staff-model plans and group-models like the Kaiser plans), the establishment of norms for clinical decision making and changes in practice patterns occur predominantly as a result of internal staff interaction, policies, and communication, with the development of formal or informal standard operating procedures for clinical practice.

However, for HMOs that contract primarily with physicians who have large fee-for-service practices, it is critical for the plan to (1) capture the attention of providers concerning the desired cost-containment goals and objectives, and (2) establish procedures whereby deviant practice patterns are identified and corrected. Techniques utilized by HMOs for this purpose include utilization review, profiling of physician practice patterns, comparison of individual practitioners to peer group norms, provider education, peer review, administrative controls, physician participation in planning and management, provider sanctions, and financial rewards and penalties. Other methods used by HMOs to control utilization include patient education (e.g., to correct inappropriate emergency room use, self-referrals, or "doctor hopping" for plans without gate-keepers), increased patient copayments or cost sharing on specific services, and mild forms of rationing through design of appointment systems and triaging procedures.

The particular set of techniques used for utilization control and cost containment differ for every HMO. Individual plans rarely rely on a single technique but use a combination of methods and procedures for controlling health services utilization and reducing or containing costs. The combination that is appropriate for one plan may not be suitable for another. In addition, the combination of techniques used by a plan changes and evolves over time in response to changing competitive conditions, relations with providers, increasing managerial sophistication, data systems capabilites, and other factors.

The fourth category of direct cost-containment methods consists of third-party recoveries. This involves systematic and determined efforts by an HMO to collect all monies legitimately due to the plan. Monies produced by items in this category can be considered either as enhancements to revenue or offsets to expenses and can include financial recoveries resulting from coordination of benefits, subrogation, third-party liability, reinsurance, Medicare, Medicaid, errors in billing and/or enrollment from major accounts, collection of patient copayments or cost sharing, and recoveries from providers or patients of payments for denied services.

Although many of these items are relatively small, together they can account for offsets of 5 to 15 percent of total expenses (depending on factors such as the level of reinsurance, proportion of members with dual coverage, and percentage of high-cost claims involving third-party liability). A key consideration involves estimation of the potential benefits versus the anticipated costs of recovery (e.g., personnel costs, related administrative expenses, and MIS costs). To achieve maximum results, a plan must be willing to commit the time, attention, and resources necessary to generate all cost-effective recoveries (e.g., the amount reclaimed exceeds the cost of recovery). A second key consideration is access to appropriate data, which is a necessary prerequisite to effective action on third-party recoveries. A plan's data system must be capable of producing whatever information is required to collect or recover the amounts owed the plan.

For many plans, however, diligent efforts at these items can result in decreases in expenses of 2 percent or more (compared to historical rates of third-party recovery). These amounts directly affect a plan's "bottom line" and can mean the difference between a profitable and unprofitable year for an HMO.

3.4 HMO Risk-Sharing Models

In general, cost-containment methods can be considered as a subset of a plan's overall risk-management program. From a business perspective, risk management is a firm's effort to identify, evaluate, and plan for risks that could result in financial loss. The objectives of a risk-management program are (1) to reduce exposure to risks that can incur a liability (which reduces the mean or expected losses), and (2) to reduce the probability of a negative outcome (which reduces the variance of losses), especially those outcomes with extreme losses, such as catastrophic illnesses, that result in large claims.

With respect to risk management, HMOs normally concentrate on medical service costs and related liabilities (e.g., medical malpractice liability) because medical service costs account for approximately 90 percent of a plan's total expenses. However, other normal business risks (outside of medical claims expense) should not be ignored.[9]

Four types of techniques are usually included in a risk-management program:

1. Avoidance (reduce incidence or number of losses)
2. Reduce severity of losses that do occur (cost per occurrence)
3. Transfer risk to another party (usually either through insurance or a contractual arrangement)
4. Assume the risk (self-insurance based on an assessment of historical loss data and projection of potential outcomes)

The first two types of risk-management techniques were discussed in the previous section regarding direct cost-containment methods. The third category, transferring risks, is usually accomplished in health plans through risk-sharing arrangements with providers by setting up risk pools and using withholds, or incentive reimbursement methods. Transferring risk can also be accomplished through reinsurance or through capitation contracts in which providers assume full risk in exchange for a fixed payment per enrollee.

The fourth category of risk-management techniques involves assumption of the risk by the health plan. Regardless of the extent to which an HMO has been successful in transferring, limiting, or avoiding risk, there is usually a substantial amount of risk that resides with the plan. The extent of the residual risk should be carefully analyzed. The decision for the plan to assume identifiable risks should be based on an analysis of historical data on the incidence of losses (frequency) and the severity of the losses (cost per occurrence). The general principle is that high-volume, low-loss risks that are highly predictable (e.g., characterized by being independent events with known mean and low variance) should be assumed by the plan as a normal risk (or cost) of doing business. For infrequent, high-loss risks that are difficult to predict, the plan should seek some level of reinsurance. Even with these risks, however, the plan should assume a level of risk that it can handle safely, from the plan's financial perspective, and use reinsurance to provide protection against losses that it could not handle (e.g., losses that could have catastrophic consequences for the financial position of the plan or that could jeopardize the plan's financial viability).

During the past five to ten years, the emphasis on risk-sharing arrangements between HMOs and providers has increased greatly. There have always been risk-sharing arrangements in the HMO industry, such as paying a fixed capitation per member per month (PMPM) to a risk-bearing medical group with an agreement to share the profits each year between the plan and the medical group as an incentive bonus. In some cases, the capitation rate is set significantly below the expected PMPM costs so that the plan has effectively transferred almost 100 percent of the risk for medical costs that exceed expected costs to the medical group. With many large HMOs, however, there is a bonus every year, and both parties are happy with the arrangement. Since the size of the bonus depends, in part, on how effectively the medical group has controlled utilization and costs, there is substantial incentive to do so. For example, the Kaiser Permanente program uses a "dual management" approach in which both health plan managers and medical group representatives jointly develop detailed annual budget projections, with risks and profits shared equally by both parties (i.e., the health plan and the medical group).

During the past few years, provider risk-sharing arrangements have become quite sophisticated with the use of withholds, fee schedules, risk pools, and incentive reimbursement formulas. This has occurred to the extent that it is now accurate to consider cost-containment mechanisms, risk-sharing arrangements, reinsurance, and other risk-management methods as a single concept (or different components under a single umbrella).

Originally, many IPA-model HMOs reimbursed participating physicians on a fee-for-service basis using a fee schedule or similar mechanism. In general, however, IPAs found that they were most successful if the participating physicians had economic incentives that corresponded to the goals of the plan. Now, IPAs use a variety of risk-sharing arrangements, including (1) paying capitation rates to primary care physicians, (2) paying on a fee-for-service basis but withholding a portion (10 to 30%) of the fees, (3) assigning primary care physicians to be gatekeepers with responsibility (and separate risk pools) for specialty care and hospitalization, and (4) establishing utilization targets (in terms of hospital days per 1,000 members per year) such that participating physicians share in bonuses or incentive compensation if aggregate targets are achieved. In addition, specific risk-sharing models can include corridor risk sharing, where potential losses are limited to specified amounts; individual stop-loss protection given to providers and pooling of high-cost cases across groups; aggregate stop-loss at specified percentages for subgroups of physicians; algorithms for distribution of risk pool surpluses; and detailed procedures to determine how losses are handled (i.e., who is responsible for what portion of each type of loss, or deficits between actual expenses and budgeted amounts).

Risk-sharing arrangements can be applied to (1) the entire group of HMO physicians (e.g., an IPA, or a medical group for a group-model plan), (2) subgroups of physician providers (i.e., primary care physicians versus specialists, different medical groups in a network-model HMO, IPAs organized as provider subgroups), or (3) individual physicians (e.g., each physician has a separate risk pool for which they are responsible and at risk). In recent years, Congress expressed concern about the appropriateness of economic incentives applied to individual providers, because of the potential for the denial of needed services or adverse quality of care (Section 9313 of the Omnibus Budget Reconciliation Act of 1986). A study found that 15 percent of HMOs had risk-sharing arrangements where individual physicians were held at risk (85 percent of HMOs have either risk-sharing arrangements for large physician subgroups or aggregate risk-sharing for the entire group of participating physicians).[10]

In summary, HMO risk-sharing models have become increasingly complex over time, as plans and provider groups attempt to determine the correct balance between economic incentives and the share of financial risks to be borne by both parties. In areas where many HMOs use the same providers or have overlapping provider panels, it is sometimes difficult for a plan to establish, or effectively implement, cost-containment methods that have the desired effect on physician practice patterns.

Risk-sharing arrangements attempt to increase the economic incentives to HMO providers to provide more cost-effective care.

Physician Incentives and Quality of Care

Just as fee-for-service medical practice may lead to overutilization, prepaid capitated revenues may create a tendency for HMOs to underutilize services. Health maintenance organizations have used a variety of approaches in attempts to increase the consciousness of physicians with respect to the financial implications of their practice patterns and clinical decisions related to utilization of medical resources. These approaches have included primary care physicians acting as gatekeepers, referral authorization, prior admission notification, second opinion surgery, concurrent inpatient review, retrospective utilization review, and profiling of practice patterns. In addition, many believe that the most effective approach to obtaining the cooperation of providers is to create a system of financial incentives, in conjunction with some or all of the above programs. This system gains the attention of providers and places them at risk financially, since part of their compensation from the HMO is dependent upon the successful attainment of specified utilization control or cost-containment objectives. A study conducted for the Department of Health and Human Services (DHHS) suggests that "the majority of the available literature supports the point that financial incentives motivate physicians to be more cost effective and to alter their practice patterns at least to some degree."[11]

Inappropriate financial incentives, however, especially in combination with inadequate monitoring of quality of care, could result in medical service reductions, limitations by providers, or denial of needed services. Thus, HMOs must achieve a balance between fiscal restraint and appropriate use of medical services. Financial incentives must be structured to accomplish the desired cost-control objectives, but they must not exert undue pressure on providers regarding the financial consequences of clinical decision making. In addition, HMOs require effective quality review mechanisms in order to ensure that appropriate medical services are being delivered.

There is little documented evidence concerning the direct or indirect effects of financial incentives on the quality of care in HMOs. However, this important issue has been raised repeatedly by Congress, employers, and other parties. As part of the Omnibus Budget Reconciliation Act (OBRA) of 1986, Congress prohibited payments by hospitals to physicians as an inducement to reduce or limit services to Medicare benefi-

ciaries. In addition, Congress applied the prohibition to HMOs and
competitive medical plans with Medicare risk and Medicaid contracts
(Section 9313 of OBRA–86). In recognition of the fact that HMOs utilize
incentive payments to physicians as part of their standard operating procedures, Congress specified an effective date of 1 April 1989 for this
provision, in order to allow time to study the issue in more detail. Congress requested a report from the Department of Health and Human
Services. A study of this topic was then commissioned with ICF, a health
care consulting firm. As part of the Omnibus Budget Reconciliation Act
of 1987, Congress extended the effective date for prohibition of HMO
incentive payments to physicians from 1 April 1989 to 1 April 1990
(Section 4016 of OBRA–87). The final report of the ICF study was
submitted to the Department of Health and Human Services on 18 May
1988.[12] In November 1989, the effective date was extended to 1 April 1991.

At the time of publication of this book, Congress had not taken
final action on this issue. Although most observers believe that Congress
will follow a course that does not place onerous restraints on the current
practices of HMOs with Medicare risk contracts, congressional action
could have a major impact on the methods that are deemed acceptable
for HMO risk-sharing and incentive arrangements with their providers.
For example, substantial attention has been given to the issue of incentive
programs involving individual physicians versus groups of physicians.
Approximately 15 percent of HMOs have incentive arrangements in
which individual physicians are at risk. It is possible that Congress will
prohibit all individual incentive arrangements, or specified types of incentive programs based on the amount or extent of risk that is assumed by
individual providers. Representative Fortney Stark, Chairman of the
Health Subcommittee on the House Ways and Means Committee,
authored the HMO physician incentives payment legislation. Stark made
the following statement regarding cost containment:

> Cost containment is a key goal, but I have been worried that some HMOs
> may give so many incentives to doctors not to order tests or refer patients
> to specialists, that the quality of care could suffer. . . . Most HMOs pro-
> vide high quality care at lower costs than the "fee-for-service" system,
> and I strongly encourage the growth of the HMO movement. It is impor-
> tant, however, that we weed out certain HMO incentive plans that could
> give the whole industry a bad name.[13]

Stark commissioned a study from the U.S. General Acounting Office
(GAO) on the topic of HMO physician incentive payments. The GAO

report examined physician reimbursement and risk-sharing arrangements used by a number of HMOs.[14] Selected results of the report are contained in Exhibit 3-2.

In terms of the relationship between incentive or risk-sharing arrangements and quality of care, many believe that physicians are guided less by financial incentives and more by nonfinancial factors such as professional ethics, esteem of peers, the threat of malpractice suits, and peer review pressures. This view holds that clinical decisions required for patient diagnosis and treatment are made independently of financial considerations. Others feel that, even if a number of physicians are oblivious to monetary pressures, some physicians respond to financial incentives directly, and still others respond indirectly, since their clinical decisions and use of medical resources are shaped to some extent by the financial implications of alternative options. Unfortunately, the literature on this topic is limited. The following limitations of available evidence were discussed in an ICF study:

> Studies of physician payment, practice patterns, cost control, and quality of care are subject to various limitations. First, most studies are relatively limited in scope, unrelated in methodology, and biased in focus. Studies have identified differences in quality but cannot attribute causes to payment, organization, controls, or financial incentives. Second, the majority of studies were conducted prior to 1982, and do not account for changes within the past five years including prospective payment for Medicare, rapidly-developing investor-owned HMOs, increased competition, and a developing surplus of physicians. Third, little research has focused on representative, multi-site samples of HMOs. Studies have centered on comparisons between, not within, prepaid groups and FFS providers, and quality is typically analyzed in the context of large, non-profit HMOs. Another limitation is the reliability and validity of questionnaires issued to derive data.[15]

Thus, a key issue for HMOs is the relationship between financial incentives and the potential for adverse quality of care. Because HMOs use a combination of financial incentives, utilization control mechanisms, and other cost-containment and quality review procedures, it is difficult to single out the causal effect of financial incentives on quality of care (e.g., to identify adverse quality of care resulting from or attributable to the structure of financial incentives in an HMO). The importance of the issue, however, guarantees that it will be a topic for discussion and possible congressional action in the future.

Exhibit 3-2: Summary of GAO Report on Physician Incentive Payments by Prepaid Health Plans

Objectives: The General Accounting Office (GAO) was asked by the Chairman, Subcommittee on Health, House Committee on Ways and Means, to (1) evaluate the potential of various types of physician incentive plans offered by HMOs serving Medicare beneficiaries to result in inappropriate reductions of services, and (2) identify plan characteristics that pose the greatest risk to quality of care.

Methodology: From January 1987 through May 1988, information was obtained from 19 HMOs concerning their financial arrangements with primary care physicians and their quality assurance plans. Seventeen of the plans were randomly selected from HMOs in California, Minnesota, and Florida while two other plans were added later: one due to its large size and long-time experience in the HMO industry and the other due to the comprehensiveness of its incentive arrangement. The 19 HMOs had a combined enrollment of over 435,000 members. The nature of the risk borne by the physicians and the distribution of incentive funds were examined. Quality assurance plans were reviewed to determine whether they might mitigate the effects of incentive plans and help assure the provision of quality care.

Results: The following table summarizes the features of the incentive plans examined in the study.

Description	No. of HMOs
Shifted risk for hospital and/or specialist services to HMO physicians and also withheld funds from the physician for distribution:	
Annually, based on group performance	2
Annually, based on combined individual and group performance	1
Monthly, based on group performance	1
Shifted risk for hospital and/or specialist services to HMO physicians without withholding funds for distribution	2
Shifted risk only for the HMO physician's own services	1
Withheld funds from physicians for distribution:	
As an annual bonus to salaried physicians, based on plan profits	1
Annually, based on group performance	5
Annually, based on individual performance	2
Quarterly and annually, based on combined group and individual performance	1
Annual bonus to salaried physicians, based on plan profits	1
No physician incentive plan	2
Total	19

Conclusions: The GAO concluded, "If the Subcommittee considers modifications to Medicare to permit certain HMO physician incentive payments, it may wish to retain a ban on arrangements that closely link financial rewards with individual treatment decisions and/or expose the primary care physician to substantial financial risk for services provided by physicians or institutions to whom he or she refers patients for diagnosis or treatment." (p. 30)

Source: U.S. General Accounting Office, *Medicare: Physician Incentive Payments by Prepaid Health Plans Could Lower Quality of Care*, GAO/HRD-89-29, Washington, DC, December 1988.

Notes

1. For additional material on prepaid group practice, see W. A. MacColl, *Group Practice and Prepayment of Medical Care* (Washington, DC: Public Affairs Press, 1966); R. Birnbaum, *Health Maintenance Organizations: A Guide to Planning and Development* (New York: Spectrum Publications, 1976); R. G. Shouldice and K. H. Shouldice, *Medical Group Practice and Health Maintenance Organizations* (Arlington, VA: Information Resources Press, 1978); and R. D. Eilers and R. M. Crowe, *Group Insurance Handbook* (Homewood, IL: Richard D. Irwin, 1965), Chapter 15.

2. See A. R. Somers, ed., *The Kaiser-Permanente Medical Care Program: A Symposium* (New York: Commonwealth Fund, 1971).

3. E. W. Saward, *The Relevance of Prepaid Group Practice to the Effective Delivery of Health Services,* Health Services and Mental Health Administration, U.S. Department of Health, Education and Welfare (Washington, DC: U.S. Government Printing Office, 1969).

4. G. Williams, *Kaiser-Permanente Health Plan: Why It Works* (Oakland, CA: Henry J. Kaiser Foundation, 1971).

5. H. S. Luft, *Health Maintenance Organizations: Dimensions of Performance* (New York: Wiley-Interscience, 1981).

6. See P. Starr, *The Social Transformation of American Medicine* (New York: Basic Books, 1982): H. N. Somers and A. R. Somers, *Doctors, Patients and Health Insurance* (Washington, DC: Brookings Institution, 1961); E. J. Faulkner, *Health Insurance* (New York: McGraw-Hill, 1960); and R. D. Eilers and R. M. Crowe, *Group Insurance Handbook* (Homewood, IL: Richard D. Irwin, 1965), Chapter 13.

7. See O. W. Anderson, *Blue Cross since 1929: Accountability and Public Trust* (Cambridge, MA: Ballinger Press, 1975); S. A. Law, *Blue Cross: What went Wrong,* 2nd edition (New Haven, CT: Yale University Press, 1976); and R. D. Eilers and R. M. Crowe, *Group Insurance Handbook* (Homewood, IL: Richard D. Irwin, 1965), Chapter 14.

8. For an excellent review of an employer's perspective on how HMOs can be used to contain health care costs, refer to Chapters 4 and 5 of G. C. Halvorson, *How to Cut Your Company's Health Care Costs* (Paramus, NJ: Prentice Hall, 1988).

9. For a comprehensive discussion of risk-management issues, from the perspective of a group-model HMO, see Chapters 2 and 3 of H. L. Sutton and A. J. Sorbo, *Actuarial Issues in the Fee-for-Service/Prepaid Medical Group* (Denver, CO: Medical Group Management Association, 1986).

10. ICF, *Study of Incentive Arrangements Offered by HMOs and CMPs to Physicians: Final Report,* Prepared for the Office of the Assistant Secretary for Planning and Evaluation, U.S. Department of Health and Human Services, 18 May 1988.

11. ICF, *Study of Incentive Arrangements,* V-9.

12. ICF, *Study of Incentive Arrangements.*

13. News release by Congressman Pete Stark, "Stark Releases GAO Report on

HMO Physician Incentive Plans," Washington, DC, 16 December 1988.
14. U.S. General Accounting Office, *Medicare: Physician Incentive Payments by Prepaid Health Plans Could Lower Quality of Care,* GAO/HRD-89-29, Washington, DC, December 1988.
15. ICF, *Study of Incentive Arrangements,* V-13.

Suggested Readings

Arnould, Richard J.; Debrock, Lawrence W.; and Pollard, John W. "Do HMOs Produce Specific Services More Efficiently?" *Inquiry* 21, no. 3(1984): 243.

Beebe, James; Lubitz, James; and Eggers, Paul. "Using Prior Utilization to Determine Payments for Medicare Enrollees in Health Maintenance Organizations." *Health Care Financing Review* 6, no. 3(1985): 27.

Berenson, Robert A. "Capitation and Conflict of Interest." *Health Affairs* 5, no. 1(1986): 141.

Burkett, Gary L. "Variations in Physician Utilization Patterns in a Capitation Payment IPA-HMO." *Medical Care* 20, no. 11(1982): 1128.

Burney, Ira L.; Schieber, George J.; Blaxall, Martha O.; and Gabel, Jon R. "Medicare and Medicaid Physician Payment Incentives." *Health Care Financing Review* 1, no. 1(1979): 62–78.

Cunningham, Francis C., and Williamson, John W. "How Does the Quality of Health Care in HMOs Compare to That in Other Settings?" *The Group Health Journal* 1, no. 4(1980): 4–25.

Deuschle, Jeanne M.; Alvarez, Barbara; Logsdon, Donald; Stahl, William; and Smith, Harry, Jr. "Physician Performance in a Prepaid Health Plan: Results of the Peer Review Program of the Health Insurance Plan of Greater New York." *Medical Care* 20, no. 2(1982): 127.

Egdahl, Richard H., and Taft, Cynthia H. "Financial Incentives to Physicians." *New England Journal of Medicine* 315, no. 1(1986): 59.

Eisenberg, John M. "Physician Utilization: The State of Research about Physicians' Practice Patterns." *Medical Care* 23, no. 5(1985): 461.

Eisenberg, John M., and Williams, Sankey V. "Cost Containment and Changing Physicians' Practice Behavior." *Journal of the American Medical Association* 246, no. 19(1981): 2195.

Fleming, Neil S., and Fleming, David G. "Approaches to Primary Care Physician Capitation." *GHAA Journal* 9 (1988): 4–12.

Fox, Peter D., and Heinen, LuAnn. *Determinants of HMO Success.* Ann Arbor, MI: Health Administration Press, 1987.

Gabel, Jon R., and Redisch, Michael A. "Alternative Physician Payment Methods: Incentives, Efficiency, and National Health Insurance." *Milbank Memorial Fund Quarterly/Health and Society* 57, no. 1(1979): 38.

Hillman, Alan. "Financial Incentives for Physicians in HMOs." *New England Journal of Medicine,* 317, no. 27(1987): 1743.

Hornbrook, M. C., and Berki, S. E. "Practice Mode and Payment Method:

Effects on Use, Costs, Quality, and Access." *Medical Care* 23, no. 5(1985): 484.

Hornbrook, Mark C.; Greenlick, Merwyn R.; and Bennett, Marjorie D. "Analytic Perspective on Data Needs of Health Maintenance Organizations." *Health Care Financing Review,* 1986 Annual Supplement: 89–94.

Luft, Harold S. "How Do Health Maintenance Organizations Achieve Their 'Savings'?" *New England Journal of Medicine* 298, no. 24(1978): 1336.

————. *Health Maintenance Organizations: Dimensions of Performance.* New York: John Wiley and Sons, 1981.

Manning, Willard G.; Leibowitz, Arleen; Goldberg, George A.; Rogers, William A.; and Newhouse, Joseph P. "A Controlled Trial of the Effect of a Prepaid Group Practice on Use of Services." *New England Journal of Medicine* 310, no. 23(1984): 1505.

Manning, Willard G., et al. "Health Insurance and the Demand for Medical Care: Evidence from a Randomized Experiment," *American Economic Review* 77, no. 3(1987): 251–77.

McClure, Walter. "On the Research Status of Risk-Adjusted Capitation Rates." *Inquiry* 21, no. 3(1984): 205.

Moore, Stephen H. "Cost Containment through Risk-Sharing by Primary Care Physicians." *New England Journal of Medicine* 300, no. 24(1979): 1359.

Scitovsky, Anne A.; Benham, Lee; and McCall, Nelda. "Use of Physician Services under Two Prepaid Plans." *Medical Care* 17, no. 5(1979): 441.

Sims, Phyllis D.; Cabral, David; Daley, William; and Alfano, Louis. "The Incentive Plan: An Approach for Modification of Physician Behavior." *American Journal of Public Health* 74, no. 2(February 1984): 150.

ICF. *Study of Incentive Arrangements Offered by HMOs and CMPs to Physicians: Final Report.* Prepared for the Office of the Assistant Secretary for Planning and Evaluation, Department of Health and Human Services, 18 May 1988.

U.S. General Accounting Office. *Physician Incentive Payments by Prepaid Health Plans Could Lower Quality of Care.* Report to the Chairman of the Subcommittee on Health, House Committee on Ways and Means. Washington, DC: U.S. Government Printing Office, December 1988.

Woodward, Robert S., and Warren-Boulton, Frederick. "Considering the Effects of Financial Incentives and Professional Ethics on 'Appropriate' Medical Care." *Journal of Health Economics* 3, no. 3(1984): 223.

Wyszewianski, Leon; Wheeler, John R. C.; and Donabedian, Avedis. "Market-Oriented Cost-Containment Strategies and Quality of Care." *Milbank Memorial Fund Quarterly/Health and Society* 60, no. 4(1982): 518.

Yett, Donald E.; Der, William; Ernst, Richard L.; and Hay, Joel W. "Physician Pricing and Health Insurance Reimbursement." *Health Care Financing Review* 5, no. 2(1983): 69.

Chapter 4

The Debate between HMOs and Employers

> While there are many problems in the healthcare market in general, I believe HMOs, particularly group practice models and well-managed IPA models, will continue to grow and thrive in spite of the intensified carrier competition, employer desire for consolidation and cost controls, and tightening regulatory pressures requiring capital. A means must be found to allay the employer fears of substantial selection in HMO enrollment, with a reasonable methodology developed to adjust for differing risk pools. The revision of the Federal HMO Law which passed on October 14, 1988 will certainly allow employers to be more flexible in adjusting their contribution rates to HMOs and, ultimately, change the marketing environment to employees. HMOs also have an extensive opportunity to try to control employers' retiree costs by creating access to retirees on a cost-efficient basis often well below the retiree cost per person currently being experienced by employers.
>
> H. S. Sutton, "The Future of HMOs in a Chaotic Environment"

4.1   Introduction

Over the past few years, there has been much debate over the methods used by HMOs to set premium rates for major employers. Although the debate is primarily between the HMO industry and many of the large employers in the United States, other participants include health benefit consultants, academic researchers, and members of the health insurance industry.

This chapter begins with a description of the key issues in the debate from the employers' perspective, and then focuses on how the HMO industry has responded to the various charges against it. In addition, the chapter includes a description of the Health Maintenance Organization Amendments of 1988, a piece of federal legislation that attempts to provide a solution to some of the major issues in the continuing controversy. The chapter ends with a summary of the key issues that surround HMO premium rate setting.

4.2   Key Issues of Concern to Employers

What are employers' major concerns and objectives in their business relationships and ongoing negotiations with HMOs? Originally, most employers had two major goals with respect to HMOs:

- Cost containment. Can HMOs be an effective instrument in an employer's attempts to restrain spiraling increases in health care costs?

- Employee satisfaction. In addition to containing costs, is it possible for employers to increase employee satisfaction by offering HMOs as alternative choices in their health benefits program?

At the present time, however, employers are more concerned about their relationships with HMOs than about either of the issues above. In addition to the changes brought about by increased competition in health care, there have also been significant changes in employers' approaches to their health benefit programs. This has included substantial efforts to contain health care costs. Employers have become knowledgeable and sophisticated purchasers of health care services. Many employers have joined together in business coalitions to develop coordinated programs to restrain health care cost increases and to expand their joint bargaining power with medical providers. Their role in the health care marketplace has increased significantly.

At the same time, HMOs have played greater roles in multiple-option health benefits programs operated by employers on behalf of their employees. This has stimulated employers to learn more about HMOs and about the legislative and regulatory processes that govern federally qualified HMOs. Some employers believe that many of the provisions originally developed to encourage the growth of HMOs now pose obstacles to the ability of employers to negotiate and contract with HMOs on a basis that makes sense for individual employers. In addition, many employers feel that some HMOs have been unnecessarily reluctant to explain their premium rate–setting methods or to provide adequate data on health services utilization and costs, thus preventing employers from assessing the cost of services used by their employees (and dependents) who enroll in HMOs. As a result, there has been increasing interest on the part of employers in exploring new arrangements and establishing new relationships with HMOs.

What do employers perceive as the key issues in the relationship between employers and HMOs? Employers argue that the issues that pose obstacles to a more effective HMO/employer relationship are as follows:

- Premium rate–setting methods used by HMOs
- Dissemination of data on HMO utilization and costs
- Quality of health care services provided by HMOs
- HMO Act requirements

The discussion of issues in this section does not represent a consensus of all employers. On any issue, some employers may feel closer to the HMO perspective while others may have stronger views than those expressed in this section, and it is likely that many employers have not focused on the issue at all. The intent of this section is to identify issues that have been raised repeatedly (usually by employer coalitions or large employers who are concerned about health costs) and to present a discussion of the issues from a generalized "employer perspective."

Premium Rate–Setting Methods Used by HMOs

The HMO Act of 1973 provided several advantages to HMOs, such as the dual-choice mandate (to increase market access) and the equal dollar contribution requirement (to protect HMOs against discrimination). However, the act also required HMOs to fulfill the following requirements for federal qualification: (1) their premium rate–setting method must use community rating, (2) their benefits must include a package of mandated health care services, and (3) they must adhere to other requirements regarding their delivery system, organizational form, quality assurance mechanisms, board of directors representation, and allowable cost-sharing and risk-sharing provisions.

The community-rating requirements have been an integral part of the HMO industry's development since 1973 (since the 1930s for the traditional prepaid group practice plans). Until the relatively recent flurry of development of nonqualified (mostly for-profit) plans offering experience-rated products, community rating was viewed by most HMO personnel as the only acceptable method for determining HMO premiums. However, the methods of implementing community rating have changed over time. Initially, community rating meant that there was only one premium based on the total experience of the whole community. More flexibility in community rating has been permitted through the 1981 HMO Act amendments, which allow community rating by class as an acceptable HMO rating method. Therefore, different premiums are often charged to different groups based on different mixes of classes of enrollees, and premiums are based on the experience of each class.

Although most small employers have health plans that are community rated or manually rated (i.e., the rates reflect specified characteristics of the group but not the specific cost experience of the group), medium-sized and large employers are most familiar with experience-rated health insurance plans. Whether they use indemnity insurance, self-insurance, or a third-party administrator, large employers are most comfortable with paying the health care costs that have been incurred by their employees (and eligible dependents).

A number of problems have arisen between employers and HMOs which derive from the use of community-rating methods for large employers. These problems include (1) cross-subsidies among employers, (2) claims of "shadow pricing," (3) claims of "skimming" or "gouging," and (4) lack of confidence in HMO rate-setting methods (brought about by the apparent lack of justification for HMO prices, which is exacerbated by inadequate explanations and documentation of pricing assumptions and methods).

In community rating, the same or equivalent premiums are charged to different groups for the same benefit package. This means that some groups enrolled in HMOs necessarily subsidize other groups. Thus, community rating implies a network of cross-subsidies between low-cost, low-risk groups and high-cost, high-risk groups. Large employers are definitely not interested in subsidizing the health care costs of other higher-cost employers.

Some employers claim that some HMOs engage in a practice that has been termed "shadow pricing," the practice of setting the price for an HMO just below that of the indemnity insurer. It is alleged that some HMOs "shadow price" in order to receive the maximum employer contribution possible. In any geographic area, indemnity premiums for large employers will vary widely across different groups, usually by a factor of two or more (the highest premiums will be twice as much as the lowest premiums, for comparable benefit packages and family composition). The magnitude of this premium differential is a function of the variation in health care costs across different groups. By law, an employer with more than 25 employees who offers his employees health insurance must also offer the option of enrolling in an HMO (if mandated by a local HMO). In addition, the employer must pay the HMO a contribution that is equal in dollars to the contribution to the indemnity plan.[1] If the HMO's community-rated premiums are significantly lower than the employer's contribution to the indemnity plan, as is the case for high-cost employer groups, then money should theoretically be "left on the table" because the HMO cannot receive more than the amount of its premium. Employers argue that, in cases like this, some HMOs artificially raise their premiums above their community rates in order to collect a higher contribution from the employer.[2]

A separate issue is whether HMOs are effective in reducing or containing health care costs for employers. Several studies have concluded that HMOs provide cost-effective health care services in an efficient manner.[3] In particular, for a given population, the practice patterns of HMO providers appear to result in lower health care costs when compared with fee-for-service medical practice.[4] However, employers argue that, in many cases, their health care costs are higher when they offer HMOs because HMOs charge premiums that are significantly higher than the costs incurred for the employer's enrolled employees.[5]

Some employers also claim that some HMOs engage in the practice of "skimming" (i.e., deliberately attempting to enroll the healthiest members of an employer's work force, whose health care costs are likely to be less than their community-rated premiums). Methods of "skimming" include (1) pricing practices that are designed to attract low-risk persons, (2) design of benefit packages to discourage sick or high-risk persons and encourage healthy enrollees, (3) marketing or advertising programs that are directed specifically at low-risk enrollees (or segmenting enrollees by risk category), and (4) other techniques to elicit a favorable selection by taking advantage of the natural selection process in multiple-option health benefits programs sponsored by employers.

Employers claim that, while they are charged premiums at community rates that assume "average" utilization of services, HMOs attract only low-risk persons who use services that are far below the average cost. In this way, HMOs receive windfall profits, and large employers are left with the high-risk employees in their indemnity plans. Because indemnity insurers base their premiums on the experience of the group, the premiums for these groups increase. As the premiums increase relative to those of the HMO, the healthier employees switch to the HMO, leaving the indemnity plan with an even worse (higher-risk) group. This is referred to as an "adverse selection spiral," and it results in the indemnity plan premiums being driven higher and higher over time.

The final problem concerns the lack of face validity to HMO rate-setting methods. Employers claim that some HMOs do not charge the same premiums to all groups for the same benefit package, although they are required to do so under community-rating requirements. Others complain that HMOs give inadequate explanations of their rating methods and that, in some cases, inaccurate or invalid assumptions are used, at the HMO's discretion, to set rates wherever the HMO wants them. In addition, employers claim that HMOs often provide inadequate documentation of pricing assumptions and the specific methods used to derive HMO premium rates. Many employers, who are primarily interested in paying the health insurance costs of their employees, perceive these methods as being unfair and arbitrary.

Quality of HMO Health Care Services

Another area of employer concern is the quality of the health care services that HMOs deliver to their employees. Although many studies have concluded that HMO care is of comparable, if not better, quality than fee-for-service medical care, employers want to see data or other documented proof of this assertion, especially for their own employees.

Employers feel that the federal qualification process is lacking in this regard. For example, although there are thorough reviews of a plan's quality assurance procedures at the time of federal qualification review, federal officials devote limited efforts to ongoing monitoring of an HMO's quality assurance program for commercial enrollees.

Employers feel that they have a responsibility to ensure that the health plan options offered to employees meet standards for quality of health care services. If an employer contracts with an accredited HMO, it should be assured that the services provided meet specified standards for quality of care. However, employers prefer a private sector approach rather than a governmental approach to accreditation. The federal qualification process is no longer the only method of assuring the quality and appropriateness of HMO services. A number of review systems have been developed by organizations such as the Joint Commission for the Accreditation of Healthcare Organizations, the Accreditation Association for Ambulatory Health Care, and the National Committee for Quality Assurance. Employers argue that these organizations have eliminated the need for the federal qualification review process.

Dissemination of Data on HMO Utilization and Costs

Employers want to receive tabulations of data on the utilization and cost of HMO services provided to their employees. They want this information as a justification of the premiums they pay to HMOs. They want to be able to determine whether the HMO represents a cost-effective method of health care delivery. And they want to determine whether the HMO has enrolled only the healthiest segment of their work force.

As the health care environment becomes increasingly competitive, employers are searching for ways to assess the efficiency and appropriateness of different forms of organizing, financing, and delivering health services. Thus, the need for adequate HMO data is a high priority for employers. In the past, some employers believed that some HMOs were reluctant or recalcitrant when requested to provide data. Employers felt that HMOs were hiding behind excuses, reporting, for example, that their computer system would not generate the requested information or that the data could not be collected in the specified format. On the other hand, HMOs feared that employers wanted to use the data as a lever in demanding lower rates or other concessions from the HMO.

Employers were strong supporters of the requirement added to the HMO Act that made it mandatory for HMOs using the new, adjusted community-rating option to maintain and disseminate certain basic types of data to employers. In addition, they believe that employers should have a say in efforts to develop standardized data collection and reporting formats. Employer groups and HMO representatives have made several efforts toward this end, including the development of a standard data reporting form by the Group Health Association of America and the Washington Business Group on Health.

Limitations of the HMO Act as Perceived by Employers

Some employers believe that their relationship with HMOs has been hampered by many of the provisions of the HMO Act. The HMO Advisory Group of the Washington Business Group on Health, one of the foremost organizations representing large employers on health issues, has studied the HMO Act in detail. They recognize that the HMO Act of 1973 gave certain advantages to federally qualified HMOs in order to stimulate the development of the fledgling HMO industry. However, they also feel that, over the past 15 years, many of these advantages have become limitations or restrictions, especially with regard to the HMO's ability to negotiate successfully with major employers. This situation has developed as a result of the rapid growth of the HMO industry and the increasingly competitive health care environment. In addition, employers have become more sophisticated purchasers of health services on behalf of their employees.

According to some employers, the following provisions of the HMO Act are no longer necessary:[6]

- Dual-choice mandate
- Employer contribution requirements
- Community rating
- The federal qualification process for HMOs

Some employers question the need for continuation of the HMO Act in any form. Given the successful growth and maturation of the HMO industry, why should HMOs continue to receive advantages such as guaranteed market access and guaranteed contributions? Why should these decisions not be determined by the marketplace? It is argued that the ultimate success or failure of HMOs (and other managed care programs) should be determined as a result of open competition in the health care marketplace, not by federal regulations or protections.

Dual-Choice Mandate

Under the HMO Act, federally qualified HMOs have the power to mandate that employers with 25 or more employees offer to their employees the opportunity of joining an HMO (at least one staff or group model and one IPA or direct contract model, if they are available in the area). The original intent of this provision was to provide HMOs access to commercial markets if employers in their area were reluctant to offer HMOs.

In principle, the mandate procedure only requires the HMO to send a letter to an employer, inquiring whether they are covered by the HMO Act and whether they currently offer the required HMOs, and requesting that the HMO plan be offered if the conditions are not met. However, in order to comply with federal regulations, HMOs must adhere to a specified timetable and must supply specific information to the employer.

Data do not exist on how many times the dual-choice mandate has been invoked by HMOs to gain access to employers. Health industry experts estimate, however, that 80 to 90 percent (or more) of all HMO/employer contractual relationships are voluntary and were not initiated through the mandating process.

Some employers argue that, although there was a need for this provision in 1973 (due to the lack of acceptance of HMOs by both providers and purchasers in many parts of the United States), conditions have changed significantly since that time. Market resistance to HMOs in most parts of the country is minimal, and HMO growth since 1980 has not been constrained by lack of access to employers. In addition, most employers want to give their employees a fair choice among different health plan options, including HMOs that are desired by their employees.

Some employers also argue that the dual-choice mandate does not make good business sense for HMOs in an increasingly competitive health care marketplace. If a mandate is used to gain access to an employer, it can create a negative climate for the entire relationship between the HMO and the mandated employer. In some cases, employers may react in ways that are not advantageous to the mandating plan. For example, the employer may delay the implementation process, choose an alternative federally qualified HMO rather than the plan that initiated the mandate, establish a pattern of employer contributions that would lead to antiselection against the HMO, or create conditions that minimize the HMO's enrollment of eligible employees.

Employer Contribution Requirements

Until the recent enactment of the Health Maintenance Organization Amendments of 1988, the regulations under the HMO Act required that employers make equal dollar contributions to HMOs (i.e., an employer must make a contribution to its HMO(s) that is equal, in dollar terms, to that made to other indemnity or self-insured health plans offered by the employer to its employees). Although it has been widely believed that all employers were subject to this constraint, this provision only applied to employers mandated under the dual-choice mandate provision. Employers not under the mandate could independently determine their contribution to an HMO they offered voluntarily, or they could negotiate terms that were mutually satisfactory to the employer and the HMO.

The Health Maintenance Organization Amendments of 1988 revised this part of the law and provided HMOs and employers with greater flexibility in determining mutually satisfactory agreements. The new provision stipulates that the method of determining the employer contribution cannot "financially discriminate" against the employees who choose an HMO option offered by the employer. The revised provisions of the Health Maintenance Organization Amendments of 1988 are described later in this chapter.

Community Rating

One of the most objectionable provisions of the HMO Act to employers was the requirement for community rating by federally qualified HMOs. Before the new amendments, HMOs were required to use community rating or community rating by class to determine premiums for enrollees in commercial groups. In particular, they were not allowed to develop premium rates based on the actual or expected cost experience of a specific employer.

As discussed previously, a primary goal for employers is to pay for the actual health care costs of their employees and covered dependents. During the past five years, there have been increasing demands by employers for group-specific rates (i.e., premium rates that reflect the actual health care utilization and cost experience of their employees who enroll in the HMO). Although federally qualified HMOs had been prohibited from experience rating or developing group-specific rates in the past, many nonqualified HMOs (including related nonqualified organizations set up by federally qualified HMOs) used experience rating in order to compete more effectively with large employers.

The Health Maintenance Organization Amendments of 1988 revised the rating requirements for federally qualified HMOs to permit "adjusted community rating." This rating option allows HMOs to develop group-specific rates based on the projected revenue requirements for specific employer groups. The provisions of this new rating method are described in more detail later in this chapter.

Federal Qualification of HMOs

The continuing relevance of the federal qualification program is another important issue in the debate over the HMO Act. To be a federally qualified HMO, a plan must meet a specific set of criteria developed by the Department of Health and Human Services. In the past, many employers interpreted federal qualification to be a measure of the quality of care delivered by an HMO. In essence, being federally qualified offered a seal of approval signifying that an HMO had passed a rigorous test of its management structure, financial soundness, and quality assurance review system.

Some employers have come to question the legitimacy of the federal government's seal of approval, especially regarding the quality of health care services provided by HMOs. For example, employers note that, after a plan has received federal qualification, ongoing monitoring of the quality of health care services delivered to commercial group enrollees is quite limited. As discussed previously, some employers believe that there are better options for evaluating HMO quality, with most of the alternative options organized in the private sector.

In summary, although groups representing employers endorsed most, if not all, of the changes enacted in the Health Maintenance Organization Amendments of 1988, they felt that the changes did not go far enough. In particular, the changes did not address the root causes of many of the present HMO marketplace inequities, as perceived by employers. The demonstrated growth and vitality of the HMO industry leads employers to question why HMOs continue to need the protection and advantages afforded by the HMO Act. If the HMO industry has matured and accomplished the primary financial and market success intended by the HMO Act, then HMOs should no longer need special support and protection by the federal government. The HMO industry should be able to stand on its record of delivering cost-effective, high-quality health care services and compete in the open market.

Summary

Employers are concerned about many aspects of their relationship with HMOs. Specific examples of current issues of concern to employers include the following:

1. Employers want to exert control over their outlays for health benefits and, if possible, to minimize their health care expenditures while maintaining employee satisfaction. They want to pay what their employees actually cost, and they want group-specific (as opposed to community-rated) premiums.

2. Employers would prefer either (1) retrospective experience rating with refunds for good claims experience, like they receive

with indemnity plans, or (2) options for self-insurance, administrative services only (ASO), minimum premium arrangements, or other forms of risk sharing between the HMO and the employer based on actual claims experience and costs.

3. Employers cannot understand why HMOs will not provide (or are reluctant to provide) employer-specific utilization and cost data to justify premium rates.

4. Some employers do not believe that HMOs always set rates according to community-rating methods. They suspect that HMOs "shadow price" the indemnity premiums, or set premiums based on "what the market will bear."

5. Employers want documentation of HMO cost savings to the employer, and evidence of efficiency and cost effectiveness of HMOs with respect to that account's employees.

6. Employers want to be assured that HMOs are not "skimming," that is, receiving favorable selection compared to the indemnity plan (especially if it is not reflected in HMO premiums).

7. Employers want to be assured that the HMO premiums they are charged are not unfairly inflated with excessive overhead loadings, especially with respect to costs for advertising, direct sales meetings with their employees, subsidizing low start-up volume for new plans, and high charges for "general administration."

8. Some employers want a more flexible benefit structure; they do not want to be locked into all of the comprehensive benefits included in most HMO benefit packages.

9. Some employers want HMOs to adopt a more flexible attitude towards patient cost sharing; they do not want to be locked into fixed limits on cost sharing imposed by most HMOs.

10. Employers want to be assured that their employees are satisfied with HMOs, especially regarding service accessibility, service quality, appointment procedures, and administrative requirements. They want effective grievance procedures in place for the resolution of employee complaints and problems.

11. Employers want to be assured of the quality of health care services provided by HMOs. They want HMOs to furnish data to demonstrate that their employees receive quality services.

12. Employers would prefer a limited number of long-term HMO relationships. They want to feel confident that (1) HMOs are good business partners, and (2) they can negotiate with HMOs on issues of major concern.

Thus, employers are concerned about many issues and aspects of their relationships with HMOs. The rest of this book will focus on the issue that draws the most attention, often resulting in fiery discussions and disagreements between HMOs and employers: HMO premium rate–setting practices.

4.3 Premium Rate Setting: The HMO Perspective

Health maintenance organizations approach the issue of premium rate setting from a different perspective than employers. Due to the nature of the HMO operation (i.e., medical service delivery and financing rather than traditional health insurance, medical claims processing, or underwriting), HMOs also view rate setting differently than do indemnity insurers or PPOs. The HMO perspective has also been affected by the community-rating requirements that are mandated for HMOs as part of the federal qualification regulations. These and other factors that have influenced the perspective of HMOs with respect to premium rate–setting practices are discussed in this section.

Changes in the HMO Competitive Environment

In most areas, the level of competition in the health care arena has increased dramatically over the last five years due to (1) a substantial increase in the number of HMOs, (2) expansion in the geographic areas served by existing HMOs, (3) the rapid development of new forms of health service delivery and financing, such as PPOs and "triple-option" plans, (4) pressure exerted by the federal government to reduce health care costs and increase competition, and (5) increased employer interest, including employer coalition activity, in containing health care costs.

As health care competition has increased, there have been several effects on established HMOs. First, competition has made both employers and employees more sensitive to prices. This has been correlated with increasing price competition between HMOs and other health care options such as Blue Cross plans, private health insurers, PPOs, and

TPAs. Second, the impact of competition has resulted in lowered inpatient utilization rates for indemnity plans. In most areas, HMOs still have lower rates, but the differential between HMOs and indemnity plans has decreased substantially, resulting in a reduction in the competitive advantage for HMOs. Third, the increase in competition has included new competitors with strategies to obtain profitable business in selected market components by such methods as seeking low-cost enrollees, using selective provider contracting, and focusing on market niches or market segmentation strategies. Fourth, there have been adverse effects on the profit margins and growth rates of established HMOs due to factors such as overcrowding of competitive market areas, providers giving discounts to other competitors in order to preserve market share, and worsening selection for established plans resulting from increasing competition for low-risk enrollees.

The overall situation for most HMOs is definitely in flux, with many changes in the number of competitors, new forms of delivery and financing, increased demands from major employers with threats to cancel (or not renew) contracts if terms are not renegotiated, and substantially increased levels of price competition. Many HMO chief executive officers (CEOs) feel that the dangers to established HMOs are real and potentially threaten the future survivability of their plans. With fixed costs in facilities and staff (and an existing membership population), it is difficult for existing staff-model and group-model plans to compete in open-ended competition with new health plans that are starting from scratch. Established IPAs, although they have more flexibility in general, have the problems of an existing membership population and maintaining effective control of health services utilization and costs.

There are obvious dangers and potential liabilities that can result from increased competition, and a plan's overall competitive position can be seriously undermined. For example, in many areas, increased competition has had the following effects on established HMOs:

- Erosion of market share and slower rate of growth
- Decrease in overall profitability (excess of revenues over expenditures—either total or per member per month or both)
- Declines in either penetration rates or profit margins (or both) of major commercial groups
- More adverse selection experienced in open enrollments
- Keener (or cutthroat) price competition

- More difficulty in maintaining the competitive position of the plan
- Gradual trend toward a higher risk level in the total enrolled membership population (as demonstrated by increasing per capita costs over time for the same population subgroups, after controlling for inflation and other relevant factors)

Determination of the true impact of increased competition on a plan's financial position requires careful analysis. It is not likely that appropriate data for evaluation of this issue will be available until a minimum of two years after the competition starts.

Advantages of Community Rating

As discussed earlier, one of the major sources of friction between HMOs and employers is the widespread use of community-rating methods by most HMOs. The remainder of this section is devoted to a review of the rationale for and the advantages of community rating from the HMO perspective.

Historically, most HMOs have used community rating as the primary method for determination of premium rates. In fact, for an HMO to be a federally qualified plan, it must adopt community rating as the basis for determination of premium rates.[7] Setting premium rates based on community-rating principles, as originally defined, involves (1) determining premium rates based on projected planwide costs and revenue requirements for the coming year, (2) offering the same premium rates to all employers for the standard benefit package, and (3) updating the fixed community rates on an annual or quarterly basis (again applying the same rates to all employers).

There are many advantages of community rating from the HMO perspective. First, community rating promotes a stable and predictable income flow for the HMO. It also spreads plan costs over the entire membership population, in effect cross-subsidizing high-risk and low-risk groups (within and between employers). Thus, community rating reduces the need for an extensive underwriting function to determine employer-specific premiums.

Second, compared to other rate-setting methods, community rating is easy to implement and monitor. In addition, community rating has been institutionalized in most HMOs. A new method would require substantial time for development and implementation.

Third, community rating facilitates projection of future revenues.

Although not the highest priority for indemnity plans, accurate revenue projection is critical for HMOs, especially those plans with fixed facilities (clinics and hospitals) or salaried physicians. With other rate-setting methods (like experience rating), it is more difficult to accurately project revenues for future accounting periods. Implementation of an alternative rate-setting system would require increased monitoring of premium revenue received over time to ensure against unanticipated shortfalls in revenue.

Fourth, community rating is linked to planwide cost-containment efforts for the entire membership population. Alternative rate-setting methods may affect the incentives of the HMO's providers for controlling utilization and costs. In most HMOs, provider reimbursement is linked to the community-rating system through capitation rates or some form of risk-sharing arrangement between the provider group and the health plan. In these HMOs, provider incentives for utilization control and cost containment are integrated with the community-rating concept.

Fifth, community rating promotes stability in premium rates. The primary alternative to community rating is to base rates on the actual utilization and cost experience of subgroups of subscribers, especially large employers. The smaller the number of subscribers (on whose experience premiums are based), the greater are the likely year-to-year fluctuations in costs. Even for relatively large enrolled subgroups (up to 500 or even 1,000 enrolled members), there can be large statistical variations in health care costs from year to year. In addition, HMOs often have many relatively small groups because they participate primarily in multiple-option programs, so they usually enroll only a subset of any employer group.

However, in contrast to group-specific experience, the utilization and cost experience of the total enrolled membership population is very stable from year to year. Thus, there is a higher level of rate stability with community rating than other rate-setting methods, and use of community-rating methods can eliminate large year-to-year fluctuations in the rates charged to employers.

Sixth, community rating eliminates the necessity for an extensive underwriting and rate-setting function within the HMO (such as the underwriting and actuarial departments found in Blue Cross plans and private insurers). Because most HMOs have relied on community-rating methods to set premiums since the start of their operations, they have not developed the staff expertise or organizational experience required to set premiums on an experience-rated basis. Thus, it is much easier for most plans to continue to use community-rating methods.

Finally, community rating places far fewer demands and requirements on the HMO's data system than alternative rate-setting systems. Because community-rated premiums are developed annually or quarterly based on planwide expenses and projected revenue requirements (possibly with adjustments for factors such as the average family size or mix of single/family contracts for individual employers), there are no requirements for detailed, employer-specific (or age- or gender-specific) utilization and cost data.

In summary, although there has been increasing pressure on HMOs to change from traditional community rating, there are many reasons to explain why HMOs have used and continue to use community-rating methods for premium rate setting. As the HMO industry has developed, community rating has been a major distinguishing feature of federally qualified plans.

Community rating is also a part of the prepayment philosophy of the original prepaid group practice plans, which emphasizes cost-effective health care services delivered within an organizational setting in return for fixed revenues paid in advance. Thus, financial incentives within HMOs operate in the direction of controlling utilization and making cost-effective decisions regarding the delivery of care. To some, experience rating based on the actual cost experience of individual groups is linked to reimbursement based on the volume of services provided (traditional "fee-for-service" medicine), which is antithetical to the underlying HMO philosophy and incentives.

In addition, the administration of a community-rating system is relatively simple compared with alternative rate-setting methods. The data requirements are minimal, and the key financial decisions are limited to a few key parameters (i.e., the annual increase factor), unlike the data requirements and the multitude of decisions required in determining premium rates for individual employer groups under an experience-rating system. Overhead expenses are reduced due to minimal underwriting functions and by not requiring data collection for the utilization or cost experience of specific commercial groups.

Finally, community rating results in greater year-to-year stability and predictability of the plan's "revenue generation process." The HMOs with large fixed costs to maintain facilities, salaried personnel, equipment, and ancillary services (primarily staff-model and group-model plans), need highly predictable prepaid revenues in order to minimize the associated financial risks. It can also be argued that the fixed costs of staff and facilities in these plans are for the benefit of the entire membership population and are not directly linked to specific units of service provided to any specific enrollment subgroup. Therefore, advocates argue that community rating enables HMOs to charge affordable rates to high-risk groups and individuals by basing premiums on a broad-based enrolled membership population that is a cross-section of the community. In this way, community rating permits internal cross-subsidization between high users and low users of services, both within commercial groups and between various membership subgroups.

Limitations of Community Rating

It is easy to see why there are so many proponents of community rating. The rates are perceived to be fair because they allow otherwise uninsurable risks to join the HMO plan at the same community rate as the majority of the population. In addition, community rating allows the HMO to concentrate its efforts on providing health care and not on nonproductive administrative details. In noncompetitive areas, where HMOs enjoy a high penetration rate, community rating has been successful, and its theoretical advantages have become a reality.

In a highly competitive environment, however, many of the advantages of community rating prove to be only theoretical, and never materialize in reality.[8] For example, community rating is thought to promote a stable and predictable income flow. However, if an HMO loses a significant portion of its enrollees (or even if its historical level of growth is curtailed) because aggressive indemnity plans (or new HMOs or PPOs) are gaining new enrollees by offering low premiums to low-cost groups, then the HMO's income flow will turn out to be much lower than predicted.[9] Although community rating facilitates the projection of future revenues, if enrollment levels change swiftly and unexpectedly, then future revenues become much more difficult to project under any rate-setting system.

Community rating is said to promote premium rate stability by preventing high levels of fluctuations in rates. If a new competitor entices a significant portion of an HMO's low-cost members, the plan could find itself raising rates very rapidly. In addition, community rating may be easy to implement and monitor, but the plan may be unable to survive with these methods for unrelated competitive reasons.[10]

Finally, the most common (and the most dangerous) misconception is that community rating eliminates the necessity for an extensive underwriting and rate-setting function. In a competitive environment, the competition is going to know the expected cost of all of its groups. By charging premiums that are related to the cost of each group, any significant changes in enrollment, because of massive enrollment or dis-enrollment of several groups, will result in similar changes in both premium income and benefit costs. On the other hand, some HMOs have little idea of the relative costs among the various groups of its membership population. Thus, whenever an HMO sees changes in its enrollment population, it is not prepared to evaluate the expected changes in the demand for its services. In many cases, it will find out only after the experience develops, and that may be too late.[11] It is important for HMOs to realize that indemnity insurers have a very good idea of the cost of each employer group and, therefore, the appropriate premium to charge the group to make a profit. For their own survival, HMOs must know the same type of information in order to make the same type of underwriting and planning decisions (whether it is necessary for their historical community-rating formulas or not).[12]

The HMO Perspective on Rate Setting

Naturally, HMOs have a different perspective on rate-setting issues than do employers. First, with respect to "charging what the market will bear," many plans establish fixed rate schedules that are applied to all employer groups for the same benefit package. The rate schedule may cover numerous benefit packages (including riders) and combinations of copayment features. However, the rate schedules of these HMOs are internally consistent and applicable to all groups. In addition, for those plans that use more flexible forms of community rating, the acceptable rating formulas are well known, and employers who are interested in investigating the derivation of their rates should be able to establish whether or not the rates conform to federal guidelines.

With respect to allegations of "skimming," HMOs believe that they have not used unfair marketing practices to attract only low-risk employees. In fact, some of the plans that converted to more flexible rating practices, such as community rating by class, did so because of the adverse selection experienced by their comprehensive, community-rated offerings competing against alternative plans. The issue of selection bias in multiple-option health benefits programs is very complex. Some HMOs have received favorable selection in particular situations; however, HMOs believe (and in some cases have documented) that they have also received adverse selection in other situations. The topic of HMO selection bias and its effects on premium rate–setting practices is discussed in more detail in Chapter 8.

Finally, HMOs understand that employers are very concerned about the increase in their health care costs and that cost containment is a high-priority issue for many large employers. In general, HMOs feel that it is unfair for them to be judged arbitrarily and seen as villains in many cases. There have been many situations where individual HMOs have responded to requests from employers regarding data on health services utilization and costs. In those cases where the employer's costs were lower than the HMO average costs/premiums, there were strong pressures for rate reductions. However, in those cases where the employer's costs were higher, employers did not want rate changes and were satisfied with the community rate. Thus, some HMO representatives believe that (1) employers are primarily interested in obtaining the lowest premium rates possible, and (2) the allegations about inconsistent HMO rate-setting practices are a subterfuge for the actual intentions and objectives of employers to obtain the most favorable rate.

The previous sections have attempted to identify and discuss the issues that are being debated by employers and HMOs. The health insurance market is definitely in transition, and it is likely that many of these issues will evolve over time before they ultimately are resolved.

4.4   The Health Maintenance Organization Amendments of 1988

On 14 October 1988, Public Law 100–517 was passed by Congress, and it was signed into law by President Reagan on 24 October 1988. Many observers believe that this legislation will profoundly affect the relationship between HMOs and employers. The committee report issued by the House of Representatives to accompany the legislation included the following statement about the background and need for the legislation:

> The bill addresses a number of issues that have arisen in recent years regarding the requirements that the federal government imposes on HMOs that seek federal qualification and on the employers that offer federally qualified HMOs to their employees. In response to the criticism that the law's requirements are too rigid, the bill would give HMOs additional flexibility in their corporate structure, the organization of their physician services, and the rating systems by which they establish their premiums for enrolled members. In response to criticism of the requirement in current regulations regarding employer contributions to HMOs on behalf of their employees, the bill would clarify for employers the level of contribution they must make on behalf of employees under their health benefits plans when employees enroll in HMOs as opposed to the other health benefits options offered by the employer.[13]

The legislation modified several portions of the HMO Act, including changes involving organizational structure, deductibles, physician services, employer health benefit plans, and restrictive state laws. Of all the legislative changes contained in the bill, there were four items that would appear to have the largest impact on the relationship between HMOs and employers: (1) additional rating flexibility, (2) employer contribution requirements, (3) allowable deductibles, and (4) authorization to allow up to 10 percent of an HMO's services to be rendered by out-of-plan physicians.

Adjusted Community Rating

Prior to passage of the 1988 HMO amendments, federally qualified HMOs were only allowed to determine premiums according to community rating or community rating by class. Section 6(b) of the bill modified the definition of community rating to permit premium rates to be established for the individuals and families of a group on the basis of the HMO's revenue requirements for providing services to the group.

This change was prompted by pressure from employers for premiums based on the utilization and cost experience of their group of employees (and dependents) enrolled in HMOs. Due to the changing competitive environment, HMOs were also interested in acknowledging the interest of employers on this topic and developing an acceptable way for federally qualified plans to respond to employer demands.

The new rating method was termed "adjusted community rating." The 1988 amendments allow HMOs the option of setting rates based on adjusted community-rating methods, which

> fix the rates of payments for the individuals and families of a group on the basis of the organization's revenue requirements for providing services to the group, except that the rates of payments for the individuals and families of a group of less than 100 persons may not be fixed at rates greater than 110 percent of the rate that would be fixed for such individuals and families under subparagraph (B) or clause (i) of this subparagraph.[14]

The final section of the above legislative language refers to premium rates for small groups. Public Law 100-517 requires that the rates for small groups under the new rating method be no greater than 110 percent of what the rates would have been under the HMO's community-rating or community-rating-by-class systems.

The House committee report provided additional guidance for interpretation of the new rating methods for federally qualified HMOs:

This amendment would allow an HMO to adopt a system of rating called "adjusted community rating." Under this provision, HMOs could determine their rates for a group based on the relationship of the group's specific utilization and intensity of service compared to overall HMO member utilization and intensity patterns. The HMO must continue to be "at risk" for providing care at that prospectively determined rate and cannot retrospectively adjust rates based on actual utilization or intensity of services. . . . The Committee notes that the general provisions which have been developed for community rating and community rating by class, such as differentials to reflect compositing or different administrative costs, apply to this new rating option.[15]

The committee report specifically forbade "experience rating" as practiced by insurance companies. The specific practice referred to in the report was "when insurance companies experience rate, they may adjust their premiums at the end of the policy year based on the actual use of health care services by enrollees." This form of rating is commonly termed "retrospective experience rating."

The committee report indicated that setting premiums prospectively, at the beginning of the policy year based on expected experience (revenue requirements), was acceptable, as long as the premiums would not be adjusted at the end of the year based on actual experience. In this way, an HMO would still be at risk for the cost of all care in excess of the premium charged for all enrolled members of the group. This form of rating was judged to be similar to the adjusted community-rating method required of HMOs that apply to HCFA for Medicare risk contracts. Although not specifically mentioned in the report, it would appear that most forms of prospective experience rating (i.e., setting premium rates prospectively, at the beginning of the policy year, based on the historical or projected cost experience of the group, but without any retrospectively determined refunds) would also be acceptable rating methods under the new guidelines.

This legislative change responded to employers' wish that HMOs would tailor their rates to specific employer groups. For example, large employers who feel that their healthiest workers tend to choose HMOs can negotiate a rate with the HMO that is specific to their employees and dependents who are enrolled in the HMO.

Disclosure of HMO Rating Methods and Data

The Senate, which considered the proposed amendments after they had been passed by the House, revised certain portions of the legislation and added some new requirements. One of the most important additions concerned disclosure of HMO rating methods and data. Public Law 100–517 contains the following language:

> If a health maintenance organization is to fix rates of payment for a group under clause (ii) [adjusted community rating], it shall, upon request of the entity with which it contracts to provide services to such group, disclose to that entity the method and data used in calculating the rates of payment.[16]

The conference committee, which met in late September of 1988 to reconcile the House and Senate versions of the proposed legislation, accepted the Senate addition regarding disclosure of HMO rating methods and data. Thus, HMOs that use adjusted community rating must be prepared to disclose their rating formulas, and the data on which the rates are based, to those employers given group-specific rates using adjusted community rating.

Employer Contributions to HMOs

Prior to passage of the 1988 amendments, most employers were required to offer federally qualified HMOs where such HMOs existed. This was referred to as the "dual-choice mandate" provision, and it applied only to employers with 25 or more employees. Thus, any health benefits program offered by an employer to its employees had to include the option of membership in federally qualified HMOs, if mandated by a local plan. In addition, federal regulations promulgated shortly after passage of the HMO Act of 1973 interpreted the act as requiring equal contributions to federally qualified HMOs, dollar for dollar, corresponding to the largest contribution made by the employer on behalf of an employee to any non-HMO alternative health benefits plan offered by the employer, up to, but not exceeding, the HMO's premium.

The Health Maintenance Organization Amendments of 1988 amended Section 1310(c) of the act to require that employer contributions on behalf of employees who enroll in an HMO must not "financially discriminate" against those employees. As discussed in the Senate committee report, this provision was added primarily in response to criticism from employers regarding "shadow pricing" (i.e., basing their premiums on what the employer pays or contributes to other plans, rather than basing premiums on HMO costs and community rates). Employers wanted greater flexibility in determining their contribution to HMO premiums (i.e., some basis other than equal dollar-for-dollar contributions based on other plan contributions).

This new provision allows employers to determine contributions to HMOs on any basis that does not discriminate against persons enrolled in HMOs. The House committee report described several proposed methods that were judged to be acceptable to the members of the House Committee on Energy and Commerce. It is anticipated that these methods will be included in the regulations as permissible ways for employers to make contributions. The methods are as follows:

1. The employer could follow the practice permitted under the existing regulations of contributing to the HMO the same amount it contributes to the non-HMO alternative. For example, an employer that contributes $80 per month on behalf of each employee who joins an indemnity plan could pay the same amount on behalf of each employee who joins the HMO.

2. Employer contributions could reflect the composition of enrollees according to attributes such as age, sex and family status, that are reasonable predictors of utilization, experience, costs, or risk. For each enrollee in a given class (based on those attributes), the employer would contribute an equal dollar amount, regardless of the plan that an employee chooses. To illustrate, one such class might be single males under the age of 30. If the employer's cost for that class is $60, the employer's contribution for HMO enrollment for each employee in that particular class would be $60. The employer would follow this methodology for each of the other classes. By calculating the contribution for HMO enrollment for each class in this way, the employer would determine its total payment on behalf of all employees enrolling in the HMO.

3. Some employers are concerned that when the HMO plan is available at no or nominal cost, employees may have an incentive to select the "free" HMO plan even though they were covered under a health benefits plan offered by their spouse's employer. In addition, as part of their employee benefits philosophy, other employers believe that all employees should contribute to their health care plan regardless of type. In such cases, if employees are required to contribute to a non-HMO plan, an employer could require employees to make a reasonable minimum contribution to an HMO. A contribution that did not exceed 50 percent of the employee contribution to the principal non-HMO alternative plan would be reasonable in such a situation. To illustrate, assume that the HMO's premium is $80, the alternative plan's premium is $100, and the employer contributes $80 on behalf of each employee who participates in the alternative plan. In such a case, employees who join the HMO have no out-of-pocket costs while employees who remain with the alternative plan would contribute $20. If the employer had a policy requiring a minimum employee contribution for health

benefits, it would be reasonable for the employer to require employees who enroll in a lower cost plan, in this example the HMO, to pay an amount not in excess of $10, which is 50 percent of the employee contribution to the non-HMO alternative.

4. Employer contributions could be made on a percentage basis whereby the employer pays the same percentage of the premium of each health plan the employer offers. For example, if an employer paid 90 percent of the premium of each non-HMO health plan the employer offered, the employer would be permitted to pay 90 percent of the premium of the HMO alternative.

5. The amendment would also permit employers and HMOs to negotiate contribution arrangements which are mutually acceptable. Such arrangements would still have to meet the standard established by this provision.[17]

The Senate bill added a provision to "sunset" Section 1310 of the HMO Act which deals with the dual-choice mandate and required employer contributions. The final legislation included a provision to repeal Section 1310 on the date seven years after the date of enactment of the amendments (24 October 1995). In the seven years prior to the repeal of dual choice, the conference agreement did not alter the current interpretation of the way in which Section 1310 applies to employers (i.e., only in the case of a mandated HMO would an employer be required to comply with the new "financial discrimination" language). Once the repeal of dual choice occurs, this limitation to mandated HMOs is changed. Beginning at that time, employers and state and political subdivisions that voluntarily offer to their employees the option of enrollment in one or more federally qualified HMOs would be required to comply with the new "financial discrimination" language for each such HMO.[18]

Deductibles and Physician Services

Prior to passage of the 1988 amendments, all basic health services were required to be provided by physicians who were either staff members of the HMO, a medical group, an individual practice association, or physicians under contract to the HMO (Section 1301(b)(3)). In addition, HMOs were allowed to charge "nominal payments" in addition to any premium (Section 1301(b)(1)). Regulations promulgated by the Department of Health and Human Services interpreted this statutory language to allow some copayments but no deductibles.

The 1988 amendments revised Section 1301(b)(3) to apply the requirement for formal or contractual arrangements with physicians only to the major portion of the HMO's physicians. Thus, HMOs are now permitted to use some fee-for-service physicians who are not under contract to the HMO and who are chosen by members at the time they need service. Section 1301(b)(1) of the HMO Act is amended to allow an HMO that offers the opportunity to obtain basic health services outside the HMO physician panel to require a reasonable deductible for those out-of-plan services.

Prior to the 1988 amendments, plans were not permitted to reimburse members for services received from non-HMO physicians, except in the case of emergency, unusual, or infrequently used services. Under the new provisions, however, HMOs have the option of reimbursing members who seek outside care on an occasional basis. Specifically, an HMO is permitted to develop and offer a health benefits package permitting up to 10 percent of basic physician services to be provided by physicians who are not affiliated with the HMO. The "self-referral" option allows members to go outside the plan for certain services and to be reimbursed for those services.

The 1988 amendments also allowed HMOs to establish a reasonable deductible to be applied to "out-of-plan" services provided by physicians who were not affiliated with the HMO. Copayments could also be applied as allowed under existing law and regulations. In the House committee report, a reasonable deductible was defined as "one that would create reasonable financial incentives for HMO members to use physicians affiliated with the HMO rather than out-of-plan physicians."[19]

Other Provisions of HMO Amendments of 1988

The following provisions were also contained in the 1988 amendments:

- Changes in requirements for HMO organizational structure
- Changes in requirements for HMO board of directors
- Changes in requirements concerning provision of organ transplants
- Changes affecting the applicability of restrictive state laws

Prior to the amendments, Section 1301(a) required that an HMO be a separate "legal entity" (i.e., it could not be part of a larger corporation or operate any other business, such as a PPO or an insurance company). The new law permits both of these corporate structures and revises the definition of an HMO by replacing the term "legal entity" with the language "public or private entity which is organized under the laws of any state."

The House committee report noted that HMOs and health insurance companies can compete more effectively if each can offer a range of coverage options. In particular, the amendments permit an HMO to set up a non–federally qualified plan without undergoing the time and expense of establishing a separate corporation. The report noted that it was confusing and unnecessary for employers to deal with separate legal entities when a single corporation could offer several options, including an HMO, a PPO, an indemnity plan, or a self-insurance administrative arrangement. It was felt that both HMOs and insurance companies would benefit from the change (i.e., insurance companies can have an HMO as a line of business, and HMOs can operate other types of health plan options).

This change will also revise some of the criteria applied by the Department of Health and Human Services during review of an applicant for federal qualification when the HMO operations are part of a component in a larger entity. Prior to the change, DHHS reviewed all activities of an entity to determine if the federal regulations were met. In contrast, when an application for a competitive medical plan is reviewed by DHHS under Section 1876 of the Social Security Act, and the CMP is an operating component of a larger corporate entity, DHHS will look only to the CMP component to determine if the applicable health care delivery system requirements are satisfied.

Prior to 1986, HMOs were required to provide as a medical service any organ transplant which was determined by the Secretary of Health and Human Services not to be experimental. The HMO Amendments of 1986 changed this requirement to include only those organ transplants determined by the secretary to be no longer experimental as of 15 April 1985. However, this provision was to be in effect only until 1 April 1988. The 1988 amendments extended the moratorium. Therefore, the current law is that HMOs must offer only those organ transplants which were required to be offered on 15 April 1985. All other transplants may be offered at the discretion of the HMO unless required under state law.

The final changes contained in the 1988 amendments concerned requirements for HMO boards of directors and restrictive state laws. Formerly, Section 1301(c)(5) mandated requirements for representation on the board of directors of a federally qualified HMO. The 1988 amendments repealed these requirements. Section 1311, which prohibited states from imposing a variety of requirements on HMOs, was revised to prohibit a state from establishing any requirement that would prevent an HMO from complying with the requirements of Title XIII. Thus, federal HMO law sets a policy that HMOs are to be encouraged and held to certain standards. State laws that are consistent with federal policy are not affected. However, state laws that would interfere with an HMO complying with Title XIII are prohibited.

Other changes made by the 1988 amendments to the HMO Act included provisions relating to evaluation of an HMO's fiscal soundness and medically necessary services. These provisions were added in the Senate version of the proposed legislation, and they were maintained in the final bill reported by the conference committee. With respect to medically necessary services, Public Law 100–517 includes a provision prohibiting the Secretary of Health and Human Services from changing regulations, policy statements, interpretations, and practices with respect to abortion services that were in effect on the date of enactment of the legislation.

Congressional Testimony on the 1988 HMO Amendments

On 30 September 1987 a congressional hearing was held on the proposed HMO amendments (H.R. 3235) by Henry Waxman, Chairman of the Health and Environment Subcommittee of the House Energy and Commerce Committee. Testimony on the proposed legislation was heard from the administration, from most of the HMO interest groups, and from interested groups representing employers. The following persons and groups provided testimony to the subcommittee:[20]

- Glenn Hackbarth, Deputy Administrator, Health Care Financing Administration, Department of Health and Human Services
- Roger Birnbaum, Chairman of the Board, Group Health Association of America and President, Rutgers Community Health Plan
- Robert Crane, Vice President, Kaiser Foundation Health Plan
- Michael Herbert, Treasurer, American Medical Care and Review Association and President, Physicians Health Services
- Leonard Wood, Senior Vice President, Blue Cross and Blue Shield Association

- Alan Peres, Chairman, HMO Advisory Group, Washington Business Group on Health and Manager, Health Care Utilization, Illinois Bell Telephone Company

The HCFA's representative, Glenn Hackbarth, presented testimony for the administration. In essence, the administration's position was that the HMO Act, while serving a very useful function in the past by encouraging the development of HMOs, had outlived its usefulness. Hackbarth gave the following testimony:

> The most important objective of the HMO Act has been accomplished; HMOs are a well-established part of mainstream American medicine. It is now time for the federal government to reduce its role and allow HMOs and employers to transact business in a competitive manner. Vigorous competition on quality and price will encourage the development of a broader array of managed-care systems designed to meet the needs of employers, unions and consumers. Thus the Administration has proposed legislation to repeal Title XIII requirements and protections for HMOs. . . .
>
> New managed-care models and new sponsoring entities continue to emerge at a record pace. Today, we have a continuum of organizations, financing and delivering health care, and many of the old distinctions are blurring or even disappearing.
>
> A basic issue that results from development of these new options is whether the law should define which entities are eligible for federal qualification under Title XIII and its related privileges, such as market access and guaranteed contributions, or whether these decisions should be determined by the marketplace. H.R. 3235 takes the position that the definition of an HMO under Title XIII should be expanded to include new models, including preferred provider organizations, and that HMOs should be allowed to expand their services to include other types of insurance, such as experience-rated products. Because each plan is different, the language of H.R. 3235 is flexible, thus leaving the federal government with the task of determining which entities would meet the new standards. We do not support a program where the federal government is left as the final arbiter of which entities can receive the benefits of federal qualification. We believe that access to market and premium decisions should be determined by the marketplace.

The Group Health Association of America was represented by Roger Birnbaum, President of Rutgers Community Health Plan and Chairman of the Board of GHAA. He emphasized GHAA's support of the HMO law and the needs of HMOs for additional flexibility in dealing with the employers that they serve.

> There continues to be enormous value in retaining the HMO Act as a kind
> of assurance of legitimacy on which the industry, employers, and con-
> sumers rely. . . . Federal qualification also has great value in assuring
> purchasers that an HMO has a quality assurance program in place. . . .
> The HMO Act provides the enforcement mechanism necessary to assure
> that appropriate care is provided. The standards under the HMO Act are
> intended to ensure that HMOs have a rigorous and comprehensive internal
> quality assurance system. . . . The challenge we face now is to amend
> the law to recognize changes in the health care markets in which HMOs
> operate while preserving the integrity of the HMO concept.

Michael Herbert, testifying for the American Medical Care and
Review Association (AMCRA), supported all of the provisions of the
proposed amendments. In particular, he emphasized the need for the out-
of-plan option. "The 'open-ended' delivery model is not available under
the current HMO Act for federally qualified HMOs. . . . Without the
ability to provide an open-ended product, my HMO plan would suffer
unnecessarily in an increasingly competitive marketplace."

Robert Crane testified on behalf of Kaiser Foundation Health Plan.
His testimony supported all of the provisions contained in the proposed
amendments. He also strongly supported continuation of the HMO Act:

> We (Kaiser) believe the HMO Act continues to perform an important
> function. It assures employers and members that federally qualified HMOs
> meet standards of fiscal soundness and quality. It sets forth 'rules of the
> game' which facilitate fair competition among HMOs. It fosters choice
> among health plans which is a key to effective competition and creates
> incentives for cost effectiveness. Finally, there are still many employers
> who do not offer an HMO option or would not do so without the Act's
> requirements. Continuation of the Act will help assure health plan choices
> for more Americans.
>
> However, the Act needs to be updated to recognize the realities of the
> late 1980's. H.R. 3235 does this and permits important new flexibility in
> HMO corporate structures, organization of services, and rating systems
> which will permit HMOs to adapt to the changing environment.

Leonard Wood testified for the Blue Cross and Blue Shield Association. He supported all of the provisions in the proposed amendments
except for the out-of-panel coverage option. The original draft of H.R.
3235 permitted HMOs to provide up to 49 percent of their services
through non-HMO physicians. Wood testified that their position strongly
opposed such a high proportion of out-of-plan services. The final bill
passed had reduced the allowable proportion of out-of-plan services to a
maximum of 10 percent of physician services.

Alan Peres testified for the Washington Business Group on Health (WBGH), one of the most active organizations representing employers on health issues. His initial comments concerned the current relevance of the HMO Act.

> The WBGH is a national organization which represents the health policy and economic interests of Fortune 500 employers. The HMO Advisory Group (HMOAG), comprised of representatives from major employers, was established in 1985 to advise the WBGH on policy issues affecting HMOs and other managed care systems.
>
> Since its inception, HMOAG has been very concerned about the HMO Act, Title XIII of the Public Health Service Act, and particularly the equal employer contribution, community rating and mandatory dual choice sections. As an indication of the seriousness of their concern, in late 1985 HMOAG members worked with HMO industry representatives to develop a proposal modifying the equal employer contribution language. The proposal, which allowed employers to negotiate contributions, make contributions based on class, or make contributions based on a group, represented the most current thinking at the time and still offers a guide for employers.
>
> The market for medical services has changed dramatically since the passage of Title XIII. Diversity in insurance products, in medical plan designs, and in the organizational and financial structures available to deliver care now represent the norm in an increasingly competitive market. Medical care itself has become much more complex with the explosion of new knowledge and new medical technologies. In light of these changes, we believe that many of the provisions of the HMO Act are now inconsistent with the market and with the benefit plan philosophies of many of the nation's companies.

Peres continued his testimony by examining each of the issues contained in the proposed amendments. In addition, he proposed an additional item for consideration:

> If the HMO Act is preserved, we would also urge consideration of a requirement that HMOs keep and disseminate certain types of data to employers, consumers and other groups. As competitive forces in the health care sector increase and purchasers are looking for ways to assess the efficiency and appropriateness of care, the need for adequate HMO data becomes paramount. HMOs have, in some cases, been unwilling to meet data requests made by purchasers, citing that their information systems don't generate the types of data requested or that different employer demands are not consistent in content or form. We feel that the data collection effort would benefit from the joint input of the HMO industry and employers as exemplified by the development of an initial standardized

data form endorsed by both the WBGH and the Group Health Association of America.

He concluded his testimony with the following statement:

In summary, WBGH and HMOAG

- could support the employer contribution legislative language prohibiting financial discrimination, if the interpretation allows an employer to utilize objective, well-reasoned methodologies in the development of the contribution.
- could support group-specific rating if employers are protected from being financially discriminated against by an HMO.
- continue to oppose the dual choice mandate.
- could support the organizational structure language if employers were not mandated to offer these new products and services.
- support exploration of alternatives to federal qualification which would provide ongoing quality oversight.
- support a requirement that HMOs keep and disseminate data.
- continue to question the overall relevance of the HMO Act in light of the success of the HMO industry and the competitive nature of the current health care market.

After the hearing, the draft legislation was revised and passed in the House in November 1987.

Senate and Conference Action on the 1988 HMO Amendments

The Senate Committee on Labor and Human Resources addressed H.R. 3235 in early 1988. In March 1988, a modified version of the bill was reported out of committee. Primarily due to a hold on the bill by Senator J. Danforth Quayle, the bill was not considered on the floor of the Senate until August 1988. Rather than incremental changes, Senator Quayle favored a repeal or sunset of the HMO Act because he believed that the HMO industry had become "fully competitive" and that the dual-choice mandate was overly regulatory.

I feel that this [dual choice requirement and nondiscriminatory employer contributions] is another example of a burdensome mandate on employer-provided health insurance with which Congress has recently been so preoccupied. Like mandatory benefit coverages and mandatory continuation of coverage, these HMO requirements simply limit employers' flexibility in providing basic health benefits to their workers. . . . For these reasons, I think the Congress should sunset the HMO Assistance Act in three years.[21]

After a compromise between Senator Edward Kennedy and Senator Quayle, the 1988 HMO amendments were introduced on the Senate floor by Senator Kennedy, Chairman of the Committee on Labor and Human Resources, on 11 August 1988.[22] The bill, with amendments by Senators Byrd, Humphrey, and Quayle, was passed the same day, and it was sent to a conference committee for resolution of the (relatively minor) differences between the Senate and House bills. The conferees for the Senate were Senators Kennedy, Simon, Adams, Matsunaga, Hatch, Quayle, and Humphrey. The House conferees were Representatives Dingell, Waxman, Wyden, Lent, and Madigan.

The conference bill was passed by both the House and the Senate and was sent to President Reagan on 14 October 1988. The legislation was signed into law by President Reagan on 24 October 1988. At the time of publication, the Office of Prepaid Health Care in HCFA had initiated work on the federal regulations to implement the 1988 amendments, but a draft of the proposed regulations was not available.

4.5 Summary

The discussions of the employer perspective, the HMO perspective, and the new adjusted community-rating option for HMOs in this chapter have identified a variety of issues related to HMO premium rate–setting methods. The following points summarize the most important issues:

1. Regarding the issue of employer requests for data and related information for justification of HMO premiums, what can employers legitimately expect? How can HMOs effectively communicate the limitations of their current data systems and the additional expense that would be required for special programming, tabulations, and other data development? Several business coalitions have been actively working with HMO representatives to determine which data should be requested by employers and developed by HMOs (a data reporting form was developed jointly by GHAA and WBGH).

2. Regarding methods for setting premiums, how can HMOs' historical use of community-rating methods be reconciled with employers' strong objection to the cross-subsidies that are a necessary part of community rating? Is it reasonable for employers to demand experience-rated premiums from most HMOs,

especially given current federal regulations for federally qualified plans? Is it reasonable for HMOs to insist on community rating, given that this is one of the highest priority concerns of many employers?

3. There has been very little published information on the overall level and distribution of HMO and indemnity premium rates, especially with respect to employer-sponsored, multiple-option health benefits programs. What is the relationship between indemnity and HMO premiums? Do HMOs set rates based on what the market will bear? Do HMOs that profess to be community rated actually practice community-rating methods when setting employer premiums?

4. How are premium rates (both HMO and indemnity) changing over time? Is there an "adverse selection spiral" occurring in indemnity premiums as a result of HMOs attracting healthier employees? Are HMOs "shadow pricing" the premium rates of indemnity plans? Is it possible for HMOs to experience adverse selection as well as favorable selection?

5. There are major philosophical differences between employers and HMOs. How, for example, can the desire of most employers for experience rating, self-insurance, or "paying what my employees actually cost," be reconciled with principal tenets of HMO philosophy—prepayment and community rating?[23]

6. In addition to the disagreements about data requests and rate-setting methods, several difficult technical issues create confusion and hamper resolution of problems related to the HMO/employer relationship. Some of these technical issues are as follows:

   • How can "selection bias" be measured? If HMOs are receiving a favorable selection of risks in multiple-option health benefits programs, how can this be quantified and incorporated into the rate-setting process?

   • How can HMOs prove that they produce cost savings for employers? Many HMOs believe that they offer employers effective managed care programs that save health care costs, especially compared to alternatives such as fee-for-service or PPOs. How can this fact be documented to the satisfaction of skeptical employers?

- How can other phenomena, such as regression to the mean, be used in the analysis of costs resulting from the interaction of HMO, indemnity, and PPO options when employers offer multiple-option health benefits programs?

There are many difficult problems that need to be addressed in order to improve the current HMO/employer relationship and create a solid foundation for the future. The recent legislation is one of the most encouraging developments that has occurred with respect to the debate between employers and HMOs over rate setting, and it should eliminate many obstacles posed by federal regulations that have prevented HMOs from considering other rate-setting methods.

Notes

1. This contribution requirement was modified by the Health Maintenance Organization Amendments of 1988, as discussed in Section 4.4.
2. In low-cost employment groups, the opposite is supposed to occur. Because the HMO premium would be significantly higher in this case, HMO enrollment would be more difficult. Consequently, HMOs may find that they will obtain a higher enrollment by lowering their premiums for low-cost groups.
3. See, for example, Harold S. Luft, *Health Maintenance Organizations: Dimensions of Performance* (New York: John Wiley and Sons, 1981); Willard G. Manning et al., "A Controlled Trial of the Effect of a Prepaid Group Practice on Use of Services," *New England Journal of Medicine* 310, no. 23(1984):1505–15.
4. The HMO cost efficiencies may benefit employees, not employers. If an HMO has a lower premium than the indemnity carrier, but the HMO's premium exceeds the contribution amount, the employer is not having any direct saving, but the employee may be getting more benefits per dollar.
5. Here, differences in benefit packages and cost-sharing provisions between alternative health plans have been ignored. Also, some employers question whether all HMOs produce lower utilization patterns and cost savings. In general, staff and group models are acknowledged to generate efficiencies, whereas IPAs are more suspect, unless they can demonstrate strong utilization control practices and effective financial incentives for participating physicians.
6. As in previous sections, this discussion of the HMO Act does not represent a consensus on the part of all employers.
7. The Health Maintenance Organization Amendments of 1988 permit federally qualified HMOs to set rates using adjusted community-rating methods based on the revenue required for individual employer groups.
8. In many areas (both inside and outside the HMO industry), there is a belief

that HMOs will be at a major competitive disadvantage in the near future if they continue to rely primarily on community rating for premium rate setting. The reasons for this belief are as follows: (1) adverse selection against HMOs will worsen as the competition increases in multiple-option health benefits programs, especially in those groups with large differences between HMO and indemnity premiums, (2) some large employers will decide not to renew contracts with HMOs that refuse to negotiate on rate-setting issues, (3) with the recent change in the employer contribution requirement, employers with high indemnity premiums may limit contributions to community-rated HMOs, which could lead to major declines in HMO enrollment as employee out-of-pocket premiums are significantly increased, (4) historically, community-rated health plans have fared poorly when there is strong competition from experience-rated rivals (e.g., the Blue Cross experience in the 1950s has lent credence to this widely held belief concerning the behavior of insurance markets), and (5) since the data are not required to create community rates, HMOs that community rate tend not to generate the data that is necessary to analyze the developments in the health care market and to make prudent "group-specific" business decisions that affect the financial viability of the HMO.

9. For example, with community-rated premiums, HMOs are now frozen out of many large employer groups with low per capita cost (e.g., a "high-tech" company that has grown rapidly and has a young, healthy workforce with extremely low indemnity premiums). Thus, a decision by an HMO regarding community rating versus other rate-setting methods will have major implications both for the plan's continued financial viability and for its overall competitive position. Some observers believe that a major disadvantage of community rating is that it restricts an HMO's capacity to compete in the marketplace. For example, indemnity health insurance premium rates of Blue Cross and private insurers typically vary widely in any metropolitan area or region. The highest premium rate for singles (or families) is commonly twice as high as the lowest premium rate offered to employers. This is the result of experience rating and variations in benefit packages. Thus, an HMO with a fixed community rate will have premium rates that are significantly higher than competitors for an employer with low experience-rated premiums. This usually leads to an extremely low penetration rate and probably adverse selection from those persons who do enroll with the HMO. On the other hand, the HMO may attract such a large enrollment from a high-cost group that the average cost of those enrolled will reflect that group's high per capita cost. Thus, for employers with high experience-rated premiums, the HMO is in a more favorable position with its lower community-rated premiums, and a higher penetration rate would be expected. However, the danger in this case is that the experience rates were set high for a good reason, and, even if the HMO receives favorable selection compared to the employer's "average" experience, it is likely to receive unfavorable selection compared to the HMO's average per member per month cost.

10. The underlying principle in this argument is that community rating is less efficient, in an economic sense, than experience rating. If insurers are able to offer healthy groups lower rates under experience rating than HMOs can under community rating, insurers will attract a higher proportion of the healthy groups and enrollees. This will leave community-rated HMOs with a higher-risk enrolled population, which will lead to higher community rates and a competitive disadvantage for HMOs. See, for example, K. S. Abraham, *Distributing Risk: Insurance, Legal Theory and Public Policy* (New Haven, CT: Yale University Press, 1986), 78.

11. As recently experienced by many HMOs, a highly competitive environment (or significant increases in competition) can lead to loss of profitability, impaired competitive position, a slower rate of growth, a gradual trend toward a higher-risk (higher cost) membership population, and erosion of market share or decreased penetration rates in major commercial accounts. Unfortunately, the true impact of increased competition is frequently not recognized, or reported in bottom-line financial results, until 18 months or more after the change in competition takes place. This results from the normal claim lags between date of service and date of payment, the time required for data processing, the time required to reflect these data in periodic reports, and other delays (e.g., scheduling and timing of MIS report generation after the end of the fiscal reporting period) before data on financial results are available for review by HMO management. Of course, depending on the marketplace and the types of competitors, an HMO may be very competitive for a high proportion of employer groups. In this case, rate setting based on strict community rating may remain the preferred method because it provides for stability of premium rates and HMO revenue, it is easy to explain and inexpensive to administer, and it spreads risk equally throughout the entire membership population. In general, however, most geographic areas have high variations in indemnity premium rates, and community-rated HMOs will suffer from adverse selection and other problems in highly competitive marketplaces.

12. This section has identified potential disadvantages of community rating for HMOs. Some arguments against community rating focus on the requirements for ''survival'' in the current competitive environment. Other observers, however, argue forcefully that HMOs can continue to operate successfully with community rating. They question the arguments offered against community rating in the future for a variety of pragmatic and philosophical reasons.

13. House Committee on Energy and Commerce, *Health Maintenance Organization Amendments of 1987: Report to Accompany H.R. 3235*, 100th Cong., 1st sess., 30 October 1987, 3–4.

14. Public Law 100–517, ''Health Maintenance Organization Amendments of 1988,'' Section 6(b).

15. House Committee on Energy and Commerce, *Health Maintenance Organization Amendments of 1987: Report to Accompany H.R. 3235*, 9.

16. Public Law 100–517, Section 6(b).

17. House Committee on Energy and Commerce, *Health Maintenance Organization Amendments of 1987: Report to Accompany H.R. 3235*, 10–11.
18. House Committee on Energy and Commerce, *Health Maintenance Organization Amendments of 1988*, H.R. Conf. Rept. No. 100–1056, 5 October 1988, 11.
19. House Committee on Energy and Commerce, *Health Maintenance Organization Amendments of 1988*, 8.
20. Excerpts from congressional testimony by Hackbarth, Birnbaum, Crane, Herbert, Wood, and Peres are taken from their statements before the Committee on Energy and Commerce, Subcommittee on Health and the Environment, U.S. House of Representatives, 30 September 1987.
21. "Additional Views of Senator Quayle," S. Rept. No. 100–304, *Health Maintenance Organization Amendments of 1987*, 22 March 1988.
22. *Congressional Record*, 100th Cong., 2d sess., 11 August 1988, S11748–52.
23. Most employers approach the topic of health benefits from the perspective of "traditional" health insurance (e.g., indemnity plans and medical claims processing, usually based on fee-for-service medical practice). HMOs strongly believe that fixed revenues (paid in advance) provide the incentives for development of an efficient health care delivery system (e.g., delivery of high quality services with the goals of utilization control, cost containment, managed care, and provider incentives). In this context, experience rating (or cost-based premiums) is equated with the practice of fee-for-service medicine, and it is antithetical to the basic philosophy of HMOs.

Suggested Readings

Bachman, Sara S.; Pomeranz, David; and Tell, Eileen J. "Making Employers Smart Buyers of Health Care." *Business and Health* 4, no. 11(1987): 28.

Bennett, Amanda. "Firms Stunned by Retiree Health Costs: Likely Result Includes Cuts in Coverage." *Wall Street Journal*, 24 May 1988.

Berwick, Donald M. "Monitoring Quality in HMOs." *Business and Health* 5, no. 1(1987): 9.

Birnbaum, Howard, and Reilly, Helena. "Retiree Health Care Costs Demand Attention." *Business and Health* 5, no. 5(1988): 28.

DiBlase, Donna, "Employers Seek Data to Study HMO Use." *Business Insurance* 20, no. 24(1986): 32.

———. "Allied-Signal Caps Its Costs with New CIGNA Health Plan." *Business Insurance* 22, no. 8(1988): 1.

Evert, David R. "Improving Indemnity Plan Is a Good Offense against HMO Costs." *Business Insurance* 20, no. 51(1986): 43.

Fritz, Dan. "Employers Changing Relations with HMOs." In *Proceedings of the 1987 Group Health Institute*. Washington, DC: Group Health Association of America, 1987.

Kittrell, Alison. "Unfulfilled Expectations: Benefit Managers Report Little Savings from HMOs or PPOs." *Business Insurance* 21, no. 53(1987): 6.

Luft, Harold S. "HMOs: Friends or Foes?" *Business and Health* 3, no.

2(1985): 5.

McClure, Walter. "Buying Right: How to Do It." *Business and Health* 2, no. 10(1985): 41.

Peres, Alan. "Is the HMO Act Good for Employers?" *Business and Health* 5, no. 4(1988): 8.

Rettig, Paul C. "Value, Not Just Costs, Need to Be Considered for Quality Managed Care." *Business and Health* 4, no. 6(1987): 64.

Stowe, James B., and Egdahl, Richard H. "Measuring Purchaser Value from Managed Care." *Business and Health* 4, no. 10(1987): 20.

Sutton, Harry L., Jr. "Community Rating: An Historical Perspective." *Business and Health* 3, no. 8(1986): 41.

Additional Readings

Employers and Health Insurance

Abramowitz, M. "End to Mandatory HMO Funding Sought." *Washington Post,* 13 January 1987.

Altmeyer, Ann S., and Phillips, John, Jr. "Corporate Benefits Strategy Supports Marketplace Reform." *Business and Health* 3, no. 2(1985): 16.

Berenson, Robert A. "A Physician's Perspective on Case Management." *Business and Health* 2, no. 8(1985): 22.

Caper, Philip; Keller, Robert; and Rohlf, Paul. "Tracking Physician Practice Patterns for Quality Care." *Business and Health* 3, no. 9(1986): 7.

Charles, Joseph G. "Using Informed Choice to Combat Health Costs." *Business and Health* 4, no. 11(1987): 36.

"Chicago HMO Consolidation: Proceeding Slowly?" *Hospitals* 62, no. 9(1988): 43.

DiBlase, Donna. "Changes Ahead for HMOs, PPOs." *Business Insurance* 21, no. 53(1987): 3.

———. "Employers Test HMOs, PPOs for Quality." *Business Insurance* 21, no. 53(1987): 10.

———. "Managed Health Care Continues to Evolve." *Business Insurance* 21, no. 44(1987): 70.

———. "More States Adopt HMO Guaranty Funds." *Business Insurance* 21, no. 53(1987): 9.

DiBlase, Donna, and Collins, Linda J. "Inflation Expected to Boost Indemnity Plan Rates." *Business Insurance* 20, no. 51(1986): 3.

DiBlase, Donna, and Huntley, Glenn. "Inflation Boosts Indemnity, HMO Rates." *Business Insurance* 21, no. 51(1987): 3.

Donlon, Thomas M. "Unbundling of Claims Services with Self-Insurance." *Business and Health* 3, no. 3(1986): 11.

Dowd, Bryan; Feldman, Roger; and Klein, John. "What Do Employers Really Want in a Health Plan?" *Business and Health* 4, no. 4(1987): 44.

Duva, Joseph W. "Employers Ask More from HMO Contracts." *Business Insurance* 21, no. 45(1987): 30.

Ellis, Randall P. "Biased Selection in Flexible Benefit Plans." *Business and Health* 3, no. 6(1986): 26.

Enthoven, Alain, and Kronick, Richard. "Competition 101: Managing Demand to Get Quality Care." *Business and Health* 5, no. 5(1988): 38.

Erlenborn, John N. "More Changes in the Offing for Employee Benefit Plans." *Business Insurance* 21, no. 44(1987): 49.

Etheredge, Lynn. "The World of Insurance: What Will the Future Bring?" *Business and Health* 3, no. 3(1986): 5.

Feldman, Sari; Fritz, Dan; and Stanfield, Charles. "Using Employee Satisfaction to Choose HMOs." *Business and Health* 5, no. 4(1988): 17.

Fletcher, Meg. "More States Offer High-Risk Health Plans." *Business Insurance* 22, no. 5(1988): 1.

Fox, Peter D., and Anderson, Maren D. "Hybrid HMOs, PPOs: The New Focus." *Business and Health* 3, no. 4(1986): 20.

Freudenheim, Milt. "Prepaid Programs for Health Care Encounter Snags: HMO Shakeout is Seen." *New York Times,* 31 January 1988, 1.

Fritz, Dan, and Repko, David V. "A Blueprint for Forging New HMO Relationships." *Business and Health* 3, no. 8(1986): 38.

Gardner, Harold H. "Putting Health Care Decisions in the Hands of Consumers." *Business and Health* 3, no. 10(1986): 22.

Geisel, Jerry. "Doctor Loyalty Deters Retiree Use of HMOs." *Business Insurance* 21, no. 51(1987): 1.

————. "Employee Benefit Costs Top $10,000 Per Worker." *Business Insurance* 22, no. 3(1988): 1.

————. "Employer Health Plan Law Taxing for Massachusetts." *Business Insurance* 22, no. 18(1988): 1.

————. "More Benefit Plans Protected by Stop-Loss." *Business Insurance* 22, no. 4(1988): 3.

————. "Most Employers Self-Fund Group Health Care Plans." *Business Insurance* 21, no. 4(1987): 3.

————. "Retiree Health Rules to Cut Profits: Study." *Business Insurance* 21, no. 47(1987): 3.

————. "Rise to Respectability: Benefit Management Gains Sophistication." *Business Insurance* 21, no. 44(1987): 3.

Ginsburg, Paul B.; Hosek, Susan D.; and Marquis, M. Susan. "Who Joins a PPO?" *Business and Health* 4, no. 4(1987): 36.

Goldbeck, Willis B. "Coalitions Treat Health Care Concerns." *Business Insurance* 21, no. 44(1987): 34.

Greenberg, Warren. "The Evolution of Blue Cross in a Competitive Marketplace." *Business and Health* 4, no. 1(1986): 44.

"Health Maintenance Organizations: Will the 'Savings' Reach Your Bottom Line?" Washington, DC: The Wyatt Company, September 1984.

Henderson, Mary G.; Souder, Barbara A.; and Bergman, Andrew. "Measuring Efficiencies of Managed Care." *Business and Health* 4, no. 12(October 1987): 43.

Hirschorn, M. W. "Cost-Cutting Methods by HMOs Increase Patient Dissatisfaction." *Wall Street Journal,* 20 August 1986.

Huntley, Glenn. "New Benefit Plan Aims at Reducing Costs." *Business Insurance* 22, no. 19(1988): 6.

Hurst, R. "Employers and a Changing Health-Care Market." *HealthSpan* 2, no. 9(1985): 18.

Kenney, James B. "Using Competition to Develop a Buyer Driven Market." *Business and Health* 3, no. 1(1985): 39.

Kenney, James B., and Riley, Patsy. "The Future of Coalitions." *Business and Health* 4, no. 2(1986): 30.

Kittrell, Alison. "Employer Cost Control Steps Include HMOs and Flex Plans." *Business Insurance* 22, no. 8(1988): 30.

_____. "Federal Health Plan Needs Reforming: Study." *Business Insurance* 22, no. 22(1988): 19.

_____. "Firms Report Health Costs Rose 7.9% in '87." *Business Insurance* 22, no. 8(1988): 3.

_____. "Flex Plans Curb Medical Costs: Study." *Business Insurance* 22, no. 19(1988): 30.

Kuhlman, Thomas J. "Employers to Define Retiree Health Benefits." *Business Insurance* 21, no. 44(1987): 63.

Lee, F. C. "Employers Cite Drawbacks, Selection Problems in Community Rated HMOs." *Business and Health* 2, no. 6(1985): 47.

Maher, Walter B. "In Spite of Savings, Employers Must Intensify Cost Management Efforts." *Business and Health* 4, no. 10(1987): 52.

"Managed Care: 1988: Lean Year for Some, Leaner for Others." *Hospitals* 62, no. 1(1988): 32.

Masotti, Iris P., and Ericksson, Nancy J. "Hidden Discrepancies in Price Focused Negotiations."*Business and Health* 5, no. 4(1988): 21.

McClure, Walter. "Buying Right: The Consequences of Glut." *Business and Health* 2, no. 9(1985): 43.

Melloan, George. "Insurers Try to Cope with AIDS Test Barriers." *Wall Street Journal*, 31 May 1988, 25.

Merrill, Jeffrey C. "Defining Case Management." *Business and Health* 2, no. 8(1985): 5.

Miller, Laird. "High-Tech Medicine Challenges Payers." *Business Insurance* 22, no. 44(1987): 46.

Milstein, Arnold. "Three Changes Expected for UR." *Business Insurance* 21, no. 44(1987): 44.

Nazemetz, Patricia M. "Health Benefits Redesigns to Stay Atop the Competition." *Business and Health* 2, no. 8(1985): 40.

Patricelli, Robert E. "Financial Risk Takes a Modern Odyssey through Health Care." *Business and Health* 5, no. 2(1987): 50.

Phillips, Kenneth. "Self-Selection Factors in Choosing a Health Plan." *Business and Health* 4, no. 10(1987): 29.

Reinhardt, Uwe E. "Quality of Care in Competitive Markets." *Business and Health* 3, no. 8(1986): 7.

Reisler, M. "Business in Richmond Attacks Health Care Costs." *Harvard Business Review* 63, no. 1(1985): 56–58, 60.

_____. "Game Plan for Business Coalitions on Health Care," *Harvard Busi-

ness Review 64, no. 6(1986): 56–59.

Rich, Spencer. "Catastrophic Insurance Bill Near Passage." *Washington Post*, 26 May 1988.

Ricklefs, Roger. "Firms Turn to 'Case Management' to Bring Down Health-Care Costs." *Wall Street Journal*, 30 December 1987.

Ripps, Jay C., and Werronen, Henry J. "Insurer-Provider Networks: A Marketplace Response."*Business and Health* 3, no. 3(1986): 20.

Rundle, Rhonda L. "Insurers Step Up Efforts to Reduce Use of Free-Choice Health Plans." *Wall Street Journal*, 11 May 1988.

Salisbury, Dallas L. "Employee Benefits in 2007 Will Be More Limited, Costly." *Business Insurance* 21, no. 44(1987): 45.

Schwartz, Ronald M. and Rollins, Pierce L. "Measuring the Cost Benefit of Wellness Strategies." *Business and Health* 2, no. 10(1985): 24.

Schmid, Stuart G., and Holmer, Martin R. "A Federal Case against Flexible Spending Accounts." *Business and Health* 3, no. 4(1986): 41.

Seeman, R. F. "Changes in Employer-HMO Relationships." In *Proceedings of the 1987 Group Health Institute*. Washington, DC: Group Health Association of America, 1987.

Shalowitz, Deborah. "New Managed Care Options Predicted." *Business Insurance* 21, no. 42(1987): 18.

————. "Self-Insurance Propels Growth of TPAs." *Business Insurance* 21, no. 44(1987): 72.

Sharkey, William H., Jr. "Insurers Finding New Niche in Cost Management Programs." *Business and Health* 3, no. 3(1986): 16.

"Standard HMO Data Form to Come." *Hospitals* 60, no. 20(1986): 70.

Stein, J. "Planning a Health Care Strategy at Weyerhauser." *Business and Health* 4, no. 11(1987): 44.

Stone, Mary Hughes. "Transforming Employees into Prudent Purchasers." *Business and Health* 3, no. 9(1986): 36.

Sullivan, Sean; Flynn, Theresa J.; and Lewin, Marion Ein. "The Quest to Manage Mental Health Costs." *Business and Health* 4, no. 4(1987): 24.

Trapnell, Gordon R. "Cost Sharing: A Prescription for Reform." *Business and Health* 2, no. 8(1985): 36.

Tresnowski, Bernard R. "Blue Cross-Blue Shield in the Future." *Business and Health* 4, no. 1(1986): 48.

Welch, W. Pete. "IPAs Emerge on the HMO Forefront." *Business and Health* 5, no. 4(1988): 14.

Weller, Charles D. "Rx for the Costly Epidemic of Health-Care Legislation." *Wall Street Journal*, 9 May 1988.

Wessel, D. "Some Large Employers Believe HMOs Overcharge and Might Not Save Money." *Wall Street Journal*, 14 September 1985.

Winsberg, Gwynne R. "The Hidden Costs of HMOs." *Business and Health* 3, no. 2(1985): 18.

Young, Art. "Managing Health Care Costs: Employers Will Purchase, Not Just Pay for, Health Care." *Business Insurance* 21, no. 44(1987): 33.

Part II

HMO Rate Setting

Chapter 5

Rating and Underwriting

Underwriting involves not only close examination of the general characteristics of the group case, but also, very importantly, the factors determining premium level. These factors include expected claims level; sales, installation and administrative expenses, commissions, taxes and risk charges; the experience rating system used in determination of renewal rates and dividends or retrospective premium credits; and the competitive posture of the market.

D. D. Cody, "Underwriting Group Medical Expense Coverage"

While the first part of this book reviewed a variety of topics related to the history and current competitive environment of HMO, Part II focuses on the theoretical aspects of premium rate setting for health care and health insurance products. The major alternative premium rate–setting methods will be described, and issues related to the rate-setting process in HMOs will be discussed.

This chapter begins with an overview of the general principles related to premium rate setting and underwriting for group health insurance. Group underwriting is the process through which an insurer determines, first, which group risks it will accept and, second, on what terms the contract will be written. In a formal sense, the underwriting function is distinct from the pricing function. However, the two functions are closely related. A pricing structure is based on an assumed level of underwriting performance. Thus, the rating process anticipates and requires an associated underwriting process. In addition, a successful group operation requires that these functions be properly integrated, effectively coordinated, and consistently performed.

Chapter 6 focuses on community-rating methods that have traditionally been the primary methods used by HMOs. Chapter 7 describes other rate-setting methods commonly used to price group health insurance products. Chapter 8 discusses the relationship between selection bias and HMO premium rate setting.

5.1 Introduction to Rating

HMOs are involved in the delivery and financing of health services for their enrolled membership population. Thus, HMOs can be viewed as a subset of two distinct industries: (1) the health services provider industry, as related to the organization, production, and delivery of medical services, and (2) the health insurance industry, as related to the financing of health services and the underwriting of HMO benefit packages sold to employers and other purchasers.

Historically, the primary emphasis in most HMOs has been devoted to development of an effective health care delivery system and implementation of the functional components related to operation of the HMO (i.e., medical/operations, marketing, budgeting, MIS, and planning). In many cases, little emphasis has been given to the traditional functions associated with group health insurance operations, such as underwriting and actuarial functions, development of detailed pricing guidelines or rate manuals, in-depth analysis of claims experience and expense allocations, and negotiation of acceptable premium payment methods and settlement formulas with large and medium-sized clients. The last item includes a variety of topics not usually considered or addressed by HMOs, such as specifying retention formulas for nonmedical expenses (claims processing, pooling or reinsurance charges, marketing and advertising, preadmission certification services, general administration) and developing dividend formulas and appropriate methods of financial participation by group contract holders in stock and mutual insurance companies.

This general pattern is changing, however, as many plans are now paying substantial attention to the insurance aspects of their business. This has come about as a result of (1) heightened competition among HMOs (and between HMOs, Blue Cross plans, and private insurers), (2) new HMO product lines that compete more directly with residual indemnity plans (e.g., PPOs and HMO-insurance combinations), (3) pressures exerted by major employer clients, (4) decreased levels of HMO profitability, (5) the growing importance of proprietary HMOs, and (6) the perceived need for increased financial sophistication.

Pricing insurance products is a dynamic and evolving process. A rating system's environment and the associated requirements change over time. Therefore, it is not possible to determine a rating structure that will remain valid indefinitely. This is especially true in the case of health insurance. For example, a health insurance rate book (the manual of standard rates used by insurers to determine the premium rates to be charged for different benefit packages and insurance classifications) may be obsolete before the end of a year. Inflation in medical care prices, changes in technology, and many other factors make it necessary to continually evaluate, update, and refine the rating structure used to set premium rates for group health insurance contracts. In addition, there are other relevant factors, such as "moral hazard" considerations, regarding the effect of increasing insurance coverage on health care utilization and costs.

Many HMOs use community-rating methods for premium rate setting. In general, this method greatly simplifies the rating process. However, it is still necessary to pay attention to all of the components of the rating process and to ensure that the pricing structure is current and competitive and that it generates the amount of revenue required to operate the plan in a sound fiscal manner. An effective rating system and adequate control of costs and expenditures are essential ingredients for maintaining a plan in strong financial condition.

Before discussing the objectives, requirements, and methods of pricing group health insurance products, some basic terms require definition. A *premium* is the consideration (money) paid for an insurance contract. To provide *insurance* is to provide coverage by contract whereby one party undertakes to indemnify or guarantee a second party against loss caused by a specified contingency or peril during a specified period of time. To *indemnify* is to reimburse or to make compensation for incurred loss or damage.

To *rate* is to fix the amount of the premium to be charged for an insurance contract or per unit of insurance coverage. A *premium rate* is a charge, payment, or price fixed according to a scale or standard, specifically the amount of premium per unit of insurance. A *premium rating system* is the process and methods for determination of premium rates to be charged to policyholders for a specific insurance product, or, more generally, the pricing methods applicable to a particular line of business in an insurance-type organization.

Objectives and Requirements for Rating Systems

The task of pricing insurance products relies heavily on the development and successful implementation of a variety of technical methods involving mathematical formulas and statistical techniques. However, the rating function must be considered in the larger context of the insurer's overall planning and management functions. In particular, a rating system must satisfy the conflicting objectives of management, policyholders, and marketing personnel (and shareholders, if the insurer is a for-profit concern). For example, the goals of management include maintaining solvency, sustaining sales growth, maximizing expected profits, minimizing operating costs, maintaining the morale of the marketing force, and maximizing service to policyholders.[1] On the other hand, policyholders are most interested in minimizing the cost of obtaining desired insurance coverage and obtaining excellent service from the insurer. The major goals of marketing personnel include low premiums (or at least very competitive rates) and maximizing sales (and compensation levels). The final group, shareholders, desires to maintain solvency to protect their investment and to maximize short-term and long-term profitability.

One might reasonably ask how it is possible for a single rating system to respond to all of these conflicting objectives. Obviously, it is impossible to achieve all of the objectives simultaneously. In many cases, it is not desirable to try to fulfill one objective while ignoring other objectives. For example, to maximize profits in the short term, it may be necessary to (1) curtail investments in future products or markets that may imperil the future solvency and profitability of the insurer, or (2) take short-term actions that have an adverse effect on patient satisfaction or quality of care.

In addition, a pricing structure that uses high rates may increase short-term profits, but it may also lead to slow sales growth, increased terminations (loss of accounts), and disgruntlement from marketing personnel. Low premiums, on the other hand, may produce a high sales growth and a satisfied sales force, but profit levels may erode and plan solvency may be threatened. In the longer run, prices may have to be raised to higher levels than would otherwise have been necessary.

In practice, pricing methods are developed, adapted, evaluated, and refined in a dynamic process that attempts to balance all of the conflicting goals and objectives. Although managers will be conscious of all these factors, they will give more weight to some than others, with decisions dependent upon the current market environment, the financial status of the particular line of business (or company at large), and other factors affecting financial performance.

Given that the goals and objectives cannot all be satisfied simultaneously, what are the most desirable characteristics for rating systems? Six characteristics are very important for rating systems for insurance products: (1) adequacy of rate structure, (2) competitiveness of rates, (3) equity among policyholders, (4) simplicity (ease of understanding and implementation), (5) flexibility/adaptability (degree of difficulty in making changes or adapting to new conditions), and (6) consistency.

The first two characteristics, adequacy and competitiveness, are primarily concerned with the overall level of rates. For an insurance product or line of business, the *adequacy* of the rate structure refers to whether the rates (the aggregate rates charged across all contracts) will cover expected expenditures and loadings (claims costs, administrative and other expenses, reserve requirements, risk premiums, profit percentage) on an incurred basis. In essence, the rate structure must be adequate, or sufficiently high, to ensure that the insurer does not experience losses. Thus, adequacy is primarily related to maintaining solvency and profitability.

The *competitiveness* of the rates charged by an insurer refers to the relative degree of attractiveness of the rates for a particular insurance product in a defined competitive market environment. For example, assuming that the benefit package and other features of a group health insurance product are satisfactory, it is also necessary that the product be priced appropriately in order for it to be competitive in the marketplace. The product must not be priced at a level that will drive consumers to another plan because of the differences in costs, especially out-of-pocket premium costs, between the plans. Therefore, an insurer's rate structure must not be substantially higher than the level of rates charged by competitors for similar products.

Although price is not the sole determinant of sales volume (quality, service, accessibility, and overall perceived value are other key factors), there is a high level of competition among HMOs, PPOs, Blue Cross plans, and commercial insurers for group health insurance business. An insurer must recognize and consider the prices of competitors in establishing a rating system. If competitive considerations prevent an insurer from charging what it feels are adequate rates in a specific market for a particular product, then that insurer may not be able to enter (or may have to withdraw from) that market.

In some cases, the rate structure is fixed by an outside agency. This occurs with Medicare risk contracts and with Medicaid contracts in many states. In these cases, the HMO does not have to develop a rate structure and evaluate its adequacy and competitiveness. Rather, the plan must determine if the fixed rates are sufficient to cover the outlays for the specified enrollees; the plan must be able to deliver the required services to the defined population without incurring losses. Other decisions must be made concerning whether optional services will be included in the benefit package, the types and amount of cost sharing that will be required, and the level of supplemental premiums that will be charged, if any.

Equity refers to the perceived "fairness" of the premium rates; that is, whether the differences among the premium rates charged to different policyholders are just, providing fair and equal treatment to all concerned.[2] The general objective of the equity principle is to make the rates equitable for all contract holders, which requires that these differences in rates have a reasonable explanation. However, implementation of this general principle in practice is often difficult because of the different perceptions of equity among different parties, including the insurer's management, the insurer's pricing officials responsible for rate making, and the different policyholders.

For group health insurance, rates may vary legitimately according to a wide range of factors such as the contract provisions (including the covered services and cost-sharing requirements), the demographic composition of the group, the prior claims experience of the group, and other group characteristics (industry, size, geographic location). At one end of the spectrum (with respect to the degree of complexity in the rating system) is a community-rating system with a fixed rate schedule in which identical rates are charged to all groups for the same benefit package. At the other end of the spectrum, an insurer may use relatively detailed and complex pricing methods that take into account not only all of the above factors but competitive and equity considerations as well.

Much of this complexity is demanded by large employers who are interested in "paying what their employees actually cost." In addition to equity considerations, this desire derives, in part, from a belief that these costs would be lower than the premiums paid under an alternative (community-rating) system. At the extreme, this desire can lead to a self-insuring arrangement whereby the insurer provides administrative services only. Thus, these employers may perceive equity in rates to be directly linked to a rating system where premiums are based on the actual experience of their group.

Related to the issue of equity is the notion that groups should be charged "self-supporting" rates. This means that the premium rates charged to a group should be approximately equal to the expected costs of the group. The basic argument is that some groups should not be charged premiums that are substantially higher than the cost of their benefits so that other groups can be charged lower, or discounted, premiums (in effect, providing cross-subsidies between groups). In fact, actuarial theory defines "equity" as charging a rate that reflects a group's actual cost. There should be no cross-subsidies, which are uneconomic in the sense that they lead to prices that do not reflect true costs.

In theory, this principle is wholly logical. However, as with many other aspects of rate making, there can be significant complications in practice. For example, in the extreme, it would mean that any group, regardless of size or other characteristics, should be charged premiums based strictly on its expected costs. Numerous examples can be constructed where strict adherence to this principle would be antithetical to the basic goal of insurance (pooling of risks), in addition to other problems. Consider a small group with one or more large hospital claims in the prior year. It is possible that the renewal rates for this group would be prohibitively high. For this reason, most group health insurers pool the experience of all small groups under a specified size and charge self-supporting premiums to the total of these groups. Although these rates are likely to vary by many characteristics of each group, this practice has some similarities with community-rating systems. (Other problems related to the random variation in health costs are discussed later in this chapter.) In this way, the principle that all groups should be charged self-supporting premiums is broadened to apply to classes of groups and covered persons, in order to get a group that is large enough to pool risks successfully. Rating structures, although pooling the experience of many small groups, can take into account various types of cost differentials between classes of groups and classes of covered individuals. For example, some industries are more expensive than others, and individuals vary in expected health costs according to characteristics such as age, sex, marital status, and family composition.

The final three desirable characteristics of rating systems are simplicity, flexibility, and consistency. *Simplicity* refers both to ease of administration of the rating system and also to ease of understanding of the rating system. All other things being equal, administrative simplicity should be a major goal in development of pricing methods. Overly complex procedures and techniques should be avoided unless they are necessary for development of an equitable rating system or other relevant reasons. In addition, the ability to easily explain the mechanics of the rating system to policyholders is a very desirable characteristic.

Flexibility refers to the capacity of the rating system to adapt to special circumstances or changing conditions. It is likely that any rating system will require changes over time, especially in a rapidly changing field such as health care. Required changes can vary from minor updates of specific rating parameters to major modifications in basic procedures, resulting from changes in policy design, contract-holders' requirements, or actions by competitors.

The final desirable characteristic for a rating system is *consistency*. In order to ensure that the objectives of adequacy, competitiveness, and equity are achieved, consistent pricing methods must be used in setting premium rates for all group health insurance contracts under a given line of business. If inconsistent methods are used (i.e., there is lack of consistency in implementation of established rating methods), the insurer faces several problems, including claims of inequity from policyholders, threats of audits from governmental entities such as the Office of Personnel Management (OPM) for the Federal Employees Health Benefits Program and the Health Care Financing Administration (HCFA) for Medicare, and increased difficulty in monitoring and evaluating overall financial experience.

Rating Systems

Three different methods of rating group health insurance are employed by most insurers: community rating, manual rating, and experience rating. Many insurers use combinations of these methods and do not rely on one method alone. For example, large groups can be experience rated, while small groups are manual or community rated. In addition, aside from rating systems, methods of financing may be even more important from an individual employer's perspective. Many large employers prefer the cash flow advantages of minimum premium plans, whereby only a portion of the normal monthly premium is paid in advance and the remaining payments are made by the employer as claims are paid by the insurer or third-party administrator. Also, many large and medium-sized employers have opted for self-insured plans.

Community rating. The use of community-rating methods for health insurance coverage, on a large scale, started with the Blue Cross plans in the 1930s and 1940s. The basic principle behind this rating method is to determine equitable rates based on community-wide experience. Under community rating, all groups are given comparable premiums for the same package of benefits. In effect, there are cross-subsidies between low-risk groups and high-risk groups. Community-rating methods have been the traditional methods used to determine premiums by HMOs. These methods are discussed in more detail in Chapter 6.

Manual rating. Manual rating is based on a set of predetermined rates applied to each prospective health insurance contract. Usually, an insurer has a rate manual or rate book that is used to determine the premium rate for a policy based on the characteristics of the policy and the characteristics of the persons (and the group) covered by the policy. The rate manual may have separate rates for each component benefit or feature included in a policy. In addition, there are usually adjustments to account for differences in the composition of the enrolled population (age, sex, and so on) and the characteristics of the group (industry, size, locations). Manual rates are also referred to as "tabular rates" or "class rates."

Manual rates are designed to reflect characteristics of the group/policy that significantly affect the health services utilization patterns and cost experience of the group. Sets of manual rates are usually established only for broad classes of risk. Thus, manual rating is significantly different from determining a premium rate for an individual policy that can take into account the detailed characteristics of the individual person being underwritten.

For HMOs, the concept of manual rating has been incorporated into the form of rating known as "community rating by class." They can use this rating method to determine premium rates based on factors such as age, sex, and other characteristics that produce differences in health services utilization and costs. However, the rates must be determined based on planwide experience and not on a specific group's experience. This form of rating is acceptable for federally qualified HMOs. Methods of community rating by class are discussed in more detail in Chapter 6.

Experience rating. Experience rating takes into account the historical and projected cost experience of a specific group. Whereas community rating is based on community-wide experience, and manual rating is based on the general characteristics of a group, experience rating attempts to determine premium rates based on the group's actual experience. Experience rating is the means by which variations in claim and expense levels, not taken into account in manual rates, can be incorporated into the cost of insurance to the policyholder.

Experience rating can be applied prospectively or retrospectively. Prospective experience rating involves setting premium rates in advance based on a group's past experience and projected future experience. With retrospective experience rating, groups with good experience (better than anticipated in the rates) are paid premium refunds or dividends. This arrangement is also referred to as a "participating" policy. The variety of possible formulas and frameworks for implementing an experience-rating system are discussed in more detail in Chapter 7.

Summary

The methods used to determine premium rates for group health insurance products may vary. However, all of the methods must be based on the basic principles for insurance rate making or pricing in general. For example, premium rates must be adequate to finance (1) medical claims incurred, (2) administrative expenses, and (3) risk requirements. In addition, the rates must be competitive in the marketplace and perceived as equitable by all classes of policyholders. They should be simple to explain and to administer, and they must be coordinated with benefit design, underwriting standards, policy provisions, and claims-processing procedures. Consistency in application of pricing methods is of high priority.

Effective planning for the current competitive situation and evaluation of possible future scenarios are critical elements of the rating process for group health insurance. The standard pricing tasks of setting rates on a group-specific basis and monitoring overall financial experience are also important. Thus, the development and implementation of pricing methods must be viewed as part of a dynamic process.

Actual claims experience must be monitored on an ongoing basis to ensure that the insurer's objectives are being met. When goals are not being achieved, the system must be evaluated and changes instituted as quickly as possible. In addition, the nature of the group health insurance environment demands quick responses to changes and new opportunities in the competitive environment.

Implementing a rating system requires the development of pricing methods, forecasting required assumptions (many of which are difficult to predict with accuracy), preparation of detailed forecasts of financial parameters and alternative scenarios, and evaluation of current experience to determine when and how changes should be made in rating practices. Specific tasks include determining the parameters of the rating process, identifying specific products and setting prices or pricing guidelines, developing the required assumptions, and monitoring the actual results to determine when changes should be made.

The rating process in an insurance organization is very closely related to the underwriting process, and it is impossible to separate the two interrelated functions. The remainder of this chapter discusses underwriting for group health insurance, in order to clarify the critical relationship between rating and underwriting.

5.2 Underwriting for Group Health Insurance

What is underwriting? To *underwrite* an insurance policy is "to set one's name to the policy for the purpose of thereby becoming answerable for a designated loss or damage on consideration of receiving a premium."[3] In other words, underwriting means financial responsibility/liability; it guarantees financial support in the context of insurance contracts. An *underwriter* is a person who works for an insuring organization, selecting risks to be solicited, rating the acceptability of risks solicited, and determining the financial terms and conditions (including premium rates) of an insurance policy.

There are many alternative definitions and interpretations of the term "underwriting." In a narrow interpretation, some refer to underwriting as a limited activity, restricted to the functions of risk selection (evaluating whether or not a case should be insured) and risk classification (if insurable, determining in which risk category the case should be placed for rating purposes). In this view, underwriting serves primarily as a screening process for prospective cases to be insured under existing insurance products. For example, the underwriting department for a life insurance product sold to individuals may focus entirely on issues such as the results of medical examinations taken by applicants; medical history and other evidence of insurability (obtained from questionnaires and interviews); demographic, lifestyle, and other characteristics of applicants; algorithms to evaluate the evidence on individual cases leading to decisions to accept or deny applications (and also to classify applicants into correct rating classes, ranging from a "preferred risk" to an "uninsurable risk"); and procedures to determine the appropriate rating category for accepted applications.

At the other extreme, many group health underwriters view the underwriting function quite broadly and include all activities related to the financial performance of an insurance product or line of business as part of the underwriter's job. In addition to risk selection and risk classification, underwriters may be given responsibility for (1) specifying the financial parameters for the coverage (including the rating basis and the contract terms regarding the financial obligations and rights of both parties), (2) making pricing decisions, including determining premium rates by using rate manuals, historical cost experience, and the underwriter's judgment concerning the competitive conditions of the case, (3) monitoring the financial performance of the line of business, (4) analyzing experience and setting trend lines and other key assumptions, (5) investigating the causes of unexpected results and the reasons for poor performance, (6) developing or revising group selection guidelines (i.e., minimum acceptable size) used for risk selection and risk classification, and (7) participating as a member of the management team regarding decisions and issues that affect underwriting policies and procedures.

Thus, depending on interpretations and divisions of responsibility, there can be a large degree of overlap between the rating and underwriting functions in an insurance operation. In this section, a variety of topics are discussed related to underwriting for group health insurance. Although some of the topics are also closely related to pricing and rating activities, they are presented in this section due to their fundamental importance to the underwriting function for insurance products.

Objectives of Underwriting for Group Health Insurance

Group underwriting attempts to (1) determine which applicants (or potential applicants) for insurance coverage should be accepted, (2) identify which potential customers should be rejected, and (3) specify and approve the financial terms and conditions for the insurance contract. The financial terms and conditions include the premium rates to be charged, agreements concerning rating methods (e.g., experience-rating formulas and dividend formulas), and other issues that could affect the financial outcome of the contract (e.g., minimum size or participation standards to be maintained by the contract holder).

The nature of losses under group health insurance is different from many other forms of insurance. Life insurance, for example, has large, infrequent losses that are fixed in size and normally beyond the control of the insured person. In contrast, health insurance involves relatively frequent losses that range in size. In addition, the losses can be controlled, to some extent, by both the person who is insured and the physician who provides the service. The size of the loss changes over time due to inflation, changes in medical technology, and a variety of other factors. Therefore, whereas life insurance fits ideal insurance standards, the nature of health insurance has very different characteristics, resulting in many demanding requirements for the successful underwriting of group health insurance.

There are significant differences between group and individual health insurance. Group insurance usually requires no medical examinations or other evidence of insurability for the persons covered by the group contract (there may be exceptions for very small groups). The insurance contract is usually between the group policyholder (usually an employer) and the insurer; the insured persons are not actually parties to the contract. In addition, the contract is usually of a continuing nature, so persons who were originally covered may leave the group and new persons may be added over time.

In underwriting for group health insurance, the insurability of each individual covered by the group contract is not usually evaluated. Nevertheless, obtaining an average selection of risks (within each risk class), consistent with the underlying underwriting and pricing procedures of the insurer, is of high priority. To accomplish this objective, the group insurance underwriter uses a variety of tools.

Major Tasks and Tools of Underwriters

Underwriting for group health insurance involves evaluating a risk, determining the conditions of its acceptability, and establishing an appropriate rating basis. The basic standard of performance for a group underwriter is the financial performance of the entire portfolio of business (the portfolio includes all group insurance contracts that have been underwritten for a defined time period or accounting period). Achieving this objective involves obtaining sufficient premiums from the insurer's policyholders to achieve the bottom-line profit goal, after accounting for all incurred claims, expenses, dividends to policyholders, and other costs during the period for which the premium is applicable.

The spreading of risk is essential in order for a group health insurance plan to operate successfully. An insurer would not be financially sound if it accepted an unreasonably high percentage of bad risks, compared to its underlying principles for rating and underwriting. To obtain a proper spread of risks, classes may be established to reflect anticipated variations in health costs due to demographic, geographic, or other underwriting or actuarial factors. In addition, a primary objective of underwriting is to obtain an acceptable cross-section of risks within each group insurance classification. This objective attempts to ensure that rates are competitive and adequate and to achieve equity among levels of risk classifications.

Since group health insurance does not usually require individual evidence of insurability (e.g., examination of health status, medical history, habits, occupation), an insurer attempts to obtain a favorable cross-section of risk by covering a large percentage of the employees of suitable employers. This is achieved by the development and implementation of underwriting methods for group selection and risk classification. The basic principles of group selection ensure that groups are stable and maintainable, and that the possibility of antiselection is minimized.[4] These general principles include (1) that the persons to be covered should be members of a natural group that is not formed specifically to obtain insurance, (2) that there should be a reasonable expectation of permanency of the group to be covered, and (3) that an adequate spread of risks should be guaranteed to compensate for the elimination of individual underwriting requirements.

These general principles are implemented through a variety of specific underwriting guidelines and procedures, including (1) setting minimum group size requirements, (2) establishing required characteristics for groups to be acceptable, (3) developing special procedures to handle particular types of groups, (4) eliminating known sources of group instability (there should be a regular flow of new and younger members into the group for stability of costs over time), (5) requiring the employer or sponsor to pay a share of the costs to encourage a satisfactory participation by eligible employees (especially relatively healthy employees who would not otherwise enroll), (6) ensuring that the types and amount of coverage provided should not be at the option of the covered individual, (7) requiring that the policyholder be a legal entity with the necessary authority to contract for coverage, (8) ensuring that the policyholder is willing and able to assume responsibility for proper administration of the policy, and (9) establishing eligibility criteria for full-time employees, dependent coverage, and so on.

In this way, an appropriate spread of risk is obtained so that unanticipated losses may be offset by incidental gains, with both losses and gains resulting from the random variation inherent in the occurrence and distribution of health costs. In comparison, losses and gains may result from biases in the rating or underwriting processes or from biased selection among the insured groups or individuals. These types of uncontrollable deviations are undesirable, and the underwriting process should guard against them.

The standard of performance for a group underwriter is the financial performance of the portfolio of business (all group health insurance contracts combined). From an actuarial perspective, a healthy portfolio of business is maintained by making sure that all insured groups have an expected value of claims consistent with the rating/premium structure. The financial performance of the portfolio is measured by the profitability of the insurance product, or line of business, that is being underwritten. Therefore, the primary goal of group underwriting is to minimize the possibility of adverse financial experience for the insurer, based on the entire portfolio of business written (to maximize profitability and to minimize losses). The job of the underwriter is to reduce the probability of loss resulting from premiums that are, in aggregate, less than the costs of incurred claims, administrative expenses, and other expenses for all insurance contracts written within a particular line of business.[5]

This means that the underwriting function has the responsibility for making the multitude of specific decisions required to maintain a profitable insurance product or line of business. This requires implementation of the insurer's pricing guidelines and principles, evaluation of the risks presented by potential customers, and determination of the appropriate basis for renewal (or termination) of current contracts that are due to expire.

To accomplish the primary task, a group health insurance underwriter must protect the insurer from antiselection (i.e., to ensure that the expected costs of each group covered by insurance can be adequately estimated and do not contain unknown adverse risks). Within a particular risk class, adverse (or favorable) selection is defined as a group of persons of higher (or lower) risk than the average (for that risk class) selecting an insurer for coverage. In this case, risk is measured by health status and other conditions related to the probability of incurring costs for future health services.

It is desirable to have predictable costs over time, since stability in a group's claims experience over time makes the underwriter's job easier. In addition, the premium rate for a group should be maintainable. If it is too high for the expected participants, it is likely to lead to an ''antiselection spiral,'' as good risks drop out of the group and poorer risks remain over time. Successful underwriting requires the development and maintenance of a healthy (i.e., fundamentally sound, stable, and profitable) "book of business," using appropriate techniques for group selection, risk classification, and rating.

5.3   The Statistical Nature of the Underwriting Process

First and foremost, the underwriter relies heavily on the statistical principle known as the "law of large numbers." Based on statistical theory, this principle states that the average of a group of independent and identically distributed random variables tends toward the mean of the underlying probability distribution as the sample size increases—that is, the sample mean converges to the true mean, with probability one, as the number of cases increases to infinity. The degree of variation in the average of the group is a function of the sample size (as the sample size increases, the variance decreases and the average becomes highly predictable). Theoretically, the assumptions required by the law of large numbers are not all satisfied in the case of group health insurance because the costs of groups and individuals covered are not identically distributed random variables. However, the basic principle underlying the law of large numbers is useful, conceptually, to facilitate comprehension of the underwriting process in an insurance context.

There is a large amount of unpredictable variation in health care costs for an individual person, a family unit, or an individual group of persons (such as the employees and covered dependents for a medium-sized employer). However, if a line of group health insurance business is large enough (i.e., covers a sufficiently large number of contracts and persons), then, under the principle of the law of large numbers, the aggregate claims experience for the entire line of business will be predictable. For example, in the best case scenario, if the insurer contracts with a very large employer group, and there are no opportunities for the individuals in the group to select against the insurer, the loss experience of the group should be predictable and stable both from year to year and also compared to the experience of similar groups. Hence, the underwriter is able to develop a premium that protects the insurer and covers the cost incurred by the members of the group.

This does not imply that the insurer expects every group to incur precisely the average amount of claims in every contract year. Rather, in any one year, there will be a large number of contracts (in the total portfolio for a particular product or line of business) that cover a much larger number of persons. The contracts will differ according to size of group, demographic composition of the group (age, sex, industry), the benefit package of the group, and factors such as cost-sharing provisions, benefit limits, and maximum payment limits. Consequently, the "expected" health care costs of the group will also vary according to these differences. The "actual" incurred claims for the group (during a one-year contract period) will also have a variance, or standard deviation, around the expected costs. The variance will be determined by the size of the group (the variance decreases as the group size increases), the incidence and severity of high-cost catastrophic cases in any one year, the inherent variation in costs among group members (which will vary from group to group), and other factors.

In this way, the insurer counts on large numbers of cases to bring actual claims close to their expected value. The goal of the underwriter is to ensure that the expected value of total claims is correct and unbiased.

In other words, the group underwriter expects that there will be differences between actual and expected costs for any one group. However, when the costs of all groups are aggregated, the law of large numbers takes effect. In particular, there should be a high degree of stability in the total costs across all groups.

Figures 5-1 through 5-6 represent the frequency distribution of the ratio of actual costs to expected costs for groups with 50, 100, 500, 1,000, 2,500, and 5,000 members, respectively (the graphs are for illustrative purposes only). The distribution of actual to expected costs would be expected to differ for each HMO based on various factors such as medical practice patterns, the relative incidence of high-cost cases, underwriting practices, the level of benefits offered, and other factors. The expected costs include adjustments for factors such as differences in demographic characteristics, benefit packages, and cost sharing among groups.

The degree of variation in the ratio of actual-to-expected health costs for groups with 50 enrollees is quite large (see Figure 5-1). Actual health costs can easily vary from a low of 15 percent to a high of more than 300 percent of the expected health costs for the group. In addition, only 14 percent of groups have actual costs within 10 percent of expected costs, and only 26 percent have actual costs within 20 percent of expected costs. Thus, approximately 75 percent of groups with 50 members can be expected to have costs that are either lower or higher than expected costs by more than 20 percent. Approximately 2.4 percent of groups with 50 members have very high actual cost experience in a year, exceeding 300 percent of the expected costs.

For groups with 100 HMO enrollees (Figure 5-2), the results have

Figure 5-1: Distribution of Actual-to-Expected Costs by
Size of Group: 50 Members

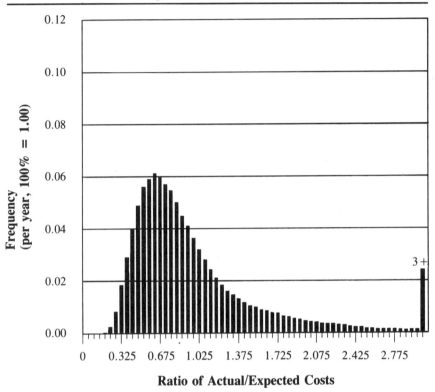

only slightly less variance than the results for groups of 50. Again, these particular figures are included for illustrative purposes; actual results will vary from plan to plan. However, they illustrate the high variability to be expected from groups with 50 or 100 HMO members. Groups of this size are common in most HMOs.

For groups with 500 and 1,000 HMO enrollees, the degree of variation in actual-to-expected costs is significantly less than for the smaller groups with 50 and 100 members (Figures 5-3 and 5-4). For example, for groups of 500, the range in the ratio is only 50 to 200 percent, compared to a range of 25 to 300 percent (or more) for groups with 100 members. In addition, 38 percent of groups have actual costs within 10 percent of expected costs, and approximately 68 percent of these groups have actual costs within 20 percent of expected costs (compared to 16 percent and 34 percent, respectively, for groups of size 100). However,

Figure 5-2: Distribution of Actual-to-Expected Costs by Size of Group: 100 Members

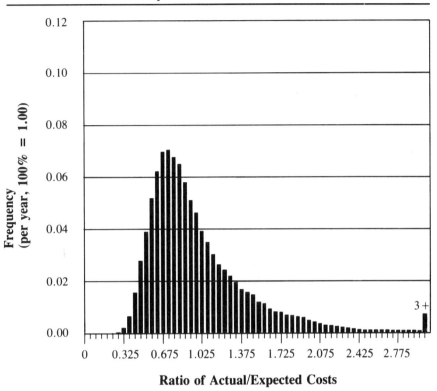

Ratio of Actual/Expected Costs

around 32 percent of these groups will still have actual costs that are more or less than 20 percent different from expected costs, and groups of 500 members are large groups for HMOs. Similar results can be seen for groups of 1,000 (Figure 5-4).

The results for extremely large groups (2,500 and 5,000 members) have a much smaller degree of variation (Figures 5-5 and 5-6). The range of actual-to-expected costs is only 75 to 135 percent. Approximately 75 to 85 percent of these large groups have actual costs within 10 percent of expected costs, and 95 percent or more of these groups have actual costs within 20 percent of expected costs. However, even in these very large groups, there is still significant variation in actual-to-expected costs, with some groups having ratios with more than 20 percent differences.

Figures 5-5 and 5-6 show large variations in the actual-to-expected ratio (the graphs have longer tails on the side of the frequency distribu-

Figure 5-3: Distribution of Actual-to-Expected Costs by
Size of Group: 500 Members

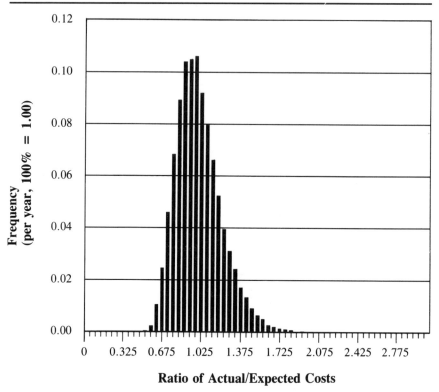

Ratio of Actual/Expected Costs

tions with the higher actual-to-expected ratios). This results from the
impact of extremely high-cost cases in some groups. The incidence and
severity of high-cost cases for individual covered persons can have a
dramatic impact on the actual costs even for large groups. These cases
also have an impact on the average, or mean, costs across all groups of
specified size. Most groups will have claims from a predictable number
of persons during a contract year because the percentage of persons with
no costs during a year is relatively stable from year to year. For any
group with indemnity health insurance, over 75 percent of total health
costs are usually incurred by only 10 percent of the covered population.
(This figure may vary for HMOs due to their broader benefits in most
instances, especially regarding coverage of physician visits, preventive
exams, well-baby care, and other outpatient services). Within an indi-

Figure 5-4: Distribution of Actual-to-Expected Costs by
Size of Group: 1,000 Members

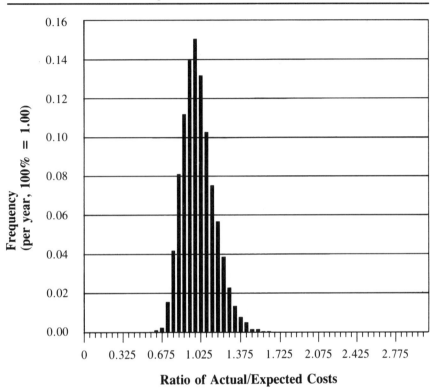

Ratio of Actual/Expected Costs

vidual group, there can be substantial variation, from year to year, in the costs resulting from the high-cost members of the group. This is the primary driving factor behind the overall degree of variation in health costs and the reason for the longer tail of the distribution for the higher actual-to-expected ratios.

If the processes of group selection, rate formulation, medical care costs, and administrative expense generation are unbiased and in accord with the underwriting standards and requirements, then the bottom-line result (i.e., total premiums less incurred claims costs, administrative costs, and other expenses) should be an aggregate underwriting profit that is in agreement with the original pricing assumptions and projections. Since few groups are sufficiently large or stable to provide highly predictable experience on their own, the group underwriting function

Figure 5-5: Distribution of Actual-to-Expected Costs by
Size of Group: 2,500 Members

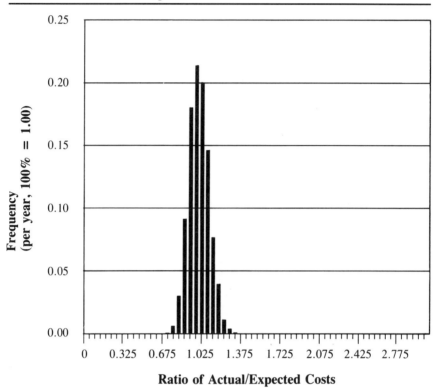

Ratio of Actual/Expected Costs

attempts to insure enough groups so that the total exposure (the total insured population, or all accumulated persons covered) will provide stability and predictability.

5.4 Marketing, Underwriting, and Rating

An insurance company's underwriting practices are based on its perception of the market and its anticipated marketing strategy. Prior to development of underwriting guidelines for a new product, each company will target a specified market (or market segment) for the product. Similarly, underwriting procedures need to be continually updated to reflect changing market conditions, especially with respect to the assumptions concerning the population of policyholders and other parameters underlying the underwriting guidelines.

Figure 5-6: Distribution of Actual-to-Expected Costs by
Size of Group: 5,000 Members

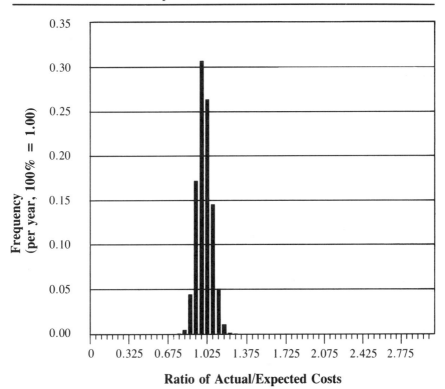

Ratio of Actual/Expected Costs

An appropriate rating system for an insurance product depends upon the anticipated marketing strategy and underwriting procedures for the product. For example, a life insurance company may decide to go after a large segment of the market with a particular product, with the anticipation that the underwriting guidelines will not be too strict for its standard coverage (i.e., policies not requiring separate rating at higher rates due to higher risks). This will normally require higher premiums than the average for the total potential population because the company would expect to attract a broad cross-section of the potential population. The company would not expect to attract a large proportion of "very good" risks because these persons would be able to find policies with significantly lower premiums, albeit with higher underwriting standards. This approach would be expected to attract a disproportionate share of those who can just meet the underwriting standards.

Alternatively, a company could structure a policy to appeal specifically to very good, or "highly select," risks (persons in excellent physical health and without any identifiable characteristic associated with higher than average mortality). For this type of policy, a company could offer very low premiums, under the assumption that policyholders would have to pass a rigorous underwriting process. The potential market for this policy would be much smaller than the market for the policy described previously, but the penetration rate may be higher, depending on the competition (total premium revenue for this product could be either higher or lower). In addition, the average premiums would be lower for this policy (per unit of insurance in force). However, this policy could have higher and more stable profit margins, as a percentage of premium, because of tighter control over underwriting and more predictable claims costs.

Both companies could expect to have profitable products in the same market, as long as appropriate underwriting and rating procedures were implemented for each product. Assuming adequate rating and underwriting, the relative success of each product would depend on factors such as the effectiveness of the marketing and sales programs, the degree of competition offered by other insurance companies for similar products, policyholder satisfaction as reflected by persistence/termination rates, and the level of antiselection experienced by the insurer (e.g., if the first insurer did not screen for HIV/AIDS, actual claims costs could be substantially higher than projected costs).

To apply this example to group health insurance, an HMO must be cognizant of the targeted market and devise appropriate underwriting and rating procedures to be successful in that market. Consider the case of an employer with a young, healthy population that represents a "very good" risk from an overall health status perspective and has a record of good experience (low claims history). If a community-rated HMO were offered in that group, one would expect that (1) the HMO's premiums would be substantially higher than the indemnity plan's premiums, (2) the HMO penetration rate would be very low in this group, and (3) the persons enrolled in the HMO would be attracted by the comprehensive benefits and would probably be in poorer health status than average (using large amounts of services in the future).

The HMO would be expected to have poor financial experience from this group because of high claims costs and enrollment that is too low to recover the required marketing, claims processing, and administrative expenses. To avoid probable losses, the HMO would be well advised not to accept this group client, primarily because the premiums generated by the HMO's rating system would not be competitive, leading to losses for such groups (i.e., groups with extremely low indemnity premiums and young, healthy populations).

If the HMO used a broad marketing strategy, similar to the first insurer described above, it might be possible for the HMO to contract with some young, healthy groups, with the knowledge that losses would most likely result, but with the intent of building a broad-based membership population for the future. However, in an increasingly competitive health care marketplace, avoiding losses will become increasingly important, and this type of strategy may have to be reconsidered.

An experience-rated HMO, on the other hand, would be able to develop competitive premiums for such a group, because the premiums would be based on the group's historical claims experience. This does not mean that experience-rated systems are better than community-rated systems, only that a plan's rating system must be consistent with the plan's marketing approach, underwriting procedures, and competitive environment in order to avoid adverse financial experience in the aggregate.

The relationship between marketing, underwriting, and rating is critical to the success of an insurance product. Underwriting guidelines and procedures should correspond directly with (1) the insurer's marketing strategy, and (2) the desired population (and characteristics) of policyholders. Similarly, the rating system must be consistent with both marketing and underwriting objectives. The rating system should be designed with an eye toward achieving the goals of competitiveness, adequacy, equity, profitability, consistency, simplicity, and flexibility.

5.5 HMO Underwriting Methods

Federal laws and regulations place restrictions on allowable underwriting practices for federally qualified HMOs. In addition, all HMOs, whether federally qualified or not, must abide by state licensure laws and regulations.

The costs incurred by an HMO depend, in part, on the plan's underwriting guidelines and the implementation of those guidelines. The selection of risks represented in an HMO's enrolled membership population is also affected by the plan's methods of underwriting. Tight and strictly controlled underwriting practices can lead to a more uniform, lower-cost enrolled population. In contrast, less well defined (or looser) underwriting practices usually result in higher costs and a less predictable population (from the standpoint of health status and medical risks).

In addition to the federal government, HMOs are regulated by state insurance departments, health departments, or both. In general, with respect to underwriting practices, HMOs have less flexibility than Blue Cross plans or private insurance carriers.

Group Enrollment

Federally qualified HMOs are prohibited from any form of selective group enrollment (e.g., medical underwriting via questionnaires or other forms of screening, use of preexisting conditions or waiting periods, or exclusions for persons with poor health status).[6] In addition, federally qualified HMOs must provide all mandated basic health services to all members of a group, regardless of the health status of any member(s) of the group.

Depending on state law, state-licensed HMOs that are not federally qualified may have more flexibility concerning the use of selective enrollment techniques. In some states, HMOs are allowed to medically underwrite individual members of a group or to establish waiting periods or limitations of coverage for preexisting conditions.

Underwriting for Small Groups

For small groups (fewer than 25 employees), private insurers typically use medical underwriting for premium rate setting, and possibly for excluding or limiting coverage for individual members of the group (or imposing substandard rates for these members).

Federally qualified HMOs are prohibited from using medical underwriting for small groups. If a group is accepted, it must be given community rates, and all members who enroll in the HMO must be given the basic benefit package. As discussed above, state-licensed HMOs have greater freedom in setting underwriting requirements for small groups.

Underwriting for Individual Coverage

All HMOs are permitted to medically underwrite applicants for individual coverage. (This does not include Medicare enrollees, for whom medical underwriting is not permissible.) However, if the individual is accepted for enrollment, federally qualified HMOs must provide all basic health services mandated by the HMO Act. State-licensed HMOs may impose preexisting condition requirements or limit the benefit package due to health status or other conditions, depending on the HMO laws of the state.

In contrast, private insurers generally impose higher restrictions on individual enrollment, and medical underwriting standards are usually higher than HMO standards. While federally qualified HMOs are forced to community rate, private insurers may employ a variety of premium rate–setting practices for individual contracts (e.g., age/gender rates, standard/substandard). In addition, for individual applicants, private insurers virtually always exclude preexisting conditions and may restrict coverage for specified services (e.g., maternity) or impose high deductibles for selected services. In contrast, federal and state HMO laws require coverage of all basic services.

In general, HMOs have less flexibility than their competitors in underwriting methods due to federal and state laws and regulations. In addition, most HMOs have been relatively unsophisticated with respect to both the use and the potential impact of underwriting practices.[7] In the past, although a small proportion of HMOs (mostly non-federally qualified plans) may have ignored applicable regulations on permissible HMO underwriting methods, many more HMOs have ignored the potential benefits to be gained from development and implementation of well-defined underwriting guidelines.

Notes

1. See, for example, R. D. Shapiro, "The Process of Premium Formulation," *Transactions, Society of Actuaries* 34 (1982): 435.
2. It is possible to distinguish between individual equity and social equity. Individual equity is based on the concept of risk classification. Each individual policyholder is expected to pay a "fair share" based on the expected cost at his or her level of risk. In the extreme, very low-risk policyholders pay very low premiums, and very high-risk policyholders are forced to pay very high premiums (or may be uninsurable). Social equity, on the other hand, focuses on an equitable spread of risks/costs throughout the insured population. In particular, efforts are made to facilitate insurance coverage of the entire population, including design of risk categories to prevent wide disparities in premiums charged to different individuals/groups for the same coverage. In the extreme, social equity is embodied in the concept of community rating.

3. *Webster's New Collegiate Dictionary,* 5th ed., S.V. "underwrite."
4. The topic of selection bias and its effects on premium rate setting are discussed in more detail in Chapter 8.
5. Again, it is difficult to draw a fine line between rating and underwriting procedures. In a narrow sense, the underwriter is responsible only for accepting and classifying applicants correctly. The task of setting the correct rates to cover the risks in each class can be considered a separate responsibility to be handled by actuaries or other financial personnel.
6. Federally qualified HMOs may use screening techniques such as questionnaires to decide if they want to contract with a group. However, once a contract is entered into, the HMO must accept all members of the group who wish to enroll with the HMO.
7. Proponents of community rating for HMOs argue that many plans have purposefully chosen this aproach on philosophical grounds. Rather than develop extensive underwriting/rating capabilities, many HMOs have decided to rely on the community-rating approach. The advantages of community rating are discussed in more detail in Chapter 4.

Suggested Readings

Actuarial Methods and Premium Rate Setting

Ang, James S., and Lai, Tsong-Yue. "Insurance Premium Pricing and Ratemaking in Competitive Insurance and Capital Asset Markets." *Journal of Risk and Insurance* 54, no. 4(1987): 767.

Barnhart, E. P. "A New Approach to Premium, Policy and Claim Reserves for Health Insurance." *Transactions, Society of Actuaries* 37 (1985): 13.

Biger, Nahum, and Kahane, Yehuda. "Risk Considerations in Insurance Ratemaking." *Journal of Risk and Insurance* 45, no. 1(1978): 121.

Bolnick, Howard J. "Experience-Rating Group Life Insurance." *Transactions, Society of Actuaries* 26, no. 4(1974): 123.

Braverman, Jerome D., and Hartman, Gerald R. "The Process of Classifying Drivers: A Suggestion for Insurance Ratemaking: Comment." *Journal of Risk and Insurance* 40, no. 1(1973): 143.

Cummins, J. David, and Outreville, J. Francois. "An International Analysis of Underwriting Cycles in Property-Liability Insurance." *Journal of Risk and Insurance* 54, no. 2(1987): 246.

Dahlby, B. G. "Monopoly Versus Competition in an Insurance Market with Adverse Selection." *Journal of Risk and Insurance* 54, no. 2(1987): 325.

Duston, Thomas E. "Insurer and Provider as the Same Firm: HMOs and Moral Hazard." *Journal of Risk and Insurance* 45, no. 1(1978): 141.

Fleischacker, Paul R., moderator. "Group Insurance Underwriting and Selection Issues." *Record, Society of Actuaries* 9, no. 2(1983): 669.

Forbes, Stephen W. "Capital Gains, Losses, and Financial Results in the Non-

Life Insurance Industry." *Journal of Risk and Insurance* 42, no. 4(1975): 625.

Green, E. A. "Medical Care Insurance Rating and Medical Economics." *Transaction, Society of Actuaries* 17, no. 3(1965): D92.

Grubel, Herbert G. "Risk, Uncertainty, and Moral Hazard." *Journal of Risk and Insurance* 38, no. 1(1971): 99.

Johnston, David R., moderator. "Risk Classification in the 1980's." *Record, Society of Actuaries* 6, no. 1(1980): 165.

Leverett, E. J., Jr. "Paid-In Surplus and Capital Requirements of a New Life Insurance Company." *Journal of Risk and Insurance* 38, no. 1(1971): 15.

Levinson, L. "A Theory of Mortality Classes." *Transactions, Society of Actuaries* 11 (1959): 46.

Pike, Bertram N. "Financial Planning and Control for Group Insurance." *Transactions, Society of Actuaries* 29 (1977): 243.

Shapiro, Robert D. "The Process of Premium Formulation." *Transactions, Society of Actuaries* 34 (1982): 435.

Shemin, Barry L., moderator. "Group Life and Health Insurance." *Record, Society of Actuaries* 9, no. 1(1983): 319.

Trapnell, Gordon R.; McKusick, David R.; and Genuardi, James S. "An Evaluation of the Adjusted Average Per Capita Cost (AAPCC) Used in Reimbursing Risk-Basis HMOs under Medicare." Paper prepared for the Health Care Financing Administration. U.S. Department of Health and Human Services, April 1982.

Witt, Robert Charles. "Pricing Problems in Automobile Insurance: An Economic Analysis." *Journal of Risk and Insurance* 40, no. 1(1973): 75.

Chapter 6

Community Rating

Health maintenance organizations (HMOs), particularly the newer plans developed within the framework of the federal HMO Act and amendments, have been legitimately concerned about requirements of federal HMO law, such as scope of covered benefits, open enrollment and community rating, that can adversely affect their ability to survive in the marketplace. There has been particular concern regarding the viability of the community rating requirement in the face of sharpened competitive pressures, including difficulties in gaining access to the market.... Health maintenance organizations represent an island of community rating in a sea of experience-rated indemnity health insurance plans. As long as employer contributions to HMOs are based on the premium levels of the indemnity plans, HMOs can and often do face severe marketing problems—with premiums that may be lower than those of competing indemnity plans in some groups while sharply higher in others.

R. W. Birnbaum, "Community Rating and Underlying HMO Reimbursement Issues"

6.1 Introduction

Most HMOs currently use community-rating methods, and a plan has to be community rated in order to be a federally qualified HMO.[1] This chapter describes some of the specific methods that are used and various options that are permissible. In addition, detailed examples illustrate the major components and optional features of a community-rating system.

Community-rating principles for health insurance were introduced, on a large scale, by Blue Cross plans in the 1930s. The earliest prepaid group practices (predecessors of present-day HMOs such as Ross-Loos Medical Foundation) also adopted community rating for premium rate setting. Originally, community-rating methods were used because they made premiums easy to determine. In addition, many believed such premiums were more equitable than those determined by experience rating.[2] In determining premiums, it was much easier to project the total premium

revenue required from all subscribers (to provide hospital insurance to
the total enrolled membership population) than to attempt to determine
premiums based on the claims experience, demographic composition, or
other characteristics of individual employer groups. To many, community-rating methods are the most equitable way of spreading health care
costs across all subscribers because premiums do not vary by such factors
as age, sex, or health status.[3]

In the 1950s, Blue Cross plans began the process of converting
from community rating to experience rating, primarily in response to
strong competition from commercial insurance companies that used experience-rating methods to set premiums for those medium-sized and large
employer groups that had lower than average costs (or lower than the
base used for the community rate). Whenever the expected cost of providing health care to the employees of a particular employer is less than
would be expected under community rating (because the employees are
younger and healthier than the average of the whole community, for
example), then that employer can usually save money by purchasing
health insurance from an insurer who is willing to use experience rating.[4]
Further, as the lower-cost groups left Blue Cross, the rate required for
those remaining increased, so that more groups were susceptible to the
competitive effects of the lower rates offered by other private insurers.
Thus, virtually all Blue Cross and Blue Shield plans were driven to use
experience rating as their primary method of premium rate setting for
medium-sized and large groups.

Today, the majority of HMOs use community rating for premium
rate setting. Recent trends have indicated that more HMOs, especially
newer plans, are using experience-rating methods, but community rating
is required for all federally qualified HMOs and is also used by many
nonqualified plans.

This chapter includes the following sections: (1) review of federal
legislation concerning acceptable rating methods for federally qualified
HMOs, (2) description of rating methods using standard community-
rating techniques, and (3) description of rating methods using community
rating by class.

6.2   Federal Legislation and Regulations

In contrast to the Blue Cross experience, most of the early prepaid group
practice plans have continued to use community rating. This was true

even before passage of the HMO Act of 1973, after which community rating was required for federal qualification, which most HMOs believed was necessary to prove that they were a bona fide alternative to health insurance.[5] Thus, historically, most HMOs have used community rating as the primary method for rate setting. These methods consist of (1) determining premium rates based on projected planwide costs and revenue requirements for the coming year, (2) offering the same, or equivalent, premium rates to all employers for the same benefits, (3) updating the fixed community rates on an annual or quarterly basis (again applying the same rates to all employers), and (4) establishing riders for additional benefits such as dental, prescription drugs, or vision care, with the riders also community rated so that premium income from riders covers the planwide costs of the additional services.

These community-rating principles were incorporated into the HMO Act of 1973. Although they have been modified several times during the past 15 years, the same basic principles govern premium rate–setting methods, not only for all federally qualified HMOs but also for the majority of nonqualified HMOs.[6] For example, according to "GHAA's 1987 Survey of HMO Industry Trends," 94.3 percent of HMOs used some variant of community rating for premium rate setting.[7] Of these plans, 63.7 percent used standard community rating exclusively, 16.5 percent used community rating by class, and 19.8 percent used both community rating and community rating by class. Experience rating was used exclusively by 5.7 percent of HMOs, while 7.8 percent of all plans used a combination of community-rating and experience-rating methods.

As would be expected, a higher proportion of staff-model and group-model plans (98.9 percent) used community rating than did IPA-model HMOs (87.8 percent). Older plans also used community rating more than younger plans—100 percent of plans over 15 years old, compared to 95.3 percent of plans 8 to 15 years old, and approximately 92.5 percent of plans under 8 years old.

The federal HMO law specifies the requirements for community rating under Section 1302. The language governing community rating in the original HMO Act of 1973 (Pub. L. No. 93–222) follows:

> The term "community rating system" means a system of fixing rates of payment for health services. Under such a system, rates of payments may be determined on a per-person or per-family basis and may vary with the number of persons in a family, but except as otherwise authorized in the next sentence, such rates must be equivalent for all individuals and for all families of similar composition:

    (A) Nominal differentials in such rates may be established to reflect different administrative costs of collecting payments from the following categories of members:

       (i) Individual members (including their families).

       (ii) Small groups of members (as determined under regulations of the Secretary).

       (iii) Large groups of members (as determined under regulations of the Secretary).

    (B) Differentials in such rates may be established for members enrolled in a health maintenance organization pursuant to a contract with a governmental authority such as States, political subdivisions of States, and other public entities.[8]

There have been several modifications to the original HMO Act of 1973 through legislative amendments and implementing regulations. With respect to community rating, substantial specificity and significant flexibility were added to the community-rating requirements of the law through the development of federal regulations from 1973 to 1980. The regulations (42 C.F.R. Section 110.105) permitted HMOs to use one of three methods to establish premium rates: (1) a fixed rate schedule, (2) rates that generate the same revenue per member per month, or (3) rates that generate the same revenue per contract (per subscriber per month). Regulations developed by the Office of Health Maintenance Organizations (OHMO), DHHS, also allowed premium rates to reflect (1) average family size, (2) the mix of single and family contracts in the group, and (3) recomposition of HMO rates to reflect the composition of in-force rates (ratio of single to family loading factors), as long as the required revenue was generated by the group's premiums.[9]

The second major change concerning community rating occurred in the HMO Act Amendments of 1981. These amendments modified the law to permit a more flexible form of community rating that takes into account differences in utilization and costs based on age, sex, and other approved factors. This form of community rating is commonly termed "community rating by class." The federal regulations describe community rating by class as follows:

    (b) Community rating system. Under a community rating system, rates of payment for health services may be determined . . . on a per group basis as described in paragraph (b)(2) of this section. . . .

       (2) A system of fixing rates of payment for health services may provide that the rates shall be fixed for individuals and families by groups. Except as otherwise authorized in this paragraph, such

rates must be equivalent for all individuals in the same group and for all families of similar composition in the same group. If an HMO is to fix rates of payment for individuals and families by groups, it shall:

(i) Classify all of the members of the organization into classes based on factors which the HMO determines predict the differences in the use of health services by the individuals or families in each class and which have not been disapproved by the Secretary,

(ii) Determine its revenue requirements for providing services to the members of each class established under paragraph (b)(2)(i) of this section, and

(iii) Fix the rates of payment for the individuals and families of a group on the basis of a composite of the organization's revenue requirements determined under paragraph (b)(2)(ii) of this section for providing services to them as members of the classes established under paragraph (b)(2)(i) of this section.[10]

As mentioned previously, further amendments to the HMO Act were signed into law on 24 October 1988. The potential impact of the new rating flexibility given to HMOs through the adjusted community-rating option should be significant. The amendments were developed with the participation of Group Health Association of America, and major HMOs representing the industry commented favorably on the amendments at congressional hearings. In addition, the initial reaction from most plans appears to be supportive of the concept, especially with regard to the potential of adjusted community rating to assist HMOs in their competitive struggles and in their negotiations with major employers.[11] However, the change to adjusted community rating is a major shift away from accepted and traditional rate-setting methods for most HMOs, and it will require substantial alterations in both the practice and the philosophy of those plans.[12]

6.3 Community-Rating Methods

In general, community rating implies that an HMO charges the same rates to all groups for the same benefits. However, federal regulations permit a number of alternative ways for HMOs to determine premium rates.[13] Federally qualified HMOs have three basic options for implementation of a community-rating system:

- A fixed rate structure (i.e., the same rates are offered to all groups)
- Maintaining the same revenue per member per month across all groups
- Maintaining the same revenue per contract (subscriber) per month across all groups

Under federal regulations, it is permissible to vary the rates to reflect different administrative charges for individual contracts, small groups of 100 subscribers or less, and groups with over 100 subscribers. In addition, rates can differ among group contracts for defined riders for supplemental benefits and differences in cost sharing (copayments). Federal regulations also allow rates to be recomposited to match the in-force rates (e.g., of the principle indemnity carrier's rates for single and family employees), as long as the basic requirement described above is maintained (fixed rate schedule or equivalent revenues per member or per subscriber). Rates can also vary according to the effective date of the group's contract (to reflect quarterly updates in rates).

Many of the traditional prepaid group practice plans used the fixed rate structure approach. The plan would have a fixed schedule of rates for the basic benefit plan and defined variations reflecting differences in riders (supplemental benefits), copayments, and individual versus group coverage. This rate schedule would be applied to all groups (new or renewal) and would be updated according to a predetermined schedule (usually annually or quarterly).

Many HMOs have taken advantage of the rating flexibility that is offered by the second option—maintaining the same revenue per member per month across groups, but varying rates to reflect differences in the mix of contracts and average family size between groups. In addition, many plans recomposite rates to match the in-force rates of the major carrier.

The third option, maintaining the same revenue per subscriber per month, has been used less often by HMOs. Basing rates on the distribution of subscribers is usually less reliable than basing rates on the distribution of members who are covered by the group policy.

There are a number of premium rate structures that are used as the basis for determining rates for group health contracts (see Table 6-1). The most common rate structures are the two-tier (single contract/family contract) and three-tier (single/two-party/family of three or more members) structures. The prevalence of different rate structures, however,

Table 6-1: Types of Premium Rate Structures

Type of Rate Structure	Description
Composite	All subscribers have the same premium rate, regardless of family size or composition.
Two-Tier	1. Single subscriber (employee only) 2. Family subscriber (2 or more members)
Three-Tier	1. Single subscriber 2. Two-party subscriber (employee and one dependent) 3. Family (3 or more members)
Four-Tier (version 1)	1. Single subscriber 2. Subscriber and spouse 3. Subscriber and child 4. Subscriber and 2 or more dependents
Four-Tier (version 2)	1. Single subscriber 2. Subscriber and spouse 3. Subscriber and 1 or more children 4. Subscriber and spouse and child(ren)
Four-Tier (version 3)	1. Single subscriber 2. Subscriber and 1 dependent 3. Subscriber and 2 dependents 4. Subscriber and 3 or more dependents
Five-Tier	1. Single subscriber 2. Subscriber and spouse 3. Subscriber and child 4. Subscriber and spouse and child(ren) 5. Subscriber and 2 or more children

varies across geographic areas. In addition, it is common for some employers to prefer specified forms of rate structures or to develop variations that take into account different characteristics of their employee work force. In some cases, health plans are free to propose their normal rate structure, even if other options offer differing rate structures. In other cases, the company/group specifies the acceptable form of rate structure(s). Thus, although the two-tier and three-tier premium rate structures are the most prevalent, the most common structure for group health policies varies from one geographic location to another. In addition, a variety of other premium rate structures are possible (based, for example, on family composition and subscriber characteristics).

Key Components of the HMO Rate-Setting Process

Figure 6-1 illustrates the overall process for HMO premium rate development. There are two primary elements in the process: (1) required data, and (2) the plan's organizational form and policies. The following data are required for premium rate development:

1. Inpatient utilization rates for the HMO's enrolled membership population

2. Hospital cost data

3. Office visit frequency

4. Physician or medical group costs

5. Ancillary services (x-rays and radiological procedures, laboratory tests, prescription drugs), utilization, and costs

6. Other data requirements (including population data by age and sex)

Data sources for these categories of required data have been discussed in detail in many publications.[14]

The second major set of factors for development of HMO premium rates is related to the plan's organizational form and policies. The plan's model type (staff, group, network, or IPA) has a substantial impact on the method used for development of the capitation rate and the plan's approach to issues such as provider risk sharing, cost-containment methods, and financial incentives. Most staff-model plans and some group-model plans use a budgeting approach to determine the plan's revenue requirements for the coming year. The budget forecast and the projected enrollment figures are used to determine premium rate increases for the plan's community rate structure. In contrast, other group, network, and IPA-model HMOs use an actuarial approach to "build up" the capitation rate on a service-by-service basis, using assumptions and parameters for utilization rates and costs per unit of service in each benefit or service category. This approach is preferred for those plans that pay claims or whose providers have a substantial amount of fee-for-service utilization.

An HMO's organizational form has a significant influence over financial decisions and the financial structuring of the plan. Three key factors are profit orientation, federal qualification status, and plan sponsorship. A for-profit plan needs to consider the goals and objectives of the investors or stockholders, and attention needs to be paid to profit generation. If consistent and steadily increasing profit streams are not produced by the plan, the value of the firm's stock will fall, resulting in

Figure 6-1: Overview of Premium Rate–Setting Practices

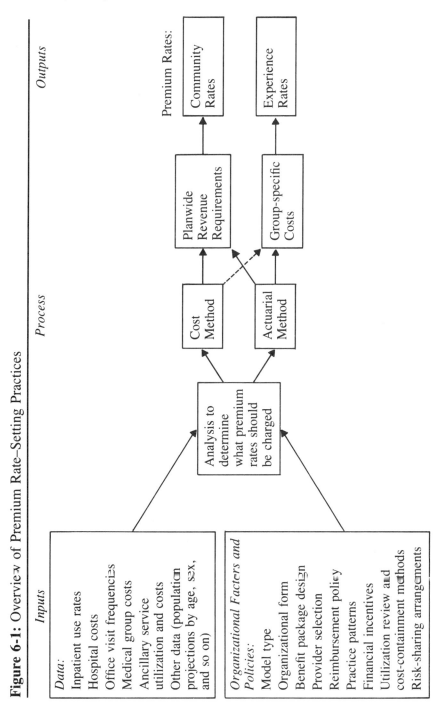

plan restructuring or replacement of plan management. In addition, access to required capital resources may be severely impaired.

If an HMO becomes federally qualified, it must abide by the current federal regulations regarding community rating and other factors related to the financial operation of the plan. As discussed previously, non-federally qualified HMOs have much greater flexibility in rating methods and other financial matters. In recent years, an increasing proportion of HMOs have decided against federal qualification. In addition, more federally qualified plans have started nonqualified subsidiaries to offer a wider variety of benefit packages and experience-rated and administrative services only (ASO) plans to employers.

Sponsorship of the HMO also affects the plan's approach to financial decisions. For example, a plan sponsored by physicians will have very different concerns about physician reimbursement and risk-sharing policies than a plan sponsored by an insurance company that wishes to contract with a medical group on the most advantageous terms possible.

A third factor is the design of the HMO's benefit package(s) and cost-sharing provisions. Federally qualified plans must offer a set of fairly comprehensive required benefits, which limits their ability to offer "very low option" plans. In addition, federally qualified plans have limits on the types and amount of cost sharing that can be included in the benefit package. Only copayments on services are allowed (no deductibles except for out-of-plan services), and the amount of cost sharing cannot exceed two times the annual premium.[15]

Selection of providers is a critical decision for any HMO. Plans with a philosophy of providing the highest quality care and using teaching hospitals and university medical centers will have very different cost experience compared to plans using lower-cost community hospitals. Also, plans such as IPAs, which contract with a broad cross-section of the community's physicians in private practice, will have different cost experience than plans that contract only with physicians or medical groups that have demonstrated cost-effective practice patterns.

Another factor affecting cost experience is the plan's policy for reimbursement of providers. Some HMOs have entered into contracts with providers on very favorable financial terms, from the plan's perspective. Other HMOs have not been aggressive in contracting. Both types of plans can be expected to evolve in the future. The HMOs that have negotiated very favorable financial terms with providers may find that they have to reduce the discounts (or raise capitation rates) as providers become less willing to take large discounts from their normal billing rates. Alternatively, plans that have not been aggressive in contracting in the past will find that they have opportunities to reduce costs by entering into mutually agreeable contracts with their major providers.

The final four items listed under organizational form and policies in Figure 6-1 concern specific issues that can have a major influence on an HMO's cost experience:

1. practice patterns
2. financial incentives
3. utilization review (UR) and cost-containment methods
4. risk-sharing arrangements

These factors are discussed in detail in Chapter 3. Each of these issues can have a significant impact on the cost structure of an HMO. If an HMO's providers do not conform to and adopt the plan's goals and objectives with respect to cost containment and the development of cost-effective methods of delivering care, then it will be reflected in the plan's cost structure and premium rates, and it will be difficult for the plan to compete effectively in today's increasingly competitive health care marketplace.

Both the data and the organizational form and policies feed into the analysis process to determine the plan's capitation rate and premium rates. As discussed above, premium rate development can follow two basic methods. The cost/budget method is used by most staff models and some group models. The actuarial/fee-for-service method is used by the other group, network, and IPA-model plans. The cost/budget method determines planwide costs and the level of revenue that is required for the plan to operate successfully during the coming year. These planwide costs and revenue requirements can also be determined using the actuarial method. To determine group-specific costs, the actuarial method is best. Community rating uses the planwide costs, revenue requirements, and capitation rates that are determined using either the cost/budget method or the actuarial method. In contrast, experience rating requires analysis of group-specific costs and the cost experience of individual employer groups. The new adjusted community-rating method is a form of group-specific rating and requires group-specific utilization or cost factors (refer to Chapter 7 for additional details on adjusted community rating).

Calculation of Community Rate Increase: The Cost/Budget Method

For HMOs using a fixed rate schedule as the basis for rate setting, all of the rates are adjusted either annually or on a more frequent basis (e.g., quarterly). Some of the rate components (rates for the major riders offered by the plan) are adjusted based on the change in costs for the specific service covered by the rider (prescription drugs, vision services, dental, or other supplemental services or contract features). However, the most significant financial decision for these plans involves determination of the rate increase for the basic coverage. This rate increase affects all of the groups covered by the HMO, and it is a major factor related to the plan's overall competitive position and financial performance. If the necessary rate increase is underestimated, then premium revenues will be insufficient to satisfy the plan's cost and capital requirements. A deficit will occur in the operating budget that will have to be met from the plan's reserves. Most HMOs do not have the level of surplus (capital) that many insurance companies do. Some staff-model plans have seen over 50 percent of their capital eaten up by two consecutive years of deficits due to poor operating results. Therefore, although projection of the necessary parameters (e.g., rate of health care inflation, rate of enrollment growth, and changes in utilization or practice patterns) is an extremely difficult task, it is critical for a plan to be able to estimate accurately the community rate increase needed to satisfy the plan's revenue requirements for the coming year.

Sample operating budget data for an HMO are included in Table 6-2. Here, we assume that we are in the middle of calendar year 1989 and are planning for calendar year 1990.[16] Actual expenditures for 1988 are known from historical data. The 1989 budget is shown, with percentage increases in each budget line item over 1988. The projected budget for 1990 has been estimated, including projected revenue requirements and plan expenses for medical center operations, other medical expenses and health plan administration.

To determine the community rate increase, a plan first prepares a detailed budget that determines the plan's revenue requirements for the coming year (Exhibit 6-1). Second, a projection of the plan's membership population is developed for the coming year. Third, minor sources of revenue such as rider income and copayments are evaluated. Fourth, after the costs and revenues due to riders and other revenue sources are accounted for, premium revenues based on the projected membership are determined under the current rate schedule. This usually results in a shortfall which must be satisfied by the rate increase. The percentage increase is determined by comparing the anticipated revenue requirements to the projected revenue under the current rates.[17]

The increase can be applied only to the projected member-months that occur after each contract renewal date. All premium revenue received prior to the contract renewal date is locked into the lower (current year) premium rates. In this example, we have assumed that there is a single annual increase that takes effect at the beginning of the calendar year (rather than quarterly increases). The new rates are applied to all groups that renew during the year. Therefore, if a group's renewal date is 1 January, then the new rates are effective for that group for the entire year. However, for a group that renews on 1 July, the old (1989) rates are in effect for the first six months of 1990, and the new rates go into effect on 1 July and remain in effect until the following 1 July.[18] If an HMO makes rate adjustments on a quarterly basis, then appropriate changes would have to be made in the community rate increase calculation (e.g., the number of effective member-months, before and after contract renewal, would have to be recalculated by calendar quarter, and the revenue estimates would need to be adjusted to reflect the quarterly rate increases). An increase of 16.4 percent is required to meet the plan's projected revenue requirements for 1990 (see Exhibit 6-1).

For most staff-model and group-model plans, there is a high level of fixed costs in staff and facilities. Thus, a careful budgeting process is required to identify the revenue requirements for the coming year (including medical service and administrative expenses, and costs related to capital acquisitions, facility construction, and debt service). In addition, due to the necessity for the plan to cover all fixed costs and provide for variable costs, a realistic forecast of changes in the membership population is required.[19]

Capitation Rate Development:
The Actuarial/Fee-for-Service Method

Whereas the cost/budget method considers the planwide costs (staffing, facility, equipment, supplies, administrative) required for plan operation, the actuarial/fee-for-service method focuses on each type of service in the plan's benefit package. This method estimates the per member per month cost of each benefit line item by projecting the utilization rate (of the membership population) and unit cost for the service.

For plans using the actuarial/fee-for-service method, the HMO capitation rate is the fundamental building block for development of premium rates under community rating. The capitation rate equals the total HMO revenue requirements per member per month for the projected time period or contract duration. All cost components must be reflected in the

Table 6-2: Operating Budget for Staff-Model and Group-Model HMOs

Category	1988 Actual	1989 Budget	Percent Change	1990 Projected	Percent Change
Revenues					
Premiums:					
Commercial	$51,975,120	$ 61,440,720	18.2%	$ 72,019,086	17.2%
Individual	6,930,875	7,902,801	14.0	8,831,334	11.7
Medicare	18,480,064	21,352,326	15.5	24,433,913	14.4
Medicaid	3,465,292	3,851,412	11.1	4,251,959	10.4
Reinsurance Payments	606,176	711,651	17.4	831,208	16.8
Third-Party Revenues	1,617,042	1,945,302	20.3	2,305,182	18.5
Interest	460,337	539,515	17.2	631,772	17.1
Copayments	808,496	959,685	18.7	1,134,347	18.2
Fee-for-service	801,575	933,835	16.5	1,078,579	15.5
Other	425,068	502,430	18.2	589,853	17.4
Total Revenues/Percent Change	$85,570,045	$100,139,677	17.0%	$116,107,233	15.9%
Expenses					
A. Medical Center Operations:					
Medical salary	$13,759,218	$ 16,125,804	17.2%	$ 18,644,675	15.6%
Other salary	10,974,655	12,818,397	16.8	14,641,157	14.2
Buildings/maintenance/rent	3,276,047	3,810,042	16.3	4,381,648	15.0
Medical supplies/equipment	1,965,601	2,333,168	18.7	2,723,143	16.7
Insurance	1,310,426	1,579,063	20.5	1,880,922	19.1
Pharmacy (in centers)	819,058	959,117	17.1	1,102,985	15.0
Other center expenses	687,961	804,226	16.9	904,860	12.5
Subtotal	32,792,966	38,429,817	17.2	44,279,390	15.2

B. Other Medical Expenses:					
Hospital inpatient	$24,360,158	$ 29,283,326	20.2%	$ 34,027,225	16.2%
Emergency/outpatient	4,209,196	5,041,596	19.8	5,848,251	16.0
Physician referral	9,660,324	11,483,258	18.9	13,340,579	16.2
Pharmacy (external)	3,368,746	4,024,589	19.5	4,648,523	15.5
Reinsurance premiums	1,360,078	1,704,892	25.4	2,027,675	18.9
Subtotal	42,958,502	51,537,661	20.0	59,892,253	16.2
C. Health Plan Administration:					
Personnel salary	$ 5,272,075	$ 6,305,402	19.6%	$ 7,251,212	15.0%
Data processing	1,160,985	1,337,455	15.2	1,578,073	18.0
Marketing	604,716	706,308	16.8	832,254	17.8
Supplies	336,592	395,832	17.6	465,207	17.5
Rent/building/maintenance	608,016	694,354	14.2	794,507	14.4
Telephone/mail	168,798	198,338	17.5	233,089	17.5
Other	252,679	297,656	17.8	352,304	18.4
Subtotal	8,403,861	9,935,345	18.2	11,506,646	15.8
Total Expenses/Percent Change	$84,155,329	$ 99,902,823	18.7%	$115,678,289	15.8%
Surplus of Revenues over Expenditures	$1,414,716	$236,854		$428,944	

Exhibit 6-1: Derivation of Community Rate Increase Factor

1. Projected revenue requirement		$116,107,233
2. Projected revenues from community rates for group and individual enrollment:		
a. Prior to contract renewals	$16,416,084	
b. After contract renewals (at current community rates)	56,053,616	
3. Other rate revenues:		
a. Medicare	24,433,913	
b. Medicaid	4,251,959	
4. Other revenues	5,739,733	$106,895,305
5. Additional rate revenue needed to meet the plan's projected revenue requirement		$9,211,928
6. Required community rate increase percentage (Item 5 as a percentage of Item 2b)		16.43%

capitation rate, including medical services costs, plan administration expenses, the value of cost sharing received by the plan or providers, other offsets to medical expenses such as coordination of benefits/third-party liability (COB/TPL), reinsurance premiums and estimated recoveries, other overhead expenses, and profit/contribution to reserves.

Medical services capitation cost.   Assuming that the HMO is contracting with a multispecialty medical group, on a capitation basis, for all physician and related outpatient services, the cost per member per month is calculated for each type of service as the utilization rate (frequency of units of service per member per year) times the unit cost (cost per unit of service) divided by 12. (The capitation rate for medical services costs is shown in Table 6-3.) The total medical services cost represents the estimated cost to the plan, on a per member per month basis, of providing the services in the basic benefit package to the enrolled membership population that is community rated.[20]

The medical services capitation is composed of per member per month costs for each type of service in the HMO's benefit package. The largest single line item cost is for inpatient hospital expenses, which is composed of two components: (1) the inpatient utilization rate, and (2) the inpatient cost per day. To estimate the inpatient utilization rate (hospital days per person per year, or alternatively, days per 1,000 members per year), a variety of methods can be used. For example, for an established plan, historical data should be used for the most recent time period for which data are available.[21] The data should be stratified by type of admission (medical, surgical, pediatric, obstetrics/gynecology, psychiatric, substance abuse), by line of business (commercial groups, Medicare, Medicaid, individual and group conversion members), and by age/sex category. Similarly, the number of member-months of exposure should be calculated for the same time period as the utilization data and according to the same categories by age/sex and line of business. The historical data should be analyzed to evaluate the utilization patterns and to determine the overall utilization rate. The historical utilization rate must also be adjusted for any change in the composition of the plan's membership population expected to occur between the time period of the historical data and the projected time period corresponding to the contract effective dates. For new plans, it is necessary to estimate the expected inpatient utilization rate based on the experience of similar types of plans, adjusted for the new plan's geographic location, projected membership population, utilization control mechanisms, and other characteristics such as the plan's physician panel.

To estimate the cost per hospital day, historical claims data should be used for established plans. For each individual hospital used by the plan, the data should be stratified by line of business, type of admission, and any other dimension that demonstrates significant variation in per diem costs. An all-inclusive cost per day should be calculated for all inpatient services provided and billed by participating hospitals. Services billed by independent providers (e.g., radiologists and pathologists) should be estimated separately. The historical cost per day then needs to be projected forward to the appropriate time period and adjusted for inflation, changes in the mix of hospitals, and other relevant factors. The provisions of current and planned hospital contracts must be incorporated into the projected inpatient cost per day, including reimbursement features (per diem, per case, DRG payments, discounted billed charges, capitation reimbursement) and any risk-sharing arrangements between the plan and participating hospitals. For new plans, the inpatient cost per day must be estimated based on the plan's projected (proportionate) use of each hospital in the community (and any specialty referral or tertiary care medical centers) and the billing rates and charge structures of these hospitals, again projected to the future time period and adjusted for discounts and other significant changes. A similar process must be followed to estimate the costs per member per month for each type of service offered by the HMO.[22]

Table 6-3: Development of Medical Service Capitation Cost
(Based on Fee-for-Service Charge Method)

Services	Frequency	Projected Average Charge	Capitation (Cost per Member per Month)
I. Hospital Services			
A. Inpatient Hospitalization			
1. In-area	.450	$493.00	$18.49
2. Out-of-area	.025	802.00	1.67
B. Outpatient Surgery	.020	647.00	1.08
C. Emergency Room	.200	74.00	1.23
D. Skilled Nursing Facility	.005	80.20	.03
Subtotal			$22.50
II. Asbury Medical Group: Prepaid Clinic Services			
A. Office Visits	3.300	23.50	6.46
B. Consultations	.060	63.50	.32
C. Inpatient Visits	.315	34.70	.91
D. Inpatient Visits—Newborn	.025	75.00	.16
E. Mental Health			
1. Inpatient	.045	46.10	.17
2. Outpatient	.200	63.50	1.06
F. Miscellaneous	1.280	16.40	1.75
G. Surgery			
1. Inpatient, in-and-out	.058	669.00	3.23
2. Office, emergency room	.200	83.10	1.38
3. Assistant	.013	201.00	.22
H. Emergency Room	.120	31.70	.32
I. Obstetrics	.025	796.00	1.66
J. Laboratory	3.710	9.80	3.03
K. X-ray	.530	50.10	2.21
Subtotal			$22.88

Continued

Projecting historical data to future periods. The following factors must be taken into account when projecting historical cost and utilization to future time periods: (1) inflation in medical costs, (2) claims incurred but not reported, (3) provider contract renewal dates, (4) delivery system changes, (5) membership population changes, and (6) changes in medical technology and other factors that affect medical costs. Future levels of medical inflation have always proven to be difficult to estimate accu-

Table 6-3: Continued

Services	Frequency	Projected Average Charge	Capitation (Cost per Member per Month)
III. Referrals, Miscellaneous			
A. Physical Therapy	.130	28.80	.31
B. Radiation Therapy	—	—	.08
C. Ambulance	.010	138.00	.12
D. Home Health	.027	32.30	.07
E. Cardiac Surgery	—	—	.23
F. Neurosurgery	—	—	.15
G. Hemodialysis	—	—	.20
H. Anesthesia	.055	231.00	1.06
I. Alcohol/Drug Abuse Treatment	.050	185.00	.77
Subtotal			$ 2.99
Total Gross Medical Services Cost			$48.37

Note: Reprinted, by permission of the publisher, from Sutton, Harry J., Jr., FSA, and Allen J. Sorbo, FSA, *Actuarial Issues in the Fee-for-Service/Prepaid Medical Group*, one in a series of seven monographs, the "Going Prepaid" series, (Denver, CO: Center for Research in Ambulatory Health Care Administration, research arm of the Medical Group Management Association, 1987), 38.

rately. Whether measured by the medical component of the consumer's price index (medical CPI), published by the Bureau of Labor Statistics, or by other indices, careful judgment is required to forecast inflation rates for medical services. In addition, there usually is a one-year to two-year (or more) time difference between the most recent historical cost and utilization data and the fiscal year for which the capitation rate must be projected.

When using cost and utilization data for a recent time period, it is likely that the data will not be complete, due to claims incurred but not reported. For accurate calculations, it is best to use data tabulated by the date when the service was rendered, rather than the date when the claim was paid. This is necessary for an accurate matching of cost and utilization data to the number of member-months of exposure for any given time period. (If membership is growing, a matching of membership data against paid claims data will result in an underestimate of utilization and cost ratios.) To avoid errors, it is necessary to estimate (1) paid claims, (2) claims in process (claims received by the plan but not yet paid), and (3) claims that have been incurred but not reported (IBNR claims). There is a substantial body of literature in the actuarial field on the problem of estimating IBNR claims expense.[23]

Provider contracting is a critical element for any HMO. Thus, in projecting historical data to future time periods, it is necessary to identify and incorporate any financial provisions in provider contracts that can have an impact on future costs experienced by the HMO. In particular, it is important to consider the effects of contract renewal dates, especially changes in reimbursement rates, into the calculations and projections. Also, if there is a change in major providers, or if there is a change in the mix of providers used, these factors must be accounted for in the projections.

Development of HMO total capitation rate. In the accompanying example (Table 6-4), it is assumed that the HMO is contracting with a multispecialty medical group that is responsible for providing all physician and related ancillary services. For other types of contractual arrangements (e.g., direct contracting with independent practitioners, contracting with a physician-sponsored IPA), it is necessary to modify the calculations to take into account the specific terms and conditions of the contractual relationship.

The first two sections of Table 6-4 show the projected costs for hospital services and medical group capitation, for the current year (Year 1) and the projected year (Year 2). To convert the medical services cost into the HMO's total capitation rate, a number of adjustments are required. First, the value of copayments needs to be calculated. For example, if the plan requires a copayment of $20 for emergency room visits, then the cost to the plan is reduced by $0.33 per member per month (200 visits per 1,000 members per year, times $20 per visit, divided by 12,000). In the example shown in Table 6-4, it is assumed that the value of all copayments equals $1.82.

A second adjustment concerns reinsurance. Most plans will purchase reinsurance for protection against catastrophic expenses, out-of-area coverage, insolvency protection, and so on. Since the services covered under reinsurance have wide variability (most years will have a low volume of reinsurance claims while relatively few years will have very large expenses subject to reinsurance), an approximate rule of thumb is to estimate that, in most years, the plan will recover $0.50 in reinsurance claims for every $1.00 that is paid in premiums. Thus, the next two entries in Table 6-4 correspond to the cost of the reinsurance premiums and the adjustment for reinsurance recoveries, respectively.

A third adjustment concerns recoveries due to coordination of ben-

Table 6-4: Determination of Total HMO Capitation Rate
(Including Medical Services Costs, Adjustments,
Administration, and Other Loadings)

	Cost Per Member per Month	
Cost Factor	*Year 1*	*Year 2*
Hospital Services	$22.50	$25.88
Medical Group Capitation:		
Medical services	22.88	25.17
(Less) discount	−2.29	−2.52
(Add) outside referrals	2.99	3.33
(Less) copayment revenue	−1.56	−1.56
(Less) reinsurance, COB	−.23	−.25
Subtotal—Medical Group Capitation	21.79	24.17
Adjustments and Loadings:		
Reinsurance premiums	1.70	1.60
Reinsurance recoveries	−.85	−.80
Coordination of benefits	−1.01	−1.17
Copayments (ER only)	−.26	−.26
Interest income	0	0
State reserve (2% of total)[a]	1.02	1.15
Administration, marketing, debt service, overhead (12% of total)	6.12	6.90
Premium tax	0	0
Profit (contribution to reserves)	0	0
Subtotal—Adjustments and Loadings	6.72	7.42
Total Cost Per Member Per Month	$51.01	$57.47

**Computation of HMO Capitation Rates (Updated Quarterly) for
Premium Rate Development under Community Rating:**

Effective Date of Contract (Year 1)[b]	*Employer Group Capitation Rates*
1st Quarter	$51.55 = [(11 × $51.01) + (1 × $57.47)]/12
2nd Quarter	$53.16 = [(8 × $51.01) + (4 × $57.47)]/12
3rd Quarter	$54.78 = [(5 × $51.01) + (7 × $57.47)]/12
4th Quarter	$56.39 = [(2 × $51.01) + (10 × $57.47)]/12

Note: Reprinted, by permission of the publisher, from Sutton, Harry J., Jr., FSA, and Allen J. Sorbo, FSA, *Actuarial Issues in the Fee-for-Service/Prepaid Medical Group*, one in a series of seven monographs, the "Going Prepaid" series, (Denver, Colorado: Center for Research in Ambulatory Health Care Administration, research arm of the Medical Group Management Association, 1987), 48.

[a]HMO is assumed to be a nonprofit corporation, 2 percent of premium is the state reserve requirement, and there is no state premium tax.

[b]Rates effective for twelve months for each employer group. Rates vary depending on effective date of contract.

efits, subrogation, and third-party liability. The total medical costs include the full cost of services delivered to enrolled beneficiaries. Any recoveries that the plan makes because of alternative health insurance coverage or the liability of a third party (e.g., workers' compensation, no-fault automobile insurance) must be subtracted from the total costs to reflect the HMO's actual exposure or liability.

Additional items in Table 6-4 must be included in the capitation rate. The first item, plan administration, includes all of the nonmedical costs of operating the plan: plan management, claims processing, data systems, marketing and advertising, health center administration, and nonmedical equipment and supplies. Any other costs for overhead should also be identified, translated to a per member per month basis, and included in the calculations.

If the plan generates interest income, it should be reflected in the calculations on a per member per month basis. If there is a state premium tax, it should also be included.

The final item is a loading factor for profit (or contribution to reserves for nonprofit plans). Since this item produces the key source of capital derived from plan operations, it should be considered carefully.

In this example, the capitation rate is shown at the bottom of Table 6-4. It consists of the estimated gross medical services costs, the adjustments to determine the net medical services costs, and the other cost elements that must be reflected in the capitation rate (administration, overhead, interest income, premium taxes, and profit/contribution to reserves).

In summary, a key ingredient for HMO premium rate development is the plan's projected *capitation rate*. Determination of the capitation rate is necessary for many common forms of community rating currently practiced in the HMO industry. The capitation rate is the revenue required per member per month to support the operation and financial requirements of the plan, and it is the primary component in the process of developing premium rates for commercial and other groups.

Flexible Forms of Community Rating: Conversion of Capitation Rates into Premium Rates

Although many HMOs use a fixed rate schedule, the majority of plans have adopted the more flexible form of community rating permitted under federal regulations. For example, premium rates can be determined using a standard cost per member per month and two-tier or three-tier rate structures (see Exhibits 6-2 and 6-3). For plans that implement community rating using a fixed revenue requirement (per member per month), although there is not a fixed rate schedule, the premium rates for all groups must generate an equivalent amount of revenue on a per member per month basis. Exhibits 6-2 and 6-3 are only concerned with the development of premium rates for the basic coverage. We have ignored differences in premium rates among groups due to riders for supplemental benefits, administrative costs, and cost-sharing provisions.[24]

Under this method, the premium rate development process starts with the HMO's *capitation rate,* that is, the plan's overall revenue requirement per member per month. As discussed above, the capitation rate includes (1) medical expenses, (2) administrative costs (including marketing and claims processing) (3) insurance premiums (e.g., reinsurance and malpractice), (4) debt service, (5) other overhead expenses, (6) reserve contribution, (7) premium taxes, if any, and (8) profit (or surplus) margin. The capitation rate also reflects other sources of plan revenue (interest income, copayments, reinsurance payments, coordination of benefits recoveries, and nonmember billings). In the accompanying examples, we have assumed that other lines of business (e.g., Medicare and Medicaid) operate on a self-supporting basis and do not require subsidies from commercial accounts.

In determining community-rated premiums, federal regulations permit HMOs to take into account differences between groups, such as (1) the mix of single and family contracts, (2) the average family (contract) size, and (3) the in-force rates of a competitor. For example, if a group has an unusually large average family size, then more members are covered for that group than are assumed in the average community rate. Thus, the adjustment for larger (or smaller) family size results in a corresponding increase (or decrease) in the group's premium. However, the formula theoretically ensures that the HMO receives an equivalent amount of revenue, per member per month, from all groups.

In Exhibit 6-2 we assume that HMO A uses a flexible form of community rating based on a fixed revenue requirement of $75.00 per member per month for all groups. Under a two-tier premium rate structure, we assume that HMO A's normal family-to-single premium ratio is 2.8:1. The *premium ratio* is a key feature of a community-rating system. In one sense, the single and family categories are risk classes, and the ratio should reflect the relative cost differences between persons covered under single and family contracts. In some areas, this is true. In others, the major health plans have long-established policies concern-

Exhibit 6-2: Flexible Forms of Community Rating: Two-Tier Rate
Structure, Standard PMPM Revenue Requirement

Assumptions:

1. HMO A uses a flexible form of community rating that is based on a fixed
   revenue requirement of $75.00 per member per month for all groups.
   Under a two-tier premium rate structure, we assume that HMO A's normal
   family-to-single premium ratio is 2.8:1.
2. Group 1 is a bank with a work force characterized by a higher proportion
   of single contracts (55%), a relatively low average contract size of 1.99,
   and an average family size of 3.2 for family contracts with two or more
   members. Group 1 has a two-tier rate structure.

Calculation of HMO A's premium rates for Group 1:

Single premium = Per member per month
revenue requirement × conversion factor

$$= \$75.00 \times \frac{(.55 \times 1) + (.45 \times 3.2)}{(.55 \times 1) + (.45 \times 2.8)}$$

$$= \$75.00 \times 1.0994$$

$$= \$82.46$$

Family premium = Single premium × 2.8

$$= \$82.46 \times 2.8$$

$$= \$230.89$$

Reconciliation to ensure that Group 1 produces average revenue of
$75.00 PMPM:

$$\text{Revenue PMPM} = \frac{\text{Average revenue per contract per month}}{\text{Average no. members per contract}}$$

$$= \frac{(\$82.46 \times .55) + (\$230.89 \times .45)}{(1 \times .55) + (3.2 \times .45)}$$

$$= \$75.00$$

ing this ratio, which may or may not reflect the current cost differentials
between single and family contracts. In many cases, it is to the HMO's
advantage to follow the prevailing pattern in major groups in order to
avoid antiselection and large premium differences among categories.

Group 1 (Exhibit 6-2) is a bank with a work force with a high
proportion of single contracts, a relatively low average contract size, and

Exhibit 6-3: Flexible Forms of Community Rating: Three-Tier
Rate Structure, Standard PMPM Revenue Requirement

Assumptions:

1. HMO B uses a community-rating method based on a fixed revenue requirement, per member per month, of $75.00. We assume that HMO B has a three-tier premium rate structure and that the normal ratio of family to two-party to single premium ratios is 3:2:1.

2. Group 2 is a manufacturing company with an older than average work force, low proportions of single and two-party contracts (30 percent and 15 percent respectively), an average contract size of 2.97, and an average family size of 4.3 for family contracts with three or more members.

Calculation of HMO B's premium rates for Group 2:

Single premium $= $ Per member per month
revenue requirement $\times$ conversion factor

$$= \$75.00 \times \frac{(.3 \times 1) + (.15 \times 2) + (.55 \times 4.3)}{(.3 \times 1) + (.15 \times 2) + (.55 \times 3)}$$

$$= \$75.00 \times 1.3178$$

$$= \$98.84$$

Two-party premium $=$ Single premium $\times$ 2

$$= \$98.84 \times 2$$

$$= \$197.68$$

Family premium $(3+)$ $=$ Single premium $\times$ 3

$$= \$98.84 \times 3$$

$$= \$296.52$$

Reconciliation to ensure that Group 2 produces average revenue of $75.00 PMPM:

$$\text{Revenue PMPM} = \frac{(\$98.84 \times .3) + (\$197.68 \times .15) + (\$296.52 \times .55)}{(1 \times .3) + (2 \times .15) + (4.3 \times .55)}$$

$$= \$75.00$$

---

an average family size of 3.2 for family contracts with two or more members.

For a case of this type, the community rate for the single premium is equal to the capitation rate (revenue requirement per member per month) times the premium conversion factor. The *conversion factor* is the average contract size (average number of members per contract) divided by the average premium unit (the average premium, expressed as a multiple of the single premium rate, weighted by the distribution of contracts). The conversion factor is used to vary premiums across groups to take into account differences in the mix of contracts and the average contract size, while maintaining a predetermined premium ratio. In this example, the single premium rate is equal to the conversion factor (1.0994) times the HMO's capitation rate ($75.00). The family premium rate is equal to the single rate ($82.46) times the family-to-single premium ratio (2.8 in this example), resulting in a family premium of $230.89.

The premium rates for Group 1 produce the desired revenue of $75.00 per member per month. The revenue PMPM is equal to the average revenue per contract per month ($82.46 times .55 plus $230.89 times .45) divided by the average number of members per contract (1.0 times .55 plus 3.2 times .45), which is equal to 75.002.

In Exhibit 6-3, we assume that HMO B also uses a flexible form of community rating, with a three-tier rate structure and a revenue requirement of $75.00 per member per month. We assume that the premium ratio for family to two-party to single contracts is 3:2:1 (the premium rate for two-party contracts is twice the rate for single contracts, and family rates, covering three or more persons, are three times the single rates). As with the premium ratio in two-tier structures, the premium ratio in three-tier structures can vary substantially between geographic areas and between groups in the same area. Usually, the two-party rate is relatively close to two times the single rate (i.e., the ratio may be between 1.8 and 2.2). The ratio of the family rate to the single rate has more variability. For example, the average family size for contracts with three or more members is usually around 4.0, and it usually varies across groups in the range of 3.0 to 5.0. However, the ratio in premium rates between family $(3+)$ and single contracts is usually in the range of 2.5 to 3.5.

Group 2 (Exhibit 6-3) is assumed to be a manufacturing company with an older than average work force, relatively low proportions of single and two-party contracts, an average contract size of 2.97, and an average family size of 4.3 for family contracts with three or more members. The single premium for Group 2 is equal to the $75.00 capitation rate times the premium conversion factor. Note that the formula for the conversion factor reflects the three-tier rate structure, although it has the same form as the one in Exhibit 6-2.

For any rate structure, the general form of the formula for the conversion factor is similar. The numerator is equal to the weighted average of the average contract size, and the denominator is equal to the weighted average of the premium ratios, with the weights for both numerator and denominator equal to the proportions of contracts in each rate category.

The premium rates for each category, in this type of community-rating system, are equal to the capitation rate times the conversion factor times the premium ratio for that category. For Group 2 in Exhibit 6-3, the conversion factor is 1.3178, and the single premium rate is $98.84 ($75.00 times 1.3178). The two-party premium is equal to $197.68 ($98.84 times 2 or, equivalently, $75.00 times 1.3178 times 2), and the family premium rate is equal to $296.52 ($98.84 times 3 or, equivalently, $75.00 times 1.3178 times 3).

The derived premium rates for Group 2 produce an average revenue of $75.00 per member per month. The average revenue PMPM is equal to the average (weighted) revenue per contract per month divided by the average (weighted) number of members per contract, with the weights equal to the proportions of contracts in each category.

Recomposition of Premium Rates to Reflect In-Force Rates

With respect to adjustments for in-force rates, an HMO will normally have a rating formula such that, in a two-tier rate structure, the family rate is a specified multiple of the single rate (usually in the 2.5 to 3.5 range). However, if the group's major indemnity plan has a distinctly different multiple between family and single rates (e.g., the indemnity family rates are 2.5 times the single rates, and the HMO's normal family rates are 3.0 times the single rates), then it is likely that, all other things being equal, the HMO's enrollment will be heavily biased with many more singles than families (due to the greater attractiveness of the HMO's single rate, as opposed to the indemnity single rate, relative to the comparison of family rates). To promote a more balanced enrollment, it is permissible for the HMO to recomposite its rates to reflect the single/family multiple in the indemnity rates. In this case, the change from the 3.0 multiple to the 2.5 multiple will increase the HMO's single rate and decrease the HMO's family rate in order to be more comparable to the single/family ratio in the indemnity rates. However, even after recompositing, the HMO's rates still produce the same revenue on a per member per month basis (assuming that the estimated enrollment is correct).

The two examples of adjusting community rates reflect the in-force rates of another health plan or carrier (see Exhibit 6-4). The two examples are drawn from Exhibit 6-2 (HMO A, Group 1, two-tier rate structure) and Exhibit 6-3 (HMO B, Group 2, three-tier rate structure). The new single premium rate for Group 1 is equal to the average revenue per contract (for Group 1 for HMO A) divided by the rate adjustment factor to match the ratio of in-force rates. The rate adjustment factor is equal to the weighted average of the premium ratios for the in-force rates, with the weights equal to the proportions of contracts in each premium category. In this example, the new family rate for Group 1 is equal to the single rate times the family ratio for the in-force rates ($76.74 times 3.1), or $237.89.

Note that the original single rate for HMO A (for Group 1) was $8.46 higher than the indemnity plan's single rate ($82.46 compared to $74.00), and the family rate was $1.49 higher for HMO A ($230.89 compared to $229.40). Since Group 1 has a high proportion of single contracts (55 percent), HMO A would have been at a competitive disadvantage with more than an $8.00 differential in the original single rates, even though the family rate was only marginally higher for HMO A. By recompositing, HMO A was able to reduce the single differential to $2.74 ($76.74 compared to $74.00). The differential in family rates increased slightly to $8.49 ($237.89 compared to $229.40), which is still within a competitive range for family contracts.

For the second example in Exhibit 6-4 the rates determined in Exhibit 6-3 for Group 2 by HMO B under a three-tier rate structure are recomposited to match the in-force rates. HMO B's original rates for Group 2 (compared to the indemnity plan) were higher for single and two-party contracts, but lower for family contracts (three or more persons). By recompositing, HMO B is able to have lower rates for all three categories (single, two-party, and family), compared to the indemnity rates.

The "revised" community rates (after recompositing) still produce the desired revenue of $75.00 per member per month. The reconciliation calculations are shown at the end of each example in Exhibit 6-4.

Different contract mixes produce different effects in the premium rates derived under a community-rating system. We can hold all other factors constant and evaluate the effect of different contract mix assumptions for five groups (see Exhibit 6-5). With all other factors held constant, the single premiums range from $87.28 to $95.54, depending on the different contract mix assumptions in the five groups. Similarly, two-party premiums range from $174.56 to $191.08, and family premiums range from $261.84 to $286.62. For these five groups, the average contract size ranges from 1.96 to 2.97, and the average revenue per contract ranges from $146.63 to $222.60. However, the average revenue per

Exhibit 6-4: Flexible Forms of Community Rating: Recomposition of Premiums to Match In-Force Rates

---

Assumptions:

1. The indemnity plan for Group 1 has rates of $74.00 and $229.40 for single and family (2 +) contracts, respectively. The family-to-single premium ratio from the indemnity plan is 3.1:1, compared to HMO A's normal ratio of 2.8:1 (see Exhibit 6-2).

2. For Group 2, the indemnity plan has rates of $97.00, $194.00 and $310.40 for single, two-party, and family (3 +) contracts, respectively. The premium ratio from the indemnity plan is 3.2:2:1, compared to HMO B's normal ratio of 3:2:1 (see Exhibit 6-3).

Recomposition of HMO A's rates for Group 1 to match the in-force rates:

$$\text{New single rate} = \frac{\text{Average revenue per contract (Group 1 for HMO A)}}{\text{Rate adjustment factor to match the ratio of in-force rates}}$$

$$= \frac{(.55 \times \$82.46) + (.45 \times \$230.89)}{(.55 \times 1) + (.45 \times 3.1)}$$

$$= \$76.74$$

$$\text{New family rate} = \$76.74 \times 3.1 = \$237.89$$

$$\text{Reconciliation:} \quad \frac{(\$76.74 \times .55) + (\$237.89 \times .45)}{(1 \times .55) + (3.2 \times .45)} = \$75.00$$

Recomposition of HMO B's rates for Group 2 to match the in-force rates:

$$\text{New single rate} = \frac{(\$98.84 \times .3) + (\$197.68 \times .15) + (\$296.52 \times .55)}{(.3 \times 1) + (.15 \times 2) + (.55 \times 3.2)}$$

$$= \$94.23$$

$$\text{New two-party rate} = \$94.23 \times 2 = \$188.46$$

$$\text{New family (3 +) rate} = \$94.23 \times 3.2 = \$301.54$$

$$\text{Reconciliation:} \quad \frac{(\$94.23 \times .3) + (\$188.46 \times .15) + (\$301.54 \times .55)}{(1 \times .3) + (2 \times .15) + (4.3 \times .55)}$$

$$= \$75.00$$

---

member per month is maintained at the desired value of $75.00 for all five contracts.

We can also examine the effects of different assumptions for contract mixes, contract sizes, and recompositing for in-force rates, using the same groups used in Exhibit 6-5 for comparison (see Exhibit 6-6).

Exhibit 6-5: Flexible Forms of Community Rating:
The Effect of Different Contract Mixes

Assumptions:

1. We assume that Groups A, B, C, D, and E have the same average contact size for family contracts (3 or more members): 4.1.

2. Under a three-tier premium rate structure, the normal ratio of family to two-party to single rates for HMO B is 3:2:1.

3. The five groups have different contract mixes as follows:

	Single	Two-Party	Family	Total
Group A	40%	20%	40%	100%
Group B	30	20	50	100
Group C	48	22	30	100
Group D	25	17	58	100
Group E	57	18	25	100

Effect of Different Contract Distributions on Premium Rates:[a]

	Premium Rates			Average Contract Size[b]	Average Revenue Per Contract	Average Revenue PMPM
	Single	Two-Party	Family			
Group A	$91.50	$183.00	$274.50	2.44	$183.00	$75.00
Group B	93.75	187.50	281.25	2.75	206.25	75.00
Group C	88.60	177.20	265.80	2.15	161.25	75.00
Group D	95.54	191.08	286.62	2.97	222.60	75.00
Group E	87.28	174.56	261.84	1.96	146.63	75.00

[a] Assumes standard revenue requirement of $75.00 per member per month. Refer to Exhibit 6-3 for other assumptions concerning HMO B.

[b] Average number of members per contract.

The HMO B premium rates are developed according to the normal premium ratio of 3:2:1 used by HMO B. Note that the range in single premiums increases from $8.26 for different contract mixes ($87.28 to $95.54 from Exhibit 6-5) to $14.90 for different contract mixes and contract sizes ($82.50 to $97.40) to $18.25 after adjustment for in-force rates ($85.05 to $103.30). Compared to an average single premium of $90.00, the above ranges are 9.2 percent (8.26/90.00), 16.6 percent (14.90/90.00), and 20.3 percent (18.25/90.00) of the average single premium. Although these calculations are based on only five sample groups, they demonstrate the increase in the relative degree of variation in premium rates as additional assumptions are added. For any HMO, however, the degree of variation in rates will depend upon a variety of factors such

Exhibit 6-6: Flexible Forms of Community Rating: The Effect of Different Assumptions for Contract Mixes, Contract Sizes, and In-Force Rates

Assumptions:

1. Contract mix assumptions for Groups A, B, C, D, and E as specified in Exhibit 6-5.
2. Under a three-tier premium rate structure, the normal ratio of family to two-party to single rates for HMO B is 3:2:1.
3. The assumptions for contract sizes and in-force rates are:

	Average Contract Size			*In-force Rates*		
	Single	*Two-Party*	*Family*	*Single*	*Two-Party*	*Family*
Group A	1.0	2.0	3.5	$ 70.00	$140.00	$199.50
Group B	1.0	2.0	3.7	85.00	153.00	212.50
Group C	1.0	2.0	3.9	90.00	180.00	288.00
Group D	1.0	2.0	4.2	95.00	180.50	266.00
Group E	1.0	2.0	4.5	110.00	220.00	308.00

Effect of Different Contract Distributions on Premium Rates:[a]

	HMO Premium Rates			*After Adjustment to In-force Rates*		
	Single	*Two-Party*	*Family*	*Single*	*Two-Party*	*Family*
Group A	$82.50	$165.00	$247.50	$ 85.05	$170.10	$242.39
Group B	86.93	173.86	260.79	100.13	180.23	250.33
Group C	86.13	172.26	258.39	83.38	166.76	266.82
Group D	97.40	194.80	292.20	103.30	196.27	289.24
Group E	91.74	183.48	275.22	94.55	189.10	264.74

[a]Assumes standard revenue requirement of $75.00 per member per month. Refer to Exhibit 6-3 for other assumptions concerning HMO B.

as the actual differences between groups in average contract sizes, contract mixes, and in-force rates.

Options for HMOs under Community Rating

There are a number of options for HMOs under community rating.

1. An HMO can base its community-rating system on (a) a fixed rate schedule, (b) equivalent revenue per member per month, or (c) equivalent revenue per contract (subscriber) per month.

2. Some groups can be excluded from the community-rating system at the HMO's discretion. For example, federally qualified HMOs can use experience rating for governmental groups such as state employees, cities, and school districts. Medicare and Medicaid eligibles can also be rated outside of the community-rating system (subject to federal and state regulations).

3. An HMO's community rates can be adjusted to match other in-force rates, as long as the basic principles for the "equivalent revenue standards" are followed.

4. An HMO can use different loading factors for administrative and marketing expenses based on (a) individuals, (b) small groups with 100 subscribers or less, and (c) groups with over 100 subscribers.

5. Community rates can be varied to reflect differences in the mix of contracts and average family size between groups.

6. Community rates can reflect differences in the effective dates on contracts (and can be updated during the year).

Thus, as prescribed by federal regulations, HMOs have some degree of flexibility in designing and implementing community-rating systems. However, the major goals and objectives for rating systems, as discussed in Chapter 4, are entirely relevant for HMOs under any form of community-rating system. In particular, they must ensure that the rating system as a whole produces sufficient revenue to satisfy the plan's financial requirements. In addition, major categories of rates should be self-supporting wherever possible (a plan's financial experience should be examined to determine if the single and family rates actually cover their expenses or if adjustments should be made to bring the rates more into line). In an increasingly competitive health care environment, great demands are placed on rating systems to facilitate enrollment growth and to meet the requirements of the marketplace. However, there are substantial dangers in the inappropriate use of the flexibility available to federally qualified HMOs under the community-rating regulations. In addition to maintaining the plan's competitive position, HMO management must also be acutely aware of the dangers of underpricing and its potential impact on the plan's overall financial condition.

6.4 Community Rating by Class

In 1981, amendments to the HMO Act permitted a new form of rating for federally qualified HMOs—community rating by class (CRC). Prior to the amendments, community rating was the only acceptable rating method for federally qualified HMOs, which meant that HMOs had to charge the same, or equivalent, rates to all groups for the same benefit package.

How does community rating by class differ from community rating? There are three major differences. First, instead of assuming that all members/groups are of equal risk, an HMO can identify a set of rating classes that correspond to different levels of risk and are based on identifiable characteristics of groups and enrolled members (age, sex, industry, family composition, and so on). Second, the plan can establish rating factors for the different risk classes that take into account their different utilization and cost patterns (e.g., males age 25 are only 60 percent as costly as the average enrollee; miners are 15 percent more costly than average, after controlling for age, sex, and other demographic characteristics; financial services companies are 10 percent less costly than average). Third, the rating factors can be used in determining premium rates for different groups, so group-specific premiums are based on the characteristics of the group's enrollees. Like community-rating regulations for federally qualified HMOs, community rating by class also prohibits setting rates based on the utilization or cost experience of an individual group (in effect, experience rating).

The fundamental elements of premium rate setting under community rating by class, as established by Section 1302(8) of the HMO Act, are as follows:

- A health maintenance organization may fix rates of payment under either a system of community rating or community rating by class or under both systems. However, the HMO may use only one such system for setting rates for any one group at any one time.
- Under traditional community rating, rates are fixed on a per person or per family basis and must be equivalent for all individuals and for all families of similar composition.
- Community rating by class allows rates to be fixed by groups for individuals and families. These rates must be equivalent for all individuals in the same group and for all families of similar composition in the same group. The three steps involved in setting the rate are:
  1. *Classification of all HMO members into classes* actuarially derived based on factors which reasonably predict differences in the use of HMO services by the individuals or families in each class.
  2. *Determination of revenue requirements for providing services to the members of each class* based upon the projected utilization of that class.

3. *For each group, establishment of a composite premium rate* for all individuals in the group and for all families of similar composition in the group. The rate would be the same for all individuals in the group and for all families of similar composition in the group.

- Under either of the acceptable rating systems, differentials in rates may be established:

    1. to reflect differences in marketing costs and the different administrative costs of collecting payments from the following categories of potential members:

        a. Individual (nongroup) members including their families.

        b. Small groups of members (100 members or fewer).

        c. Large groups of members (over 100 members).

    2. for members enrolled in an HMO: (1) Under a contract with a governmental authority under section 1079 of Title 10 ("Armed Forces"), United States Code, (2) under any other governmental program (other than the health benefits program authorized by chapter 89 of Title 5 (FEHBP), United States Code), or (3) under any health benefits program for employees of States, political subdivision of States, and other public entities. It is important to note that community rating is not required for these groups of members.

    3. for separate regional components of the organization upon satisfactory demonstration to the Secretary of the following:

        a. Each regional component is geographically distinct and separate from any other regional component; and

        b. Each regional component provides substantially the full range of basic health services to its members, without extensive referral between components of the organization for these services, and without substantial utilization by any two components of the same health care facilities. The separate rate for each regional component of the HMO must be based on the different costs of providing health services in the respective regions.

- Experience rating is clearly prohibited.
- The Secretary (of DHHS) is required to review the factors used by each HMO to establish community rates by class. If the Secretary determines that any factor may not reasonably be used to predict the use of health services, then the factor must be disapproved.

Definitions

Factor: A factor is a characteristic of individuals or families that reasonably predicts differences in the use of HMO services by the individuals or families. Age, sex, income, marital status are all examples of factors. Consistent with the administration's policy, race will not be an acceptable factor. Based on permissible factors, HMO members are divided into categorics, e.g., age: under 65 and 65 and over, sex: male and female.

Class: A class is a sub-population of an HMO's members, usually representing more than one group, all of whom fall into the same category. Under a community rating by class system, an HMO would establish "classes" of individuals and families. The purpose of these classes is to put all individuals and all families who are expected to have similar utilization experiences (and thus similar costs to the HMO) into the same class, regardless of group identification. A class would be actuarially derived or developed by the HMO based on factors which reasonably predict differences in the use of HMO services by individuals or families in the class. The number of factors and classes established is left to the discretion of the HMO. Males ages 30-35 is an example of a class where two factors, age and sex, are used to predict differences in the utilization of services. The following classes are prohibited:

- A class may not be a group, i.e., one employer's employees.
- A class may not be a combination of two or more groups.
- A class may not be an occupation, defined as that activity which chiefly engages one's time; one's trade, profession or business.
- Because race is not an acceptable factor, classes may not be defined by race.[25]

The group-specific premiums determined under a CRC system are different from those of an experience-rating system. With community rating by class, the risk classes are defined with respect to the demographic and other characteristics of enrollees, and the rating factors are based on planwide utilization and cost experience.

As of February 1989, acceptable factors for determining rating classes under community rating by class were (1) age, (2) sex, (3) marital status, (4) family size, (5) industry, and (6) smoking/nonsmoking status.[26] Any factor that can be shown to result in differential health services utilization patterns (based on an HMO's planwide experience) can be utilized in a CRC system. However, new factors have to be submitted for approval to the Office of Prepaid Health Care, U.S. Department of Health and Human Services.

Factors denied by DHHS for use in CRC systems include (1) race, (2) occupation, and (3) geographic area/region. In addition, factors cannot be used if they apply only to a single group, effectively experience rating that group.

When the CRC rating factors are applied to a specific group, the resulting premiums reflect the planwide risk levels based on the class characteristics, but the premiums do not reflect the actual utilization or cost experience of the specific persons enrolled in the group, as they would under an experience-rating system (see Section 7.4 for more details about experience rating).

In essence, community rating by class is a *manual-rating system.* In this form of rating system, risk classes are established together with a set of manual, or tabular, rates. Most private insurers use the manual rates for determination of premiums for groups that are too small for experience rating or for which the historical experience is unknown (refer to Section 5.1 for additional details about manual rating). On the other hand, community rating by class permits HMOs to set premiums on a group-specific basis, in a way that is not permissible under community rating. With community rating by class (or manual rating), premium rates reflect the most salient characteristics of the group and its enrollees, but the rating factors are based on the total (planwide) utilization and cost experience of all persons/groups covered by the insurance product, rather than group-specific experience.

The flexibility in federal regulations for community rating also applies to community rating by class. This includes the methods for determining premium rates discussed in the previous section. Federally qualified HMOs may use community rating for some groups and community rating by class for other groups. Other provisions include (1) different administrative expense ratios for individual contracts, groups under 100 subscribers, and groups with 100 or more subscribers; (2) exemptions for governmental units, Medicare, and Medicaid; (3) premium ratios can be varied to match in-force rates; and (4) rates can be varied according to contract mix and average contract size.

The following three examples illustrate the different forms of community rating by class. The first example uses a limited set of age/sex factors applied to HMO members. The second example uses factors derived for different classes of subscribers. The third example integrates demographic profile data and CRC relative cost factors.

Example 1

This example follows from material presented in "Guidance for Community Rating by Class."[27] Community rating by class factors are limited to age and sex, producing six classes:

1. Males under age 19
2. Males age 19–44

3. Males age 45–64
4. Females under age 19
5. Females age 19–44
6. Females 45–64

The capitation rate (e.g., revenue requirement per member per month) is disaggregated into major rate components. For each class, relative utilization and revenue requirements are determined. Next, each class-specific relative utilization rate is calculated by dividing the utilization rate for the class enrollees by the overall utilization rate for all enrollees. Then, the revenue requirement for each class is determined by multiplying the relative utilization rate by the per member per month community rate components. Next, the individual rate is determined by weighting the class-specific revenue requirements by the number (or proportion) of HMO enrollees in each class, and the tiered premium rates can be composited.

The calculations for Example 1 are displayed in Table 6-5, including the major components of the community rate (capitation rate per member per month), and the development of the revenue requirement for each class for inpatient and outpatient services. It is assumed that Class 1 (males under age 19) have a hospital utilization rate (inpatient days per 1,000 members per year) that is 48 percent of the inpatient rate for the total enrolled membership population for the HMO, and an outpatient visit rate equal to 97 percent of the HMO's average rate. The class-specific revenue requirement for Class 1 for inpatient services is equal to the relative utilization factor (.48) multiplied by the hospital component of the capitation rate ($14.50), or $6.96. Similarly, the outpatient revenue requirement for Class 1 is $20.37 (.97 multiplied by $21.00). Note that the total relative utilization factors are 1.00 (representing a weighted average across risk classes, with weights equal to the proportion of members in each class), and the revenue requirements for all classes (weighted average) are equal to the community rate components for the entire HMO population.

Note that Group A of the two sample groups (Section III, Table 6-5) has a significantly younger distribution of members than Group B (Group A has 10 percent of its members over age 44, compared to 45 percent for Group B).

The premium rate development process for Group A and Group B includes several steps (Section IV, Table 6-5). First, the community rate by class (the adjusted capitation rate reflecting the distribution of members across classes) is computed for each group. Next, the contract mix

Table 6-5: Community Rating by Class: Example 1

I.   Per Member per Month "Community Rate"[a]

Hospital Services	$14.50
Medical Services	21.00
Other	4.50[b]
Total	$40.00

II. Relative Utilization and Revenue Requirements

Classes	Inpatient Utilization Factor[c]	Outpatient Utilization Factor[c]	PMPM Revenue Requirement	
			Inpatient	Outpatient[d]
1	.48	.97	$ 6.96	$20.37
2	.54	.68	7.83	14.28
3	2.01	1.05	29.14	22.05
4	.44	.99	6.38	20.79
5	1.44	1.16	20.88	24.36
6	1.82	1.33	26.39	27.93
All Classes	1.00	1.00	$14.50	$21.00

III. Percentage Distribution of Members

Classes	Group A	Group B
1	20%	10%
2	25	15
3	5	20
4	20	10
5	25	20
6	5	25
All Classes	100%	100%

IV. Per Member per Month "Community Rate by Class"[e]

	Group A	Group B
Hospital Services	$12.62	$19.11
Medical Services	20.38	22.51
Other	4.50[b]	4.50[b]
Total	$37.50	$46.12

Continued

assumptions for both groups are displayed. Note that, in this example, we assume that there is a four-tier rate structure with categories: single party, adult and child, two adults, and family with three or more members.

Table 6-5: Continued

V. Development of Four-Tier Premium Rates

Assumption for premium ratios: 3.0:2.0:1.5:1.0 for Family: Two adults:
Adult and child: single party rates

Contract mix and size assumptions:

Premium Category	Group A %	Group A Size	Group B %	Group B Size	Premium Ratio
Single party	35%	1.00	40%	1.00	1
Adult & Child	5	2.00	10	2.00	1.5
Two Adults	15	2.00	15	2.00	2
Family (3 +)	45	4.56	35	4.57	3
Total	100%	2.80	100%	2.50	

$$\text{Conversion Factor A} = \frac{(.35 \times 1) + (.05 \times 2) + (.15 \times 2) + (.45 \times 4.56)}{(.35 \times 1) + (.05 \times 1.5) + (.15 \times 2) + (.45 \times 3)}$$

$$= \frac{2.80}{2.075} = 1.3494$$

$$\text{Conversion Factor B} = \frac{(.40 \times 1) + (.10 \times 2) + (.15 \times 2) + (.35 \times 4.57)}{(.40 \times 1) + (.10 \times 1.5) + (.15 \times 2) + (.35 \times 3)}$$

$$= \frac{2.50}{1.90} = 1.3158$$

Premium Rates:	Group A	Group B
Single Party	$ 50.60	$ 60.68
Adult & Child	75.90	91.03
Two Adults	101.21	121.37
Family (3 +)	151.81	182.05

Source: U.S. Department of Health and Human Services, "Guidance for
Community by Class," Office of Health Maintenance Organizations,
22 March 1982.

[a]Projected per capita cost and capital requirement.

[b]Assumed, for illustrative purposes, to be $4.50 for each member, regardless
of class.

[c]Each entry equals the utilization of the class divided by the utilization of
all members. Hospital days per 1,000 members and doctor office visits
per 1,000 members are surrogates for inpatient and outpatient utilization, respectively.

[d]Utilization multiplied by the relevant community rate component.

[e]PMPM revenue requirements weighted by the percentage distribution of members.

Finally, the premium rates for each group are calculated. In this
example, we assume that the premium ratios are 3.0:2.0:1.5:1.0 for the
four rate categories of family, two adults, adult and child, and single
party, respectively. First, the conversion factor (i.e., the average contract

size divided by the average premium ratio) is computed for each group (refer to Section 6.3 for further explanation of the formula for the conversion factor). Next, the premium rate for each category is determined as the product of the community rate by class (adjusted capitation rate) multiplied by the conversion factor multiplied by the premium ratio for that category. Note that the adjusted capitation rate for Group B ($46.12) is 23.0 percent higher than the adjusted capitation rate for Group A ($37.50), whereas the single premium rate for Group B ($60.68) is only 19.9 percent higher than the single premium rate for Group A ($50.60). This difference is due to the different contract mix and average contract size between the two groups. For other groups, the relationship could go in the opposite direction.

The final step in the premium rate development could be recomposition of the rates to match the in-force rates of another carrier. The process for accomplishing this step under community rating by class is the same as that described in the previous section for community rating.

Example 2

Focusing on analysis of subscriber units, the factors here are age, sex, and industry. The classes are five-year age/sex cells for single-party and family $(2+)$ subscribers, respectively. The industry adjustment factor reflects differences in use of health services by members of different industries, after controlling for age/sex differences; this factor is applied after the age/sex calculation is completed.

Section I of Table 6-6 contains the age/sex relative cost factors for the single and family subscribers in each five-year age/sex category. An example of the CRC calculations is shown in Section II for a sample group. Note that the composite age/sex adjustment factor is .975 for single contracts and 2.728 for family contracts. In this example, we assume that the industry adjustment factor is .95 (this industry is 5 percent less costly than average, after controlling for age/sex and contract mix differences between industry groups). Therefore, the single premium rate is equal to the capitation rate ($75.00) multiplied by the age/sex factor (.975) multiplied by the industry factor (.95), or $69.47. Similarly, the family premium rate is equal to the capitation rate ($75.00) multiplied by the age/sex factor for family contracts (2.728) multiplied by the industry factor (.95), or $194.37. The final step in this example could be to recomposite the rates to match the in-force rates of another health plan using the methods described in Section 6.3.

Table 6-6: Community Rating by Class: Example 2

I. Community Rating by Class Factors, by Age/Sex Category of Subscriber

Males	Single	Family	Females	Single	Family
Under 25	.55	3.05	Under 25	.95	2.50
25–29	.65	3.40	25–29	1.00	2.75
30–34	.75	3.15	30–34	1.05	2.50
35–39	.85	2.90	35–39	1.10	2.25
40–44	.95	2.65	40–44	1.15	2.00
45–49	1.05	2.75	45–49	1.20	2.10
50–54	1.25	2.90	50–54	1.25	2.20
55–59	1.45	3.05	55–59	1.30	2.30
60+	1.65	3.20	60+	1.35	2.40

II. Development of Premium Rates for Group A, Two-Tier Structure

	Single			Family		
	#Ee's	Factor	Product	#Ee's	Factor	Product
Males						
Under 25	35	.55	19.3	30	3.05	91.5
25–29	40	.65	26.0	55	3.40	187.0
30–34	25	.75	18.8	75	3.15	236.3
35–39	20	.85	17.0	70	2.90	203.0
40–44	15	.95	14.3	60	2.65	159.0
45–49	15	1.05	15.8	45	2.75	123.8
50–54	10	1.25	12.5	30	2.90	87.0
55–59	10	1.45	14.5	20	3.05	61.0
60+	5	1.65	8.3	10	3.20	32.0
Females						
Under 25	40	.95	38.0	20	2.50	50.0
25–29	40	1.00	40.0	25	2.75	68.8
30–34	30	1.05	31.5	40	2.50	100.0
35–39	30	1.10	33.0	40	2.25	90.0
40–44	25	1.15	28.8	35	2.00	70.0
45–49	20	1.20	24.0	30	2.10	63.0
50–54	15	1.25	18.8	25	2.20	55.0
55–59	10	1.30	13.0	20	2.30	46.0
60+	5	1.35	6.8	15	2.40	36.0
Total	390		380.4	645		1,759.4
Age/Sex			.975			2.728
Industry			.95			.95
Premium			$69.47			$194.37
Rate						

This method of implementing community rating by class is useful if information is known about the potential subscribers from groups but not about the characteristics of all family members or enrollees. The CRC factors are developed from the planwide experience of the total enrolled membership population in the HMO. The method can be implemented, however, using only information about the characteristics of the subscribers (employees) who are expected to enroll.

Example 3

A more detailed form of community rating by class starts with a profile of the HMO's membership population (Table 6-7). The expected cost per member per month for each age/sex category corresponds to the CRC rating factors for this example. Note that distinctions are not made according to family composition. For example, females age 30–39 have the same CRC factor whether they belong to a single contract, two-person contract, or family contract. This is an approximation. Other plans have found it useful to develop CRC factors by age, sex, family composition, and industry. The basic calculations, however, are the same as the examples in this section.

The CRC factors from Table 6-7 can be used to determine average medical service costs (per member per month), by contract category, for a sample employer group, Ajax Box Company (see Table 6-8). According to the demographic profile for this group, the weighted average cost for single contracts is $65.62. For two-person and family contracts, the weighted average costs are $62.79 and $44.56, respectively. Note that the community rate for the HMO is $44.29 (Table 6-7). Compared to the planwide average, this group has a significantly lower proportion of childen as enrolled members, with a correspondingly higher average cost PMPM ($54.61 versus $44.29).

The CRC premium rates for Ajax Box Company can also be calculated (see Table 6-9). The average medical service cost for each contract type is multiplied by the average number of members per contract to determine the cost of care per contract. The nonmedical service costs, adjustments, and loadings are then factored into the premiums. Using this method, the total premium rate is $75.82 for single contracts, $145.97 for two-person contracts, and $164.27 for family contracts. As described in Section 6.3, these premiums can be recomposited into alternative premium rates to reflect different step-loading assumptions.

Summary

Community rating by class offers an HMO a more flexible form of rating. In particular, a limited form of group-specific rating is permitted. The group-specific rates determined under community rating by class are not based on the historical experience of the group, but the premium rates do reflect the most salient characteristics of the group and its HMO enrollees.

Acceptable factors for determining rating classes under community rating by class include age, sex, industry (as long as it is not limited to a single occupation or a single group), family composition (e.g., family size, marital status), and smoker/nonsmoker status. Any factor that can be shown to result in differential health services utilization patterns (based on an HMO's planwide experience) can be used in a CRC system. However, new factors have to be submitted for approval to the U.S. Department of Health and Human Services, as discussed above. In addition, factors that isolate an individual group cannot be used, since the identified group would be experience rated.

If a community-rated HMO decides to introduce a CRC system, several factors should be considered. First, the HMO's data system must be capable of producing the detailed data that is required to implement such a system. Data must be sufficient to (1) analyze the HMO's experience according to the desired rating classes, (2) determine appropriate rating factors for the defined risk classes, and (3) permit examination of the effect of a proposed change in rating systems on major groups.

Second, community rating by class is more complex than standard community rating for an HMO. It is likely that a plan will use community rating by class for a set of the larger groups, but will continue to rely on standard community-rating methods for small groups. In this case, it is necessary to determine the adjustments that are required in community rates to ensure sufficient revenue (e.g., if all of the groups rated under community rating by class result in 2 percent less revenue than would have been generated under community rating, then this revenue shortfall must be made up by an increase in the community rates for the remaining groups). Thus, it is likely that an HMO using community rating by class will encounter increased needs for monitoring the revenue generation process within the plan to ensure that revenue requirements are met under the more complex system. The basic criterion to be monitored is the expected premium income, which must be sufficient to meet the antici-

Table 6-7: Baseline Data for Community Rating by Class
Using Age/Sex Factors: Example 3

Age/Sex Category	*(1)* Planwide Distribution of Enrollment	*(2)* Expected Cost per Member per Month	*(1) × (2)* Weighted Average Cost per Member
Male			
Under 30	7.4%	$27.459	$ 2.032
30–39	9.5	34.621	3.289
40–49	5.6	45.875	2.569
50–59	4.5	65.067	2.928
60–64	1.5	87.200	1.308
Female			
Under 30	12.2	72.492	8.844
30–39	11.6	65.043	7.545
40–49	6.3	62.921	3.964
50–59	4.9	68.714	3.367
60–64	1.3	75.615	.983
Child	35.2	21.199	7.462
Total	100.0%		$44.291

Membership by Contract Type and Age/Sex Category

Age	Single Male	Single Female	Two-person Male	Two-person Female	Family Male	Family Female
Adult						
Under 30	52	130	67	84	52	68
30–39	40	79	47	40	133	150
40–49	18	46	19	20	92	79
50–59	13	39	34	38	57	37
60–64	7	11	15	10	13	8
Totals	130	305	182	192	347	342

	Single	Two-person	Family
Total Adults	435	374	689
Total Children	0	26	788
Total Members	435	400	1,477
Total Contracts	435	200	365

Continued

Table 6-7: Continued

Contract Size Assumptions

	Single	*Two-person*	*Family*
Adults	1.00	1.87	1.89
Children	0	.13	2.16
Total	1.00	2.00	4.05
Distribution	43.5%	20.0%	36.5%

Note: Reprinted with the permission of the publisher, from E. L. Schafer and M. E. Gocke, *Management Accounting for Health Maintenance Organizations* (Denver, CO: Center for Research in Ambulatory Health Care Administration, research arm of the Medical Group Management Association, 1984), 180–81.

pated expenses of the HMO's total enrolled membership population on a fully incurred basis. If premium revenue falls short of projected requirements, then it may be necessary to formulate and implement effective remedies (e.g., reduce nonessential categories of expenditures, increase community rates at the next opportunity) in order to avert a serious negative impact on the financial position of the HMO.

Third, a plan must be careful in designing the CRC system. Which groups are going to be rated under community rating by class and which groups will continue to be community rated? The pressure from employers (and probably also from the marketing department) will be for the lowest possible rates. If the decision-making process for rating groups is not well disciplined, there will be a tendency for community rating by class to be applied to groups that result in lower premiums. This can cause problems. First, revenue shortfalls might develop if the reduced revenue from the lower premiums is not offset by raising rates for groups with higher indicated rates (or the community rate for all other groups is not adjusted upward to compensate). Second, if the HMO participates in the Federal Employees Health Benefits Program, then U.S. Office of Personnel Management auditors will demand the lowest rates produced by both rating systems if the plan does not have objective criteria for deciding which groups will be rated under each system. The safest position for an HMO is to develop clear and unambiguous criteria for iden tifying how groups will be rated (e.g., based on group characteristics such as size, industry, or other factors).

Fourth, federal regulations provide guidance regarding specific features or aspects of a CRC system for federally qualified HMOs. If desired by the HMO, different classes can be established for different subsets of

Table 6-8: Derivation of Medical Service Cost for Ajax Box Company Using Community Rating by Class: Example 3

Age/Sex Category	Cost per Member per Month[a]	Distribution of Contracts (%)			Weighted Average Cost[b]		
		Single	Two-person	Family	Single	Two-person	Family
Male							
Under 30	$27.459	3.33	3.60	2.78	.914	.989	.763
30–39	34.621	5.55	6.00	5.00	1.921	2.077	1.731
40–49	45.875	6.67	9.60	6.67	3.060	4.404	3.060
50–59	65.067	6.67	8.80	5.00	4.340	5.726	3.253
60–64	87.200	8.89	14.00	7.22	7.752	12.208	6.296
Female							
Under 30	72.492	7.78	15.00	8.33	5.640	10.874	6.039
30–39	65.043	12.22	11.00	6.67	7.948	7.155	4.338
40–49	62.921	13.33	7.00	3.33	8.387	4.404	2.095
50–59	68.714	17.78	10.00	6.12	12.217	6.871	4.205
60–64	75.615	17.78	9.00	4.44	13.444	6.805	3.357
Child	21.199	0	6.00	44.44	0	1.272	9.421
Total		100.00	100.00	100.00	$65.623	$62.785	$44.558
Total Members		450	500	900			
Total Contracts		450	250	300			
Average Contract Size		1.00	2.00	3.00			

Note: Reprinted, with the permission of the publisher, from E. L. Schafer and M. E. Gocke, *Management Accounting for Health Maintenance Organizations* (Denver, CO: Center for Research in Ambulatory Health Care Administration, research arm of the Medical Group Management Association 1984), 182–85.

[a]Cost of medical services per member per month by age/sex category of member.

[b]Weighted average cost equals PMPM times % of contracts in each category.

Table 6-9: Derivation of Premium Rate for Three-Tier Contracts Using Community Rating by Class: Example 3

Costs	Single	Two-person	Family
		Type of Contract	
Medical Services Cost:			
Per member per month cost of care	$65.623	$ 62.785	$ 44.558
Multiplied by contract size	1.00	2.00	3.00
Per contract per month cost of care	$65.623	$125.570	$133.674
Adjustments and Loadings:			
Reinsurance premium	1.70	1.70	1.70
Reinsurance recoveries	− .85	− .85	− .85
Coordination of benefits	− 1.01	− 1.01	− 1.01
Copayments	− .26	− .26	− .26
State reserve (2% of total)	1.52	1.52	1.52
Administration, marketing, debt service, overhead (12% of total)	9.10	9.10	9.10
Additional revenue and expense per member per month	10.20	10.20	10.20
Multiplied by contract size	1.00	2.00	3.00
	$10.20	$20.40	$30.60
Total Premium Rate per Contract:	$75.823	$145.970	$164.274

Note: Reprinted, by permission of the publisher, from E. L. Schafer and M. E. Gocke, *Management Accounting for Health Maintenance Organizations* (Denver, CO: Center for Research in Ambulatory Health Care Administration, research arm of the Medical Group Management Association, 1984), 189. The above rates are community based and adjusted for the age and gender mix of Ajax Box Company.

services (e.g., one set of age/sex classes can be used for inpatient hospital services and a different set applied to outpatient services). As under community rating, composite premium rates can be developed for single contracts and all reasonable categories of family contracts (i.e., rates can distinguish between rate categories, such as two adults; adult and child; adult, spouse, and child; adult and two or more children). Minimum and maximum rates or rate changes cannot be established under a community rating by class system. In addition, community rating by class rates cannot be phased in over time to avoid large rate changes. However, a group can be switched between the two rating systems at the HMO's discretion. As discussed above, though, it is advisable to have objective criteria for classifying groups for rating purposes, and groups should switch rating systems only if their characteristics change (e.g., a group's enrollment exceeds the size threshold to be rated under community rating by class). All nongroup enrollees (e.g., individual pay, group conversion contracts) can be characterized as a group for rating purposes under community rating by class, but all individuals and families of similar composition in this "group" must be charged equivalent rates. Supplemental benefits can be rated under a different rating system than the basic benefits for the same group (e.g., the basic benefit package can be subject to CRC methods, while supplemental benefits, or riders, can be community rated).

Finally, introduction of a CRC system is likely to have other, possibly unintended, effects for the HMO. For example, if risk classes are established for rating purposes, it may generate requests from providers for risk-adjusted capitation rates.

Moving to risk-adjusted capitation rates may be logical and make sense in the context of a plan's overall relationship with its providers. However, care should be taken to ensure that inconsistencies are not introduced between the rating (revenue-producing) system and the provider reimbursement (expenditure or cash disbursement) system. If providers are paid on a risk-adjusted basis for all enrolled members, the actual enrollment pattern may result in an increase in the relative proportion of higher-cost members in community-rated groups. This would require more funds to be paid out to providers (in risk-adjusted capitations), but average levels of premium revenue would be collected by the plan (under community rates), resulting in reduced profit margins or financial losses for the HMO. This is an example of one of many possible situations that could jeopardize the financial stability of the plan.

In any event, there will be differences between the actual enrollment pattern and the assumptions that were used to set premium rates. Short-term imbalances that are relatively minor in nature should be expected and are not problematic. However, key financial indicators should be monitored closely by the HMO, and corrective actions should be taken if adverse experience is encountered. In addition, the increased complexity introduced by a more detailed rating system requires that the plan adopt a more sophisticated approach to financial issues and financial planning, as compared to the historical approach used by most HMOs with reliance on standard community-rating methods.

Community rating by class requires more attention to group-specific membership forecasting and analysis. The potential increased variation in premium revenue generated under a CRC system should be evaluated on an ongoing basis by the plan's financial personnel. Unexpected revenue shortfalls should be identified and corrective actions taken (e.g., updating of revenue forecasts at groups' contract renewals to incorporate more current information on group demographics). In addition, if an HMO is not performing according to its revenue budget, it may be necessary to reevaluate the CRC factors and change the community rate or the current budget, or to institute cost-reduction procedures.

Notes

1. The new "adjusted community rating" option introduced by the HMO Amendments of 1988 is considered an acceptable form of community rating for use by federally qualified HMOs.
2. Many HMOs are nonprofit organizations that have tax-exempt status with the IRS. Community rating has been recognized as an important factor in maintaining the tax-exempt status of some organizations.
3. Of these factors, health status is the one that generates the most controversy, since persons in poor health can be cared for in a socially responsible way by spreading their costs over a large group. Other factors, such as age and sex, are starting to be viewed as unnecessary in preserving the community-rating principle. Recent changes allow community rating by class, which allows differences in rates for these factors.
4. A plan that uses experience rating has a price advantage (over a community-rating plan) that can be used to attract groups that are healthier, or lower-cost, than average. This process could, theoretically, continue until there are no groups left in the community-rated plan, except groups with approximately equivalent risk levels far above the average (in this case, the community rate would approximate the experience rate for these groups).
5. Public Law 93-222.
6. Until the effective implementation of the HMO Amendments of 1988.
7. Group Health Association of America, *1987 Survey of HMO Industry Trends* (Washington, DC: Group Health Association of America, 1987).
8. Title XIII of Public Health Service Act, Section 1302, Paragraph 8 (Pub.L.No. 93–222, 29 December 1973).
9. Other topics related to community rating have been specified in the legislation and regulations: (1) nominal differentials in rates may be established to reflect differences in marketing costs and the different administrative costs of collecting payments from the following categories of potential subscribers: individuals, small groups of 100 subscribers or fewer, and large groups of over 100 subscribers; (2) separate rates may be established for employees of states, political subdivisions of states, or other governmental or public employers; (3) an HMO may establish a separate community rate for separate regional components of the organization; (4) the community-rating requirement will not apply to an HMO during the 48 months follow-

ing qualification if it provided comprehensive health services on a prepaid basis before it became a qualified HMO; and (5) an HMO may require supplemental payments for optional services, under the condition that payments for optional services on a prepaid basis shall be fixed under a community-rating system.

10. 42 Code of Federal Regulations, Section 110.105, February 1986.

11. However, many HMOs continue to believe that community-rating methods are the fairest and most equitable pricing methods. For philosophical and other reasons (i.e., ease of administration), it is likely that many plans will continue to community rate.

12. The advantages, disadvantages, and limitations of community rating are discussed in Section 4.3 of Chapter 4. Readers who bypassed Part I of the book may want to review Section 4.3 before reading about rating methods.

13. For additional information on community-rating requirements for federally qualified HMOs, readers should contact the Office of Prepaid Health Care, Health Care Financing Administration, 200 Independence Avenue, SW, Washington, DC 20201. Information on community-rating requirements is contained in two papers available from that office, "Establishing Prepaid Rates for Federally Qualified Health Maintenance Organizations under a Community Rating System" and "Guidance for Community Rating by Class." For additional details on actuarial methods for estimating HMO costs and developing premium rates, interested readers are referred to H. L. Sutton and A. J. Sorbo, *Actuarial Issues in the Fee-for-Service/Prepaid Medical Group* (Denver, CO: Medical Group Management Association, 1986). This book covers more topics than can be covered in this section.

14. See Sutton and Sorbo, *Actuarial Issues*; the OHMO Guide to HMO Development; and R. Birnbaum, *Health Maintenance Organizations: A Guide to Planning and Development* (New York: Spectrum Publications, 1976).

15. The cost-sharing requirements for federally qualified HMOs were changed in the 1988 HMO Amendments. Plans can require deductibles on services provided by non-HMO physicians (up to 10 percent of total physician services provided by the HMO).

16. Note that rates for the Federal Employees Health Benefits Program (FEHBP) for the year starting 1 January 1990 had to be submitted to the U.S. Office of Personnel Management by 31 May 1989. Thus, for many plans, new community rates must be established at least seven months before the year starts, and they remain in effect for twelve months after that date.

17. Because periodic losses are inevitable in any insurance operation, sound rates should also include a margin to accumulate reserves/surplus.

18. In some cases (e.g., New York), calendar year rates are required (e.g., non-calendar year renewals have a portion of months at an approved rate and a portion of months at an anticipated rate).

19. If the enrolled membership population is projected to grow, a corresponding increase must be projected in required personnel, supplies, and so on. An allowance for replacement or expansion of facilities must also be incorporated in the projections.

20. The procedures for estimating the required utilization and cost assumptions are discussed in detail in Sutton and Sorbo, *Actuarial Issues*; and Department of Health and Human Services, Office of Health Maintenance Organizations, *Guide to HMO Development* (Washington, DC: U.S. Government Printing Office, 1979). Separate calculations are required for optional or additional services and also for separate enrollment groups such as Medicare and Medicaid eligibles.

21. It is very important to verify that the data are complete. For example, for a recent time period, it is likely that all claims have not been paid for hospital admissions during the period. Therefore, it is necessary to estimate the claims incurred but not reported for the period and add them to the paid claims. Estimation of IBNR claims is an extremely important topic and is discussed in more detail later in this chapter.

22. For a more in-depth discussion and additional details relevant to the cost-estimating process, refer to Sutton and Sorbo, *Actuarial Issues*.

23. See, for example, Chapter 7 of Sutton and Sorbo, *Actuarial Issues*.

24. For additional information, see R. V. Anderson and N. Auger, "Community Rating in the Kaiser-Permanente Medical Care Program," *Topics in Health Care Financing* 8, no. 2(1981): 35–49; and Sutton and Sorbo, *Actuarial Issues*.

25. U.S. Department of Health and Human Services, "Guidance for Community Rating by Class," Office of Health Maintenance Organizations, 22 March 1982, 2–5.

26. Don Kollmorgen, Division of Qualification, Office of Prepaid Health Care, HCFA, personal communication, 2 February 1989.

27. U.S. Department of Health and Human Services, "Guidance for Community Rating by Class."

Suggested Readings

Blumberg, Mark S. "Inter-Area Variations in Age-Adjusted Health Status." *Medical Care* 25, no. 4(1987): 340.

Bragg, J. M. and Green, E. A. "Health Insurance Claim Reserves and Liabilities." *Transactions, Society of Actuaries* 16, no. 3(1964): 17.

Handley, Thomas L. "Developing Premium Rates for a Preferred Provider Organization (PPO)." *Transactions, Society of Actuaries* 37 (1985): 187.

McClure, Walter. "On the Research Status of Risk-Adjusted Capitation Rates." *Inquiry* 21, no. 3(Fall 1984): 205.

Stiefel, Matthew, and Cooper, William J. "The ACR Methodology: Medicare Prospective Capitation in an HMO." *The Group Health Journal* 5, no. 1(1984): 8.

Sutton, H. L. "Community Rating: An Historical Perspective." *Business and Health* 3, no. 8(1986): 41.

Sutton, H. L., and Sorbo, A. J. *Actuarial Issues in the Fee-For-Service/Prepaid Medical Group.* Denver, CO: Center for Research in Ambulatory Health Care Administration, 1986.

Chapter 7

Alternative Rating Methods

The goal of this legislation [Health Maintenance Organization Amendments of 1988] is to give HMOs and employers the additional flexibility they need to respond to the ever-changing health care marketplace. HMOs compete with a vast array of health care insurers and plans that offer a multitude of different benefits and financing arrangements. Employers are faced with the difficult job of identifying the good plans that can control unnecessary hospital use while offering the best quality of care.

Representative Henry Waxman, Report No. 100–145, Committee on Energy and Commerce, U.S. House of Representatives

The bill [HMO Amendments of 1988] makes a number of important changes. . . . Most important, the rules on community rating of premiums and equal contribution of employers to premiums will be revised to more closely reflect the actual cost of serving employees who choose to enroll in an HMO. This modification will benefit HMOs by allowing them to compete more effectively in the health insurance marketplace, and it will benefit employers by allowing them to pay an HMO premium that more closely reflects the characteristics of the employer group that chooses to enroll with the HMO.

Senator Edward Kennedy, *Congressional Record*

7.1   Introduction

In the last chapter, the traditional community-rating methods used by HMOs were reviewed and discussed. This chapter identifies alternative methods for premium rate setting. The following methods will be discussed:

- Adjusted community rating
- Experience rating
- Group-specific rating

195

All of these methods deviate from the basic principles embodied in traditional community rating (i.e., charging all groups the same, or equivalent, rates for the same benefit package, in effect spreading the risk and costs of health services equally throughout the entire membership population of the HMO).

The final section of this chapter includes a discussion of other factors and considerations that affect (1) an HMO's approach to rating, (2) the feasibility of alternative rating methods, and (3) the key decisions that must be made for development and implementation of the most appropriate rating system for a given plan. These factors include underwriting considerations, HMO data system considerations, the need for pricing flexibility, and HMO financial analysis capabilities.

Due to the historical development of prepaid group practice plans and federal requirements for community rating by federally qualified HMOs, many HMOs have not explored rating options beyond the "tried and true" community-rating methods. However, pressure from employers and an increasingly competitive health care environment have forced the HMO industry to reevaluate its position on this critical issue. In particular, the HMO Amendments of 1988 provide a radical departure from tradition by allowing federally qualified HMOs to use the adjusted community-rating option, which is basically a form of prospective experience rating.

In approaching the topic of HMO rating, it should be acknowledged that premium rate setting for health insurance plans, including HMOs and other managed care plans, is partly a science and partly an art. Some aspects rely heavily on accounting (i.e., the expected revenue over all groups must match the expected outlays on an aggregate basis). Although community rating provides a relatively simple and easy-to-understand method for determining premium rates, other rating methods are substantially more complicated from a technical standpoint and require a significant amount of judgment by underwriters and rating personnel. In addition, data requirements to support more complex rating methods are greatly increased, and the organization might be forced to hire additional financial personnel (underwriters, actuaries, financial analysts, or other technicians) to implement a new or refined rating process. There are also increased requirements for client interaction (e.g., explaining the mechanics of the new rating methods to employers).

Although many HMOs may be reluctant to depart from community rating, there are strong forces acting in the opposite direction, encouraging HMOs to become more sophisticated with respect to premium rate setting and product pricing. These forces include (1) employers' growing sophistication as knowledgeable purchasers of health care for their employees and as critics of the advantages and disadvantages of offering HMOs, (2) trends toward increasing use of self-insured options and plans administered by third parties, (3) the development of flexible benefit plans,[1] (4) the new legislation that permits employers to negotiate group-specific rates with HMOs, rather than being forced to accept community rates, (5) increasing complaints from employers regarding shadow pricing and charging what the market will bear, (6) additional competition between HMOs and PPOs, managed care indemnity programs, triple-option plans, "sole-sourcing" arrangements, and other HMOs, resulting in fierce price competition in many areas, and (7) the maturation of the HMO industry, including loss of profitability for many established plans and what appears to be the beginning of a major shakeout and consolidation period for the industry. In response to these forces, many HMOs will be required to review and seriously consider changing their approaches to premium rate setting.[2] Key needs and concerns include the following:

1. The need for pricing flexibility. Traditionally, HMOs have offered few benefit packages and options, in part because they lacked the capability to price out various combinations and options. However, HMOs need to evaluate the design of their products compared to what is offered in the marketplace. If the HMO is constrained, or at a competitive disadvantage, because of its limited offerings, then there is a need to evaluate the issue of pricing flexibility (i.e., the ability to price out a larger variety of benefit packages, cost-sharing options, riders, and so on) as part of the analysis of different rating options.

2. Data requirements. In order to implement a more sophisticated rating system, the HMO's MIS system should be fully capable of supporting the data requirements of the rating system. For example, if the current MIS system cannot provide the group-specific cost data required to implement an experience-rating system, it will be necessary to consider only those approaches that require more limited data, which can be provided reliably from the MIS system. Feasible rating options are constrained by the data elements that are captured by the MIS system. In addition, it is likely that a new rating system will require substantial MIS development work to produce new reports and data tabulations from existing data files.

3. Financial analysis and underwriting capabilities. Because they

rely on community-rating approaches, many HMOs have had little incentive to develop the types of financial analysis and underwriting capacities that are necessary for the more complex rating systems (normally found in insurance companies). For example, a prerequisite to any of the more complex rating systems is the ability to obtain, evaluate, and project utilization and cost data on a group-specific basis. In other words, in order to set group-specific premium rates, it is necessary for an HMO to have (1) the capacity to produce historical data for individual employer groups, and (2) the ability to perform an in-depth analysis of the resulting cost and utilization patterns (including determining the "credibility" of a group based on its size and the number of HMO enrollees). This could mean that an HMO will be required to hire additional specialized personnel or to upgrade the internal capabilities for financial analysis. In particular, it is likely that additional control procedures will need to be implemented over the process of developing and approving the premium rates for different categories of groups.

Many HMOs were able to get established and to succeed in the 1970s and early 1980s by tightly controlling inpatient utilization and by relying on discounts from major providers (hospitals and physicians). However, the potential for significant savings from provider discounts or hospital use differentials, relative to other plans, has greatly diminished in the late 1980s. In addition, easy access to capital in the past made pricing decisions less critical. Now, however, it is necessary for most HMOs to compete on the basis of price in addition to quality and "value." Many view an HMO's approach to rating, including the development and implementation of effective pricing methods, as an essential ingredient for financial stability and long-term survival.

It is not easy to institute a new rating system. The process of evaluating past financial experience and developing projections of future cost assumptions is technically demanding, with many opportunities for error. Many cost components are not fully under the control of the plan. There can be significant errors due to statistical and random variations, even for large groups. Determining trend factors for health care cost increases over time can be a very difficult task, especially during times of rapid increases in health costs due to inflation, technological advances, malpractice premiums, or other factors. In addition, competition has increased dramatically, and the margin for error keeps getting smaller.

This chapter describes alternative methods for premium rate setting and analyzes many of the above issues in more depth.

7.2 Adjusted Community Rating

The Health Maintenance Organization Amendments of 1988 made it possible for federally qualified HMOs to use a new rating method termed "adjusted community rating" (ACR). Adjusted community rating permits an HMO to establish premium rates based on the expected revenue requirements for individual groups and to take into account a group's historical utilization, intensity, or cost experience in setting premium rates. It is a particular form of prospective experience rating, which will be discussed in more detail in the next section.

The ACR rating option was patterned after the approach used to determine the adjusted community rates for HMO Medicare risk contracts.[3] Under the approach used for Medicare, the starting point was the HMO's community rate for non-Medicare enrollees, which was "adjusted" for differences in benefits, volume, and intensity of services in order to calculate appropriate rates for Medicare eligibles who were enrolled in the HMO. For example, it is necessary to adjust for differences between the plan's basic benefit package and the set of Medicare-covered services, and also for differences in the volume and complexity/intensity of services used by Medicare enrollees compared to non-Medicare enrollees. In the rate calculation for HMO Medicare risk contracts, the base community rate is broken down into line item components by type of medical service for calculation of the various adjustment factors.

Until the 1988 amendments, the federal HMO Act permitted only two methods of setting premium rates—community rating and community rating by class. Previous federal requirements for community-rating procedures prohibited establishing rates based on the utilization or cost experience of individual groups. Although community rating by class allows variations in premium rates between groups based on factors such as age, sex, family status, and industry, rating based on group-specific factors such as utilization or cost differences is not allowed under CRC.

As defined by the legislation, adjusted community rating methods determine premiums for the individuals and families of a group on the basis of the organization's revenue requirements for providing services to the group. Under this provision, HMOs could determine their rates for a group based on the relationship of the group's specific utilization and intensity of service compared to overall HMO member utilization and intensity patterns. However, the HMO must continue to be "at risk" for providing care at that prospectively determined rate and cannot retrospectively adjust rates based on actual utilization or intensity of services.

Representatives of established HMOs advocated changing the HMO Act to include the adjusted community-rating option for the following reasons:

1. Adjusted community rating is responsive to the desires of some employers to make only payments related to the HMO costs incurred by their employees and dependents. Not being responsive to this concern may cause employers to drop their HMOs or promote non-HMO alternatives.

2. Adjusted community rating is a known rating methodology and has been accepted as a reasonable method for paying HMOs for the costs of risk-basis Medicare members.

3. If ACR was permitted for federally qualified HMOs, some employer opposition to HMOs because of HMO Act community rating constraints would be reduced.

4. Adjusted community rating helps maintain "rules of the game" so that government and employers have standards to judge HMO rating practices. This should be of special interest to employers who offer large numbers of HMOs and who are concerned about an increasing inability to evaluate the reasonableness of HMO rates.

5. Fixed, prospective rating, such as ACR, is compatible with employer interests in having predictable, stable payments and having HMOs accept risk.

6. Continuing a defined set of rating rules for HMOs should enhance their ability to predict revenues in relation to costs, thus maintaining or improving their financial stability.[4]

The basic ACR approach is to set fixed, prospective rates for groups that reflect projected differences between groups in their utilization of health care services or cost experience. Under the 1988 amendments, the ACR option would be applicable for setting premium rates for commercial groups. In its most simple form, an ACR methodology can be based on developing a single "adjustment factor" that represents the difference in volume and intensity of services for a particular group compared to the HMO's overall service utilization pattern. For each group that is rated using ACR, a factor is developed corresponding to the average utilization for the specific group's enrollees, relative to the average planwide utilization for all HMO enrollees. This factor would then be used to adjust average rates (based on planwide experience) to derive the group-specific rate for the particular group in question. In essence, the adjustment factor represents the difference between the "best estimate" of the plan's revenue requirement for that group and what the group would have been charged under the plan's standard community-rating system (an aggregate adjustment factor of 94 percent would imply that the group's cost/revenue requirement is 6 percent less than the plan's average cost/revenue requirement).

In general, ACR can be thought of as a form of prospective experience rating. Although the federal regulations governing the adjusted community-rating option have not yet been promulgated, it is anticipated that many forms of prospective experience rating would be allowed by the regulations.[5]

The 1988 HMO amendments and accompanying congressional reports state that experience rating using retrospective adjustments, refunds, or dividends would not be an acceptable form of adjusted community rating. In particular, the HMO's rates must reflect the projected revenue requirements for the group, and the HMO must be at risk with respect to the fixed, prospectively determined rates.

Example: Adjusted Community Rating

A simplified ACR calculation is shown in Table 7-1. This form of ACR is especially appropriate for: (1) HMOs with limited data systems, or (2) plans that desire to implement a relatively straightforward, group-specific rating system that is easy to explain and administer. More detailed forms of group-specific rating systems are discussed later in this chapter. We assume that the HMO has 50,000 members and that the community rate is $75. The budget projection anticipates the following distribution of expenses for inpatient hospital, outpatient services, and administration: 40 percent, 50 percent and 10 percent, respectively.

We assume that the HMO has established guidelines for determining which groups will be given group-specific rates under ACR (i.e., all groups with 750 or more enrollees). As a result of the application of the guidelines, the seven largest groups in the plan have been selected. We

Table 7-1: Example of Adjusted Community Rating

I. HMO's Budget and Community Rate:

	PMPM	Percent of Total
Inpatient Hospital	$30.00	40%
Outpatient Services	37.50	50
Administration	7.50	10
Total	$75.00	100%

II. Group Selection for ACR Rating:

		Utilization per 1,000		Relative Intensity	
Group	Members	Inpatient Days	Visits	Cost/Day	Cost/Visit
Group A	4,200	325	3,975	$650.00	$35.00
Group B	3,140	440	4,570	680.00	35.00
Group C	2,700	340	4,250	625.00	35.00
Group D	1,250	285	3,725	705.00	35.00
Group E	1,025	360	4,260	670.00	35.00
Group F	905	275	3,520	710.00	35.00
Group G	780	460	4,750	640.00	35.00
ACR Groups	14,000	357	4,173	$661.37	$35.00
Non-ACR	36,000	361	4,211	$680.55	$35.00
Total HMO	50,000	360	4,200	$675.00	$35.00

III. ACR Adjustment Factors:

	Inpatient			Outpatient		
Group	Utilization	Intensity	Total	Utilization	Intensity	Total
Group A	.903	.963	.870	.946	1.000	.946
Group B	1.222	1.007	1.231	1.088	1.000	1.088
Group C	.944	.926	.874	1.012	1.000	1.012
Group D	.792	1.044	.827	.887	1.000	.887
Group E	1.000	.993	.993	1.014	1.000	1.014
Group F	.764	1.052	.804	.838	1.000	.838
Group G	1.278	.948	1.212	1.131	1.000	1.131

Continued

have assumed that the seven groups have 14,000, or 28 percent, of the plan's membership. There are three large groups (Groups A, B, and C) ranging in size from 2,700 to 4,200 members. The four other groups selected for ACR group-specific rating are smaller and range in size from 780 to 1,250 enrollees. In this example, the HMO does not have Medicare or Medicaid groups, and the remaining 36,000 members belong to groups that are community rated.

Table 7-1: Continued

IV. ACR Rate Calculation:[a]

Group	Hospital	Outpatient	Administration	Total (ACR Rate)	Ratio (to CR)
Total (CR)	$30.00	$37.50	$7.50	$75.00	1.000
Group A	$26.10	$35.48	$7.50	$69.08	.921
Group B	36.93	40.80	7.50	85.23	1.136
Group C	26.22	37.95	7.50	71.67	.956
Group D	24.81	33.26	7.50	65.57	.874
Group E	29.79	38.03	7.50	75.32	1.004
Group F	24.12	31.43	7.50	63.05	.841
Group G	36.36	42.41	7.50	86.27	1.150
Subtotal: ACR groups				$73.91	.985

V. Recalculation of Community Rate for Non-ACR Groups:

Numerator = HMO's revenue requirement that must be obtained from non-ACR Groups
$$= (50,000 \times \$75.00) - (14,000 \times \$73.91)$$
$$= \$2,715,260.00.$$

Denominator = $50,000 - 14,000 = 36,000$

Revised community rate for non-ACR groups = $75.42 PMPM

[a]For each component, the group-specific rate is equal to the community rate (for that component) multiplied by the group's composite adjustment factor (as calculated in section III above). For example, for inpatient hospital services for Group A, the ACR rate is equal to $30.00 times .870, or $26.10. In this example, we have assumed that there are no differentials in per member per month administrative costs across groups.

The data on utilization and relative intensity of services for these groups are also shown in Table 7-1, including subtotals for the ACR and non-ACR groups, and a grand total for all HMO members. The ACR groups in aggregate have slightly lower utilization rates than the non-ACR groups (357 inpatient hospital days, per 1,000 members per year, compared to 361 days, and 4,173 office visits compared to 4,211 visits, for inpatient and outpatient utilization, respectively).

The ACR adjustment factors for each group are calculated in Table 7 1 as the product of the relative volume and intensity factors for inpatient and outpatient services, respectively. For example, the adjustment factor of .903 for inpatient utilization for Group A equals 325 (days per 1,000) divided by the average for all HMO members of 360 (days per 1,000). Similarly, the inpatient intensity adjustment factor of .963 for Group A equals $650 divided by $675. Note that we have assumed that there is no intensity differential between the groups for outpatient services (i.e., that there is no difference in the average cost per outpatient visit between the groups). This assumption could be relaxed to increase the accuracy of the calculation, assuming that appropriate data were available.

Next, the adjustment factors are applied to the community rate components (inpatient, outpatient, and administration in this example) to determine the ACR rate for each of the major groups. For each component, the group-specific rate is equal to the community rate (for that component) times the composite adjustment factor for each component (Table 7-1). In this example, we have assumed that there are no differentials in per member per month administrative costs across groups (in general, there should be an increased loading for smaller groups because of higher marketing and administrative costs, on a per member per month basis).

Note that the group-specific rates range from 84 percent to 115 percent of the community rate. In this example, four groups have lower rates under ACR, while three groups have higher rates.

Any HMO contemplating the introduction of ACR should conduct a detailed study of the likely impact of a change in the plan's rating methodology on the major groups served by the plan. The major groups are likely to be the groups selected for group-specific rating, depending on the decision criteria for group selection. In the example portrayed in Table 7-1, the implementation of ACR would have differential impacts on the three largest groups (groups A, B, and C). In this example, the rates for two of the groups (A and C) are lowered by 8 percent and 4 percent, respectively, while the rates for Group B would be raised by approximately 14 percent under ACR. Therefore, it is necessary for any plan contemplating a rating method change to consider the potential impact on major groups from both a policy and a competitive standpoint.

Finally, it is necessary to recalculate the base community rate for all HMO enrollees not included in the seven major groups under ACR. The combination of the revenue from the ACR groups and the revenue from the non-ACR (community-rated) groups must be sufficient to achieve the HMO's revenue requirements in the aggregate. In effect, the seven groups are taken out of planwide calculation (for the remaining groups) for the revised community rate. The recalculated community rate is $75.42. Thus, in this example, one effect of implementing ACR for selected groups is to raise the community rate slightly for the non-ACR groups. It should be noted, however, that if the application of ACR significantly lowers the rates charged to the ACR groups, in aggregate, then the revised community rate will have to increase proportionately to compensate.

It is anticipated that all nongroup enrollees (e.g., direct pay, group conversion) and their family members will make up a group for the purposes of computing an ACR rate. However, it is likely that all individual contracts and family contracts of similar composition will have to be charged the same rate. (Refer to the federal regulations for additional details on this and related topics.)

Summary

Some view ACR as a form of "risk rating," which is sometimes differentiated from experience rating. In general, experience rating is equated with the rating methods commonly practiced by insurance companies and performed by large underwriting/actuarial departments using detailed claims systems (and usually involving calculation of retroactive refunds for groups with good experience). Risk rating generally refers to the determination of prepaid rates based on the group's revenue requirements or a measure of the level of risk represented by the group. Community rating by class is also a form of risk rating.

Whereas CRC attempts to project a group's risk based on demographic factors such as age and sex (a key assumption is that all members of a "class" will have the same risk or expected utilization, and a rate is developed for the group based on the composition of the group and the associated level of risk), ACR attempts to establish premium rates based on extrapolations of the group's own cost and utilization experience. In most cases, ACR develops more accurate premium rates than CRC, in terms of the actual costs resulting from a group's experience (primarily because ACR uses the actual historical experience of the group, rather than approximations of risk levels represented by the risk classes under CRC).

Like other types of rating systems, ACR will result in actual premium income and actual costs for a group that are dependent on the actual enrollment pattern, rather than on the assumptions used for premium development. In addition, if the distribution of enrollments changes under ACR, from groups whose rates are increased to groups whose rates are decreased, total revenue per member will decrease. However, the total size of the HMO's membership population may increase under ACR because of the more competitive rating structure. The HMO's portfolio of business is likely to be healthier, from an underwriting stand-point, with self-supporting rates for larger groups (since there will be fewer major groups with large underwriting gains or losses, a condition of instability where the HMO is vulnerable in a competitive marketplace).

Adjusted community rating allows HMOs much greater flexibility in premium rate setting, and it maintains the stability and predictability of income and revenues. In addition, ACR permits federally qualified HMOs to compete more effectively with nonqualified competitors. It is also compatible with employers' interest in paying what their employees actually cost. In comparison with claims-driven, experience-rating systems (and the associated data requirements), ACR may be much more feasible for HMOs.

7.3   Kaiser Permanente's Adjusted Community-Rating System

This section explores examples of adjusted community-rating methods, focusing on the methods that are currently under development by Kaiser Foundation Health Plan.

Kaiser Permanente is the largest HMO in the United States, with over 5.6 million members as of 31 December 1988. There are 12 Kaiser regions, all operating relatively autonomously. The Kaiser corporate office is located in Oakland, California. The corporate staff provides a range of centralized services to the regions, including legal, strategic planning, facilities planning, medical economics, actuarial, financial, and human resources services.

Kaiser has used traditional community-rating methods since its beginnings in the 1940s. Although there are some variations according to region, Kaiser's basic rate schedule uses three-tier rates for a set of basic benefit packages and riders for specific supplemental services. The basic benefit packages can include different cost-sharing features (copays for outpatient visits) and benefit combinations.

Over the past few years, however, Kaiser has been actively exploring different rating options. For example, community rating by class was implemented on a trial basis in its Northwest region in 1987. In addition, Kaiser management has closely followed the development of the HMO Amendments of 1988, including the new adjusted community-rating option permitted to federally qualified HMOs by the amendments. In early 1987, a decision was reached to begin development of group-specific rating methods, assuming that the amendments would be passed and signed into law. The decision was based on the belief that, to ensure the future competitiveness of the Kaiser plans, it might be necessary to use group-specific, risk-based rates to satisfy large employers. If a change from community rating was to be made, it would be a change to an approach embodied in ACR (at least for large groups). Subsequently, work began on the specifications of an ACR-based system, and all of the Kaiser regions began to "gear up" to develop the capability to implement group-specific rating. At the outset, this preparation was expected to last several years. Even the decision to begin preparations was not reached easily, since Kaiser has historically been one of the most vocal advocates and supporters of community-rating methods for HMOs.

Eventually, each region will have the capability to implement Kaiser's ACR system in a way that is compatible with their needs, data capabilities, and current operating procedures. Preparations for regional capability to use ACR have begun in earnest throughout the Kaiser system. It is a major task, one requiring new data collection systems, cost accounting capabilities, and additional technical staff resources.[6]

Goals of Adjusted Community Rating

As described in the HMO Amendments of 1988 (Pub. L. No. 100–517), adjusted community rating permits federally qualified HMOs to set premium rates for commercial groups according to each group's expected use of plan resources. The primary goal of Kaiser's ACR system is to institute rating methods that will have each major group "pay its own way" while maintaining rate stability and predictability. The ACR system uses a combination of ACR, community rating by class, and community-rating methods for determining group (and individual) rates. These group-specific rates reflect Kaiser's best estimate of the services a group will use for the upcoming contract year. The ACR system is constructed so as to maintain rate stability and to continue to serve all segments of the community.

ACR for Groups with 1,000 or More Members

Adjusted community-rating methods are applied to all groups with 1,000 or more enrollees (credibility factors are applied for smaller groups). For each eligible group, utilization data are assembled for three historic years. The utilization is adjusted for "intensity" of the services provided (e.g., a hospitalization for heart surgery uses more resources than a hospitalization for a normal vaginal delivery). After adjustment for such differences, Kaiser refers to it as "intensity-adjusted" utilization. Each group's intensity-adjusted utilization, on a per member per month basis, is compared to that of the overall membership for each type of service (e.g., inpatient hospital, outpatient visits, and ancillary services) and indexed (i.e., the average across all groups equals 1.00).

These indexed relative "costs" per service (utilization multiplied by intensity) are averaged with weighting by the proportions of the budgeted community rate devoted to each service. (The resulting index for each of these years, if multiplied by the community rate, is similar in concept to the Medicare risk ACR.) The resulting indexes for the three years are then used to project each group's ACR for the upcoming rate year. The ACR is also expressed as a per member per month index relative to the health plan average. The ACR is then translated into group-specific rates by multiplying it by (1) a "member-to-contract" adjustment, and (2) the health plan standard contract rates.

Smaller Groups under the ACR System

As described above, each group with 1,000 or more members is given full credibility in the ACR system (the group's rates are based entirely on the ACR calculations and a group-specific rate is determined). For groups with under 1,000 members, the year-to-year fluctuations in health care cost and utilization make it necessary to incorporate credibility factors into the rate-setting formula. This is accomplished by using demographic-based CRC estimates of group risk and by pooling small groups' experiences together in a small group "community rate."

Data Requirements for ACR

In contrast to traditional community rating, ACR requires that a plan have access to detailed information about the services provided to each member. These services are then linked with data rgarding the resources, or costs, required to perform each service. The data must be readily available and easily manipulated and assembled. This type of data is not generally kept by many HMOs. Computer capabilities, data collection routines, and trained analytic staff are all prerequisites for ACR.

The limited availability of member and group-specific data is particularly acute in outpatient services. Typically, capitated physician arrangements have been attractive to all parties because providers need not keep track of services on a member-specific basis. Under ACR, "cost" details and procedure information, for each provided service, must make their way to the HMO in order for each group's relative adjusted outpatient utilization to be determined.

Other Methodological Issues

Other methodological issues considered by Kaiser during development of the basic outline and structure of the ACR system included the following:

- How to handle rate development for "new groups"
- How to account for double-covered members, over-age members, retroactively added/deleted members, and interregional members
- How to incorporate inpatient professional fees, capitated specialists, and other negotiated provider contracts
- How to accurately assign resource use (costs) to specific services
- Whether and how to incorporate appropriate stop-loss adjustments
- How to handle missing data
- How to provide for a reasonable transition from traditional community rates to group-specific rates

Kaiser analysts believe that these issues are critical to the development of an acceptable and effective ACR system by a federally qualified HMO.

Although it is not possible to go into detail about each of the major issues identified above, this section will describe how Kaiser resolved two issues: stop-loss adjustments and assignment of resource use and "cost" to specific services. For each issue, the options that were considered and the resolution of the issue will be discussed.

Stop-loss adjustments. Providing groups with an appropriate adjustment for their share of high-cost cases and, at the same time, protecting them against extraordinary high-cost events poses a problem for HMO risk-based rating. Groups need protection against catastrophic random incidents (e.g., a severe burn case), yet even seemingly random events may have a higher probability of occurring among certain categories of people and, hence, in certain employer groups. The challenge under ACR is to identify and give groups appropriate credit for their experience. Hence, the ACR system has the following goals:

1. To protect groups against high-cost cases that may be beyond their control

2. To credit groups with their appropriate share of risk

One option for meeting these goals is to eliminate from group-specific experience all cases above a certain cost threshold or of a certain case type (e.g., specific DRGs). These high-cost cases would then be spread evenly as a "risk charge" across all groups. This option satisfies the first goal at the expense of the second goal (crediting groups with differences in their underlying risk for the high-cost cases).

The option at the other extreme (i.e., having no stop-loss protection and using all cases, regardless of cost or condition, to assess group-specific risk) has the opposite effect. It meets the second goal but fails to protect groups against the highest cost cases.

In most ACR or experience-rated systems, some form of stop-loss protection is incorporated into the system. The major issues are how much protection to give and how to apply it.

Kaiser decided to handle this problem by crediting groups with all of their cases, but to limit the cost of each case to a specific maximum dollar amount (e.g., $25,000). Although establishing the magnitude of the stop-loss can be somewhat arbitrary, this approach provides protection against the extreme high-cost portion of the distribution of cases by cost. In addition, it eliminates "outlier" costs as DRG weights generally do. It may reflect dampened DRG weights if such are used in intensity calculations and if the extreme weights represent cost in excess of the dollar stop-loss limit.

How to assign cost per case.   Historically, many HMOs have had poor data with which to devise group-specific cost-management information. This poses a significant block to implementing a good group-specific rating system. The ideal approach to assigning costs per case and suggested proxies to use on a more temporary basis are described below, along with some points of distinction between ACR and experience rating.

The objective of ACR is to reflect differences in risk between groups. In addition to risk, cost differences among groups may indicate which providers are used by a group's members for a given condition. Different providers within an HMO are likely to be paid different amounts. For example, suppose that obstetrician A is affiliated with the HMO and paid on a discounted fee basis at $50 per visit, whereas

Obstetrician B is paid under capitation and has an "equivalent" visit cost to the HMO of $40. Assume that Group X members see Obstetrician A and Group Y members see Obstetrician B at the same utilization rate. Obviously, the two groups' costs are different. However, their risk is the same, and, therefore, their ACR for this service should be the same.

To emphasize this point of distinction between risk and cost, the following points can be added:

1. Members of HMOs do not generally have control over whether they go to the efficient versus the inefficient provider.
2. To the extent that marked differences in "input" costs may exist within an HMO service area, these can be reflected in geographically distinct rates and should not obfuscate ACR adjustments.
3. Cost differences may be a function of the particular contract arrangement in effect at one point in time, changing when the contract renegotiations occur. Members who see the provider for the same condition just before or after any contract term changes will have different costs assigned to them if cost, not risk, is the area of focus.

The challenge to assigning cost or intensity to specific services includes establishing the average HMO cost for each service type rather than the actual cost for a specific service rendered to a particular member. One vehicle for this approach for inpatient care is a DRG weight, or relative cost per DRG. Ideally, these weights should come from an HMO's internal cost-accounting system. Often, this is not possible for a variety of reasons, including (1) lack of access to appropriate information (e.g., when the HMO-hospital contract includes an all-inclusive, per diem payment arrangement), and (2) no means to collect, store, or manipulate member-specific data.

Even if the data are available, the use of the data may be complicated by a small plan size. In these cases, all DRGs may not be represented with sufficient frequency to construct plausible weights for all classifications.

Alternatively, external sources of DRG weights may be used. All payer states have these available. Versions can be constructed from statewide hospital charge data in some states. (The presumption here is that relative charges per case are a decent measure of intensity.) Use of these DRG weights also presumes the existence of member-specific DRG discharge data.

Similarly, for outpatient and physician services, weights for CPT-4 or other appropriate coding systems must be developed. Hence, the same issues arise. However, data availability becomes more of a problem for most HMOs since outpatient services may be provided by physicians and other providers closely affiliated with the HMO, as opposed to a community hospital which generates bills or other standard information for patients regardless of their HMO affiliation. Assuming that external weights are available, the requirement for member-specific CPT-4 data for each encounter-procedure continues to pose a significant data collection problem for many HMOs.

Revenue Forecasting and Revenue Sufficiency

Under the ACR system, the revenue forecasting process is more complex. Projected ACR rate adjustments for the rate-setting year, as well as those in effect for the current year, must be included in the rate revenue forecast.

Group-specific rating introduces more variation into expected rate revenues. However, this variation in expected revenue from group to group should not materially affect the financial performance of a health plan, if sufficient care is taken in forecasting rates and membership. It may be prudent for smaller plans to consider larger reserves as part of an ACR strategy. Other financial effects of ACR are as follows:

1. The community rate or standard base rate used as the basis for ACRs will not necessarily equal the traditional community rate.

2. Group-specific rating requires more attention to group-specific membership forecasting.

Over time, if the ACR system introduces excessive variation into the revenue generation process, modifications can be made to promote greater rating and revenue stability.

Subsidies under ACR

Implementation of an ACR system will not eliminate all rating subsidies. Subsidies are inherent in any rating system, even retrospective experience-rating systems. However, there are likely to be more explicit, intentional subsidies in ACR systems, including the following:

- The capping of groups' year-to-year rate adjustments to achieve rate stability, to ease the transition from other rating methods (e.g., traditional community rating), or to ease the year-to-year changes in rate adjustments

- The per case stop-loss used in the calculation of groups' ACRs to spread the high-cost cases over the community
- Blending of rates (credibility-related adjustments applied to mid-sized groups' rates)
- A limit on the small groups' rates of 10 percent above the community rate (an HMO Act requirement)
- Need-based rate reductions for certain conversion and other individual members and small groups
- Limits on rates for other needy groups and members (One example of this may be Medicare risk members for whom the reimbursement rate falls below the "cost" of the members. Similarly, prepaid Medicaid contracts in some states have reimbursement rates below the cost or the ACR for Medicaid numbers. In these cases, a subsidy is needed in group rates to make up the difference.)

To ensure against unanticipated shortfalls in revenue, any explicit subsidies in an ACR system (e.g., the shared cost of capping and the stop-loss protection) must be absorbed in the basic community rate or reflected in the other groups' adjustment factors.

7.4 Experience Rating

Experience rating, in the group health context, refers to a form of premium rate setting that takes into account a group's utilization and cost experience. To many employers, experience rating is equated with the concept of "paying what my employees actually cost" with respect to the health services utilized by the employees and their dependents. In contrast, community-rating methods set premiums based on the average, planwide cost experience, and the premium rates that a group is charged may be quite different from the group's actual cost experience.

Private insurance companies have used experience rating for decades as the primary method of determining premium rates for group health insurance policies for large employer groups. Many Blue Cross plans, which originally used community-rating methods, switched to experience rating in the 1950s and 1960s, mainly in response to competitive pressures. Thus, the health insurance industry has many years of experience and much expertise in applying experience-rating techniques to group health insurance products, and in responding to the competitive environment and the interests of employers.

During the past five years, there have been increasing demands from employers for group-specific premium rates. With the passage of the HMO Act amendments, it appears that experience rating, in the form of adjusted community rating, will begin to be considered seriously by many HMOs. This does not mean that all HMOs are expected to switch to experience rating (nor should they—there are many serious issues and implications related to an HMO's conversion from community rating to experience rating). Rather, it is likely that there will be a gradual but significant shift in the HMO industry as a whole from community rating to experience rating, as individual plans adopt various forms of experience rating or adjusted community rating.

Once an HMO has decided to use alternative rating methods, some operating changes will make it difficult or impossible to turn back or to reverse the decision. Commitments made to employers are one factor. In addition, there will be a substantial impact on the managed care systems that have been developed at each plan. To some degree, the change will redefine and refocus the marketing, pricing, and data systems at each plan.

There are many forms of experience rating, and there are many different ways of implementing the basic experience-rating concepts. Although experience rating is commonly referred to as a generic rating method (for example, as an alternative to community rating, with the implication that there is a choice between only two methods), the experience-rating systems employed by the major private insurers and Blue Cross plans differ significantly.

The General Approach Used in Experience Rating

The purpose of an experience-rating system is to determine premium rates on a group-specific basis, with the premium rates reflecting the health services utilization and cost experience of each group. Groups are usually divided into two or more categories. Large groups will have their rates based primarily on their own experience. Small groups (usually under a size threshold of 50 to 250) will generally not be experience rated, due to the high degree of random variation in health care costs for small groups from year to year. These groups will usually be community rated (or rated by age, sex, or industry). In some cases, there will be an intermediate category for medium-sized groups, with premium rates established partially on the basis of experience and partially on age/sex or other manual rates. The amount of "credibility" to be given to the experience of a medium-sized group is usually based on the size of the group (and possibly other factors such as industry, geographic location, and number of years under contract) and is usually established in the underwriting guidelines that govern the insurer's experience-rating system.

A variety of data are needed for implementation of an experience-rating system. Experience rating requires cost data on a group-specific basis. Thus, an HMO wishing to implement experience rating will require the capability to monitor group-specific claims experience. In experience-rating systems, costs such as administrative, marketing, claims processing, and other expenses are also allocated on a group-specific basis. Thus, methods are required to distribute administrative, marketing, and other costs among employer groups.

Reporting requirements also increase under experience rating. It is likely that agreements with employers will stipulate that the HMO will provide the employer with a detailed account of premium revenue received, claims paid, estimates of claims incurred but unpaid, and administrative and other expenses charged to the account. In addition, the HMO will have to report the profits (or losses) for each group and to justify the renewal rates in light of this data disclosure. Other aspects of retention accounting and reporting will also need to be considered.

A change to experience rating gives an HMO the potential to improve relations with employers. For example, the capacity to produce group-specific rates should enhance a plan's ability to negotiate with major employers. An important component of the process is to have a contractual agreement between the HMO and the employer concerning the "ground rules" that will govern the rate-setting process. Will prospective or retrospective experience rating be used? At the present time, only adjusted community rating (a form of prospective experience rating) is permissible for federally qualified HMOs. Alternatively, if retrospective rating methods are to be used, will there be any "pooling" mechanisms? How will retention be calculated? How will claims incurred but not paid be estimated? How will surpluses/deficits be handled?

The impact of a change in rating methods on the groups and individuals enrolled in the HMO must also be considered. In underwriting terms, this is referred to as portfolio transition and reconstruction. For example, it is likely that a change from community rating to experience rating will result in a different approach to the marketplace. The increased flexibility of group-specific rating will permit the HMO to market to new groups and to expand into untapped markets. To some extent, the change in rating methods will precipitate a selection process that will change the content and composition of the HMO's "book of business." Ultimately, there should be an evolution to a portfolio that is stronger and higher in quality (with respect to the commitment between the groups and the HMO), with lower risk in terms of bottom-line profitability. The down side is that some groups may cancel, and some valued relationships may be strained due to the change in rating methods (e.g., the case of a long-term client with high-cost enrollees who resists the increased premiums charged under experience rating). However, it can be argued that increased cancellations are the price to be paid for a more healthy portfolio with increased profitability and improved bottom-line results. In addition, the HMO has to consider the implications of not changing rating methods and ignoring the demands of employers for group-specific rates.

There are two basic types of experience-rating methods— those that set rates *prospectively* and those that operate *retrospectively* (e.g., where total premiums are determined retroactively after a group's cost experience is known, or can be estimated accurately, for the period in question). This characteristic is one of the key distinguishing features of alternative experience-rating methods.

With prospective rating methods, a group's historical cost experience is used as a basis for determining future premiums. The rates are set at the beginning of the year (or contract/reporting/accounting period), and the insurer is at risk for any differences between the actual cost experience and projections. Thus, the plan incurs a loss if premiums are inadequate in any contract year, and the plan experiences a gain if premiums exceed expenses and a surplus accrues. With prospective experience-rating methods, there are no adjustments at the end of the year to reflect the results of actual claims experience.

Experience-rating methods operating on a retrospective basis take into account a group's actual experience in determining the total premiums that the insurer is due for providing group health insurance coverage to the particular group. For example, if a group's actual experience, in aggregate, is lower than the total amount of premiums paid during the year, then the group will be paid a refund or dividend, or will receive a rate credit that will be used to reduce future premiums. In some cases, surpluses may go into a reserve (or rate stabilization) fund that is used to stabilize and smooth out year-to-year fluctuations in premium rates.

If retrospective methods are used and a group incurs a deficit (e.g., claims, administrative, and other expenses exceed the amount of premiums paid during the year), then an adjustment is made to recover the loss. If a reserve fund has been established, then the deficit is subtracted from the fund. Under some rating systems, the group is assessed the additional costs, usually up to a limit (expressed as a percentage of premium) agreed to and specified in the contract. In some cases, the deficits are carried forward, and future premiums are increased to recover the costs.

Thus, retrospective methods, like prospective experience-rating methods, also use a group's historical experience to set premium rates. Retrospective methods, however, employ end-of-year settlements to determine the amount of surplus/deficit for each group, and cash payments or adjustments are made to reflect the group's actual cost experience.

Finally, experience-rating systems place a much heavier emphasis on group underwriting than do community-rating systems. To implement experience-rating methods, underwriting personnel assume great responsibility in evaluating prospective groups and determining appropriate rates for new and renewal groups. Inherent in the process of underwriting with experience rating is greater recognition of the unique characteristics of groups, prospective and in-force, including all characteristics (i.e., age/sex composition, industry, history, experience, positioning, disposition, and other factors that influence a group's cost experience) that must be taken into account to develop appropriate and competitive rates for the group.

It is commonly said that the rating/underwriting process is both an art and a science. It is scientific in the sense that specific methods and techniques are used in determining the premium rates. It is considered an art in the sense that underwriters are required to exercise judgment in setting rates for a particular insurance product or line of business.

Although this section does not delve into great detail regarding the "art" of the pricing/underwriting process, it is a crucial part of the business. The multitude of individual decisions that are required force the underwriter to develop an overall perspective to ensure that the basic goals of consistency, adequacy, competitiveness, and equity are accomplished. The standard of performance for the underwriter is the level of profitability of the insurance portfolio, or book of business. Under an experience-rating system, it is unwise to mechanize all aspects of the rate-setting procedures. Rather, it is necessary to rely on the underwriters and rating personnel to apply appropriate skills and to exercise judgment in efforts to guide the process and to achieve the overall goals and objectives.

It is essential to have a flexible and adaptable process for rating and underwriting. The same general techniques and methods are generally used for determining rates and evaluating the past experience of all groups. However, the underwriter must be aware of the unique circumstances of each major group (including associated factors such as the competitive environment, recent actions by major competitors, changing trends, and subtle aspects of the client relationship) and to adapt to changing conditions and competitive requirements.

This does not mean that the underwriter is exempt from controls and monitoring by plan management. Relevant control procedures (including checks and balances) must be installed to measure and monitor the success of the rating/underwriting function over time. An experience-rating system will rely heavily on underwriting/rating personnel (much more than will community-rating systems). In addition, it will be necessary to establish an appropriate balance between a degree of freedom for the underwriter in exercising his or her skills and judgment, and the needs of the HMO for adequate monitoring and control over the rating/ underwriting process.

7.5   Group-Specific Rating*

Group-specific rating is a particular form of prospective experience rating that takes maximum advantage of the rating flexibility contained in the 1988 HMO Act amendments. The purpose of the rating strategy is to identify, as precisely as is feasible, the current areas of cross-subsidies between groups and to determine appropriate adjustment factors so that group-specific rates for major employer groups will be self-supporting.

Group-specific rating will enable HMOs in competitive market-places to survive on a profitable basis, despite the threatening financial pressures. The strategy is a synthesis of traditional group insurance rating techniques and community rating by class. It appears to be fully consis-

---

*Section 7.5 was adapted from Gordon R. Trapnell and Charles W. Wrightson, "HMO Pricing Issues from an Actuarial Perspective," in *Proceedings of the 1988 Group Health Institute* (Washington, DC: Group Health Association of America, 1989). Reprinted with the permission of Group Health Association of America, Inc., 1129 20th Street, NW, Washington, DC 20036.

tent with the standards for adjusted community rating set forth in the 1988 HMO Act amendments, although the final regulations governing ACR for federally qualified HMOs had not been published by HCFA at the time of this writing.[7] Although the proposed group-specific rating methods are generally consistent with the 1988 amendments and the congressional intent, some modifications may be necessary to the methods discussed in this section in order to conform to the final regulations.

The essence of the strategy is to assess the adequacy of the rate to be charged to each group separately, and to determine that the expected cost of the group for claims (plus a proportionate share of average administrative costs) is below the premium rate to be charged to the group (on a prospective basis). The claim cost must include both the expected average claims given the characteristics of the group and, to the extent that size permits, the actual claims experienced in the past projected to the period covered by the premium rate on a fully incurred basis (i.e., by date of service).

The principal concept is that the premium rates for each group must be self-supporting (i.e., the rates are set at levels that are expected to be sufficient to cover the group's medical expenses and administrative costs), at least at the level of expectation, or credibility. (For groups of sufficient size, the actual cost experience of the group is used to set the rate. For smaller groups, the group's actual experience is partially used to determine the rate.) Implementing the strategy requires both adjusting rates and culling unprofitable groups. Since, as a practical matter, HMOs cannot raise rates significantly beyond those charged by competitors in any rating class (assuming that employers pass on all marginal increases in the form of additional employee contribution rates), the implication of this group-specific rating approach is a policy as follows:

1. Determine accounts for which the HMO must either

   - Incur a probable *loss* because competitive rates will not produce enough income to cover the expected claims and administrative costs of the account, or
   - Incur an unacceptable risk of *adverse selection* if rates are raised enough to at least break even on the account.

2. Offer a reduced benefit package to such accounts, with a premium that is higher relative to the value of the benefits than feasible for present coverage; or discontinue the group.

The rationale behind this strategy can be illustrated with respect to open-panel HMOs. In general, competition forces an insurer (and HMOs are a special type of insurer) to charge rates that are expected to be fully self-supporting for all accounts large enough for the experience to be fully credible, and rates that reflect the expected average cost for smaller accounts. If an insurer tries to charge a higher amount than the self-supporting or expected cost rate, another insurer can duplicate the service network and charge a lower premium for essentially the same coverage. Futher, in open enrollment competition, the healthiest employees and families will tend to switch to the low premium insurer (if rate differentials are fully reflected in employee contribution rates). The resulting antiselection will reduce or eliminate the margin in the rates charged.

In most groups, an insurer will be inhibited by competition from charging rates that are significantly higher than the expected rates. If there were a systematic pattern of such higher rates, another insurer could again duplicate the service network and enter the groups with the higher profit margin, undermining the original insurer.

As a practical matter, of course, new insurers cannot just enter markets and duplicate the existing networks. However, a similar effect is created by the many HMOs, especially the open-panel models, that sign up virtually the same physicians in many areas. Even closed panels generate similar pressures with differential rates. Further, the selection impact for closed-panel plans could be even greater, since employees with no family members undergoing treatment tend to change HMOs in greater numbers than others.

Thus, an insurer can expect to lose money if it sells at a loss to a significant number of employment groups. Employers being charged rates that are lower than expected will be delighted with their bargains, but those with rates that are higher than expected will go to competitors.

The situation for an open-panel HMO is more complex, but similar pressures produce a similar conclusion. Other IPA-model HMOs can duplicate the service network well enough that a substantial number of employees, especially those with the healthiest families, will find it advantageous to change if a lower rate is charged. Since the HMO must lower its rates to the level of expected costs, to meet competition on cases with a surplus, it must raise them on any with a deficit, to avoid an aggregate loss.

The fact that their situation is complicated by the impact of the delivery system, internal risk-sharing arrangements, or discounts with providers does not free HMOs from competitive pressures they face as insurers. The same general principles apply.

This group-by-group rate adequacy criterion is at the opposite extreme from traditional community rating. Community rating produces rates that will be profitable in some groups and produce losses in others. The community rates (whether per capita, by demographic category, or by class) must be adequate over all groups to support the HMO as a whole. But profits on some groups are offset by losses on others (i.e., there is a pattern of internal cross-subsidies within the plan).

Determination of Expected Costs by Case

Group-specific rating requires determining an expected rate for each group, regardless of size. The expected cost of a group enrolled from any employer will depend on a number of factors, including (1) proportions of singles, doubles, and families, (2) age/sex distribution of enrollees, and (3) the health status of the enrollees, relative to that of all persons of comparable age, sex, and marital status enrolled in the HMO.

Most HMO rate structures correct for the first of these factors (at least for cases where three-tier rates are used), but not for the other two. In other words, revenue will increase in proportion to risk if more families enroll than singles. Many HMOs now also use community rating by class, at least in the aggregate for larger groups, which adjusts revenue for the second factor as well. But since many HMOs do not use age/sex specific rates, there is no protection against enrolling groups that are older or have more married females at childbearing ages. Similarly, there is no protection against enrolling groups that have more persons with chronic conditions, attracted by the limits to cost sharing available in the HMO coverage. Thus, HMO rates typically do not reflect all factors that are important in determining the expected cost of any group of enrollees.

Group insurance actuaries have found through experience that the most accurate basis for computing the expected costs for any group of persons (of sufficiently large size) is a relatively short-term projection from what the specific group actually cost to service in a past period. Such calculations must be made for a period for which relatively complete data are available on an incurred basis (i.e., with all services tabulated by date of service). This means that the base period used to determine the experience rate must end long enough before the analysis that data relating to most of the services performed for members of the group will have been processed. This may take several months or longer, depending on the length of time required for the flow of claims in an administrative system. It also requires the use of actuarial techniques to determine the completeness of the data used in the analysis.

The primary lesson to be learned from the experience of group insurance actuaries is that the most accurate way to measure the impact of health status is from the experience of the specific group of persons involved in some past period. A convenient technique is to determine the ratio of the cost of the enrollees from a specific employer to the average cost for all of the HMO's enrollees with the same benefit package, adjusted to have the same distribution by age, sex, and marital status. This ratio, called the "actual-to-expected" (or "actual-to-tabular") is the backbone of all group health insurance experience-rating systems.

Health insurers have found through many years of experience that there is a high degree of correlation between the actual-to-expected ratio in one year and the same ratio in the next year. One would expect this to be the case, since the health status of enrollees in a group tends to change slowly. Higher costs are associated with having more than a random share of persons in a group in poor health.

Thus, where there are enough enrollees for the experience of the group to be credible, the best estimate of cost for a future year can be obtained through the following steps:

1. Determine the actual-to-expected ratio for the enrollees from an employment group in the most recent past period for which adequate data are available on an incurred basis. This is the ratio of (a) the actual cost for the enrollees from the group to (b) an expected cost obtained by multiplying the number of enrollees in each actuarial rating cell by the community rate in the HMO for that class in the period corresponding to the data for the group (i.e., reflecting the composition of the group by age, sex, and marital status).

2. Determine the average expected rate for the future period based on the projected composition of the group (allowing for any changes in demographics or benefits that are expected to take place in the group).

3. Multiply (1) and (2).

The rate obtained is an experience rate for the specific enrollees from the employment group. This is a vital step toward an actual rate, and should be the actual rate if (1) the group is large enough for full statistical credibility, (2) competitive conditions permit actually charging the rate, and (3) there are no other overriding considerations that must be taken into account. The rates charged to all groups, weighted by the enrollment in the groups, must reproduce the total revenue that would be obtained if the experience rates were charged to all groups.

There are many practical difficulties in the application of this conceptually simple technique. The most important guiding principle is to maintain consistency between the various numerators and denominators. For example, a staff-model HMO may not have charge data or even complexity-weighted encounter data for visits to the HMO's clinics. The most important rules in calculating an actual-to-expected ratio are (1) that the numerator and denominator be defined and calculated in a consistent manner, and (2) that the average weighted actual-to-expected ratio for the entire HMO be unity.

The basis for the expected rates is the traditional community rate for the HMO, preferably calculated by demographic category (and best if calculated by age/sex group and any other subgroups of the HMO enrollment that have different costs). These average planwide rates provide the basis for determining the actual-to-expected (A/E) ratios.

Example

Suppose the following facts pertained to an employment group with a renewal date of 1 January 1989, which we can refer to as the XYZ Corporation:

1. The group has 450 employees enrolled in the HMO as single adults and 550 as families during 1988 (and for simplicity, none leave or enter during the year).
2. The group was charged the HMO's monthly community rates of $92 for single employees and $230 for families during 1988 (which includes allowances of $80 and $200, respectively, for the cost of medical care and an additional 15 percent for administration and the cost of capital).
3. In October 1988, the HMO made the following projections:
   - Based on experience through July 1988, the HMO's community rates should have been 2.5 percent higher (based on hindsight the HMO should have been charging rates of $1.15 \times \$82.00 = \$94.30$ and $1.15 \times \$205.00 = \$235.75$ during 1988).
   - The community cost for medical care in 1989 is projected to be $88 for singles and $220 for families; that is, 7.3 percent

higher than the (estimated) actual cost in 1988 and 10 percent higher than charged for 1988.

- Administrative and other loadings were projected to be 14 percent in 1989, relative to the projected claim costs.

4. Based on experience through July, the plan projected that the total costs incurred for XYZ employees in 1988 would be $1,975,380. The following adjustments were made to arrive at that figure:

- The services provided to the employees and dependents of the XYZ Corporation, as recorded in the data base through July, were adjusted for services provided through July but not so recorded, and

- The total was adjusted by the rate of increase in medical costs per capita for services provided through the plan from the January through July period through the calendar year 1988 level.

The analysis would proceed as follows. The actual (as projected) claims of $1,975,380 would be divided by the expected or average claims for all enrollees (or what claims would have been if XYZ enrollees had cost the same as all enrollees) as follows:

$$\frac{\$1,975,380}{[(450 \times \$82) + (550 \times 205)] \times 12} = 1.100$$

This shows that enrollees from XYZ were 10 percent more expensive than all enrollees in the HMO in the base period. We refer to this ratio as a "relative experience ratio" (RER). It is a form of the actual-to-expected ratio.

The central feature in experience rating is the assumption that any large group of enrollees will tend to have the same relationship to the average cost over all enrollees over time (or over all persons in employment groups in the community); that is, the RER for any large group of enrollees changes slowly over time. There are many reasons to expect a high degree of correlation in the RER from one time period to the next in a large group of enrollees. A high proportion of the cost of providing medical care to a group of enrollees relates to the persisting chronic conditions among those enrollees, and these tend to change slowly from one year to the next. Further, patients normally use the same physicians, and the cost of treatment will reflect their styles of practice. In any event, this high degree of correlation has been overwhelmingly confirmed by the actual experience of the insurance industry, which found it feasible to use the RER approach as a basis for virtually all renewal rating decisions for large health insurance groups.

Thus, in the above illustration, the HMO's 1989 rates for enrollees from the XYZ Corporation would be based on the same RER, the community rates for 1989, and the expense-loading factor for 1989, as follows:

$$\text{Singles: } 1.10 \times \$88.00 \times 1.14 = \$110.35$$
$$\text{Families: } 1.10 \times \$220.00 \times 1.14 = \$275.88$$

For the sake of simplicity, the illustration did not include demographic differences between the particular group and the total HMO enrollment. But an age/sex/family composition factor is easily introduced. For example, suppose that the age/sex composition of the above group increases the expected cost by 5 percent (i.e., the age/sex weighted rate for the group is 5 percent higher than the community rates). The age/sex factor would be obtained by weighting each age/sex group by a relative cost factor and dividing by a factor derived in a similar manner over the entire HMO enrollment. The calculation could be made for all enrollees together or separately for singles and families. An additional factor, family size, could be included in calculating the family rates.

The RER relative to age/sex specific rates for the group would then be $1.100 \div 1.050 = 1.048$. But if the same demographics are projected for the group in the following year, the age/sex factor will simply cancel out in calculating the appropriate rates for the following year: $1.048 \times 1.050 \times \$88.00 \times 1.14 = \$110.39$ (which differs only by the effect of rounding the age/sex factor).

This arithmetic shows that introducing the age/sex factor will not affect the results unless some change is forecast in the age/sex composition of the group that would change this factor for the following year. For example, suppose a new low-cost HMO will be offered during the next open enrollment period. It is feared that some of the youngest enrollees may defect to that HMO and that, as a result, the age/sex factor is projected to rise to 1.075 in the next year. Incorporating this factor, rather than the current one, will directly increase the projected cost of the group. In this case, the appropriate rates would be as follows:

$$\text{Singles: } 1.048 \times 1.075 \times \$88.00 \times 1.14 = \$113.02$$
$$\text{Families: } 1.048 \times 1.075 \times \$220.00 \times 1.14 = \$282.55$$

An equivalent way to reach the same conclusion is to look at the actual loss ratios compared to those anticipated. In the illustration, the projected loss ratio for 1988 is as follows:

$$\frac{\$1,975,380}{[(450 \times \$92) + (550 \times 230)] \times 12} = .9804$$

This contrasts with the original loss ratio $(1 \div 1.15 = .870)$, which was established when setting the premium rates but which was based on a premium now projected to be 2.5 percent too low. Taking all of this into account, the experience rate relative to the community (or average) rates is calculated as follows:

Relative Experience Ratio = Actual Claims ÷ Average Claims

$$= \frac{\text{Actual Claims}}{1.025 \times (\text{Premiums} \div 1.15)}$$
$$= \frac{1.15}{1.025} \times \text{Loss Ratio}$$
$$= \frac{1.15}{1.025} \times .9804$$
$$= 1.100$$

This follows since the average claims were projected to be 2.5 percent above the estimates on which the premium rates were based (and were loaded 15 percent for administrative expenses), and the loss ratio is the ratio of actual claims to premiums.

This formulation may be more convenient from a practical perspective. It permits the computation of the relative experience ratio from two numbers: the claims incurred and the premiums accrued (premiums collected during the year adjusted for premiums earned but unpaid at the beginning and end of the year). There is no need to determine the average numbers of singles and families enrolled, which may be burdensome when these are constantly changing, especially if there are more than two demographic categories (e.g., three- or four-way rate systems). In fact, sometimes the best way to estimate the persons enrolled is to divide the premiums collected by the known premium rates and the average mix of singles and families. This method also provides a check on the consistency of the data provided for a particular group.

In the illustration, significantly higher rates are needed for the XYZ Corporation for 1989. For reasons discussed earlier, it may not be advisable to charge rates that are that much higher. It may be possible, however, to substitute a lower option. The appropriate rates for a lower option are based on the projected planwide 1989 rate *for that option* multiplied by the RER. (If the community rates for the low option are computed over different enrollees, a further adjustment is needed to estimate what the RER would have been over enrollees in the low option. For the sake of simplicity, let us assume that the community rates for all options are set with respect to the entire HMO enrollment.)

For example, suppose that the HMO offers a low option with projected 1989 community rates of $65 for singles and $165 for families. The premium rates needed for the low option for the XYZ group are calculated below:

$$\text{Singles: } 1.100 \times \$65.00 \times 1.14 = \$81.51$$
$$\text{Families: } 1.100 \times \$165.00 \times 1.14 = \$206.91$$

These will be self-supporting rates for that option if there is no further antiselection against the HMO. Whether the rates should be offered or not depends on a judgment concerning the likelihood of significant antiselection as present enrollees react to the loss in coverage from the high to the low option.

A limitation of the relative experience ratios is that they do not allow for any regression to the mean (see Chapter 8 for a discussion of this concept). This will not normally be a major factor if the RER is within 10 percent or so of unity. But at extreme values, it may reflect a temporary situation. A very high ratio may be explained by several extraordinarily expensive conditions. As these patients die, the RER will tend to regress toward unity. It is advisable to examine RERs more than 15 percent from unity to determine whether there is some reasonable explanation for such a large deviation, and where there are grounds for believing that it will change.

Adjusted community rates represent a formal method for calculating relative experience ratios. In effect, the various adjustments permitted disaggregate the RERs into component parts. For example, in calculating the ACR for Medicare risk contracts, the HMO is permitted to adjust the HMO-wide community rate by factors representing the relative utilization of persons over age 65 and the relative intensity of the services used by Medicare eligibles. The HMO can use data from its own experience to establish these factors. Taken to the extreme, there would be factors that explained all the differences between the cost of a target group of enrollees and the HMO-wide averages.

For staff- and clinic-based HMOs without a large fee-for-service practice to provide the basis for determination of the cost of services furnished to specific groups, factors such as those allowed by HCFA in ACR calculations may be helpful in estimating the cost for different groups. But where more direct measures are available, such as the charges of the clinic or individual physicians in an IPA (up to the fee maximums recognized by the HMO), the steps in a formal ACR calculation do not add a significant degree of insight. Further, their impact would be the same as the age/sex factor illustrated above. Note that ignoring the age/sex factor altogether did not change the answer (assuming that the age/sex composition of the group did not change from one period to the next).

Any factor incorporated explicitly into the rate calculations should have the following properties:

- The magnitude of the factor can be estimated with reasonable accuracy and cost (e.g., how much the rates are changed by including age or gender as factors).

- The characteristics to which the factor must be applied must be readily available for specific employment groups, so that the impact of the factor can be readily incorporated into the rate calculation.

- Changes in the factor from year to year can have a significant impact on the rates for different employment groups.

These conditions indicate that the factor is worth incorporating (i.e., that it improves the accuracy of the estimate of the RER at reasonable cost).

Small Groups

The most difficult problem in applying this basic rating principle is the small size of most HMO enrollment groups. (Although large groups constitute a significant proportion of total HMO membership, the vast majority of HMO groups have fewer than 100 enrollees.) Rating by age, sex, and marital status (and perhaps by industry, occupation, employment status of spouse, and actual number of children) may solve a major portion of this problem. But only partial consideration, or credibility, can be given to the past actual-to-expected experience of a small group of enrollees. Insurers have developed a variety of techniques to cope with this problem.

One technique is to combine several years of experience for a group.

This can help if turnover is low. But there is a danger that turnover within the group may undermine the validity of the measure, or that recent, bad experience can be attributed to recent, persistent illnesses.

Another technique is to weight the actual-to-expected ratio by the "credibility" of the size of the group. The credibility factor is a number between zero and one that allows for the possibility that good or poor experience is attributable to fluctuations expected in a small group of enrollees. Traditionally, group insurers would give full credibility to groups of 1,000 or more members (i.e. they would project the actual-to-expected ratio from the most recent past period to the future without further adjustments). For smaller groups, the actual-to-expected ratio would be weighted with unity by a credibility factor. For example, suppose the insurer had credibility factors as follows:

Size	*Credibility*
Less than 100	None
100	10.0%
101	10.1%
102	10.2%
. . .	. . .
999	99.9%
1,000 or more	100%

Suppose also that a group of 400 had an actual-to-expected ratio of 110 percent in the most recent past period, and that the average rates were the same as for XYZ Corporation above. Then the credibility factor for the group would be as follows:

$$1 + (40.0\% \times 10\%) = 1.04 \text{ [or } (.6 \times 1.0) + (.4 \times 1.1)]$$

The following rates would be charged:

$$104\% \times \$88.00 \times 1.14 = \$104.33$$
$$104\% \times \$220.00 \times 1.14 = \$260.83$$

In order to add the impact of the age/sex distribution, suppose that the weighted age/sex composition factor in the past period was 1.05 and that, for the future period, it is expected to be 1.075. Then the actual-to-expected ratio, adjusted for credibility, would be as follows:

$$(1.0 \times .60) + (1.10/1.05 \times .40) = 1.019$$

And the following rates would be charged:

$$\text{Singles:}\quad 1.019 \times [.6 + (1.075 \times .4)]$$
$$\times \ \$88.00 \times 1.14 = \$105.29$$
$$\text{Families:}\ 1.019 \times [.6 + (1.075 \times .4)]$$
$$\times \ \$220.00 \times 1.14 = \$263.23$$

Thus, the rates charged would reflect both the past experience of the group and the projected change in the age/sex distribution of the group.

Open Enrollments

An additional, crucial consideration applies to HMO rates in competitive open enrollment situations: the effect of rate differentials on antiselection. The actual-to-expected factor will not be valid if there is a substantial change in the specific persons enrolled. The number of persons changing health plans is particularly sensitive to contribution differentials. For example, if another HMO is offering comparable coverage at a significantly lower rate, some of the healthiest persons in the group can be expected to switch to that HMO. (Some of the least healthy members may also switch, but on balance the selection can be expected to go against the more costly HMO.) Further, if the rate is raised to allow for this, the antiselection may only get worse. Thus, the HMO cannot charge a rate outside the competitive range.

An alternative strategy is called for in these situations. The HMO can either cut benefits by offering a lower option where the cost comparison with competing HMOs is not so poor, or terminate the group's policy. To continue with the example above, suppose the low-option rates in the future period are $65 for singles and $165 for families. Then the correct rates would be as follows:

$$\text{Singles:}\quad 1.04 \times \ \$65.00 \times 1.14 = \ \ \$77.06$$
$$\text{Families:}\ 1.04 \times \$165.00 \times 1.14 = \$195.62$$

Other factors that need to be considered for group-specific rating include (1) provider incentives, (2) capitation reimbursement for primary care physicians, (3) other provider risk-sharing arrangements, and (4) the relationship between group-specific rating methods and the HMO's utilization control and cost-containment procedures.

Group-Specific Rating and Adjusted Community Rating

The method of setting rates outlined above is a form of prospective experience rating. It meets the specific objectives of ACR rates:

- The rate is set in advance and is not affected by the actual experience of a group of enrollees during the specified period.
- It reflects the experience of a group only to the extent that such experience provides a guide to the future cost of the group.
- No dividends or other considerations are made retroactively to reflect actual experience.

The principal difference between this form of group-specific rating and the present practices of insurers relates to the use of surpluses or deficits in the operation from year to year. The normal practice in the insurance industry is to keep a strict accounting of claims incurred, to subtract these and formula-determined administrative and "risk" charges from premiums accrued, and to pay a dividend (or apply a "rate credit") equal to any surplus. If the resulting calculation is negative (claims and other costs are higher than premiums), deficits are accumulated and applied against future surpluses. The procedure may be complicated by procedures such as "pooling" large claims (charging average or expected claims rather than actual claims above some threshold such as $25,000 or $50,000); combining the experience for life, disability, or accidental death and dismemberment (AD&D) coverages with health; and accumulating the dividends in a "rate stabilization reserve."[8]

The ACR calculations required by the Health Care Financing Administration for Medicare differ from the methods discussed in this section primarily by prescribing in detail exactly how each step of the Medicare calculation must be made. If Medicare is regarded as one large group, the goals of the Medicare ACR calculation are very similar to those of group-specific rating described above. The difference is in the orientation. The federal procedures are designed to make sure that the HMO does not make a higher profit margin than on private groups and to place the burden of proof on the HMO for each step of the calculation that might increase what the federal government or beneficiaries must pay. HCFA has a very limited list of adjustments that will be allowed and it prescribes the precise conditions under which they may be calculated.

Other forms of ACR rating are feasible. The primary difference between the recommended procedures and other forms of adjusted community rating is in degree rather than kind. Group-specific rating may be thought of as a series of steps toward the most accurate projection possible of the expected cost to provide health care through a particular HMO for a specific group of persons. Other methods make partial adjustments. For example, the approach to ACR described in Section 7.2 would adjust the general community rate only for significant utilization and intensity differences between the specific group's experience and the average HMO experience. This form of ACR would be applicable to any HMO, even plans with limited data systems capabilities. However, if an HMO has a detailed claims-based data system, it would probably be worthwhile to explore the advantages (and disadvantages) of a more detailed group-specific rating system.

7.6 Rating and Data Analysis Strategies

For a plan to implement more competitive rating strategies, it must know, year by year, the profitability of each service and each group of enrollees. With this knowledge, an HMO has much more flexibility in its rating strategies and a much better sense of how to develop a more sophisticated rating approach. Based on the ideas and concepts discussed previously, the development of a more effective rating strategy should proceed along these lines:

1. Develop the strategy for rate increases.
2. Conduct a feasibility study for using adjusted community rating or another form of group-specific rating.
3. Conduct a study of the profitability of major employer clients.
4. Conduct a study of the profitability by line of business.
5. Analyze the ''portfolio'' of group business.
6. Analyze the cost structure and cost experience of the plan.

In order to develop more competitive and sophisticated rating approaches, an HMO must usually improve its data systems and data analysis capabilities.

Rate Increase Considerations

The choice of the aggregate rate increase factor (trend factor) may be the most important financial decision made by the plan each year. All pertinent factors relating to this decision need to be considered, including revenue requirements based on various enrollment scenarios, the projected rate increases by competitors, and the overall competitive position of the plan. For staff-model plans, the overriding consideration is the financial stability of the plan, the need to guarantee that future revenue will cover the fixed costs of facilities, equipment, salaried physicians and support staff, and administrative expenses. Given the underpricing that has occurred in many areas in recent years, most plans should take a conservative position on this decision and consider the largest possible increase generated by the alternative revenue requirement forecasts that is also consistent with the overall competitive market environment.

Although HMO enrollees have demonstrated high loyalty to the plan in the face of premium increases, this does not guarantee that plans are immune from high disenrollments following consecutive years of high rate increases. However, if raises in rates are kept within reasonable levels, especially compared with the actions of competitors, then HMOs should not experience large disenrollments solely based on price. Price competition, however, could have a significant impact on the drawing power of the plan for new enrollees. Previous research has confirmed that, all other things being equal, the single most important factor in an employee's choice of health plan is the level of the employee contribution rates (out-of-pocket premiums paid by employees) among competing options.[9]

Group-Specific Rating Considerations

Most HMOs can benefit from detailed analysis of cost and utilization data and exploration of alternative premium rate-setting strategies. In addition, in order to be able to respond to inquiries from employers regarding group-specific utilization and cost data, most plans would benefit from studies of the experience generated by their largest groups. For example, an analysis could be conducted to determine the profit/loss status of all commercial groups with 100 or more members. For each employer/group, the analysis should compare premium revenue received by the plan with expenditures incurred for each of the last eight calendar quarters. Although detailed ambulatory encounter data may not be available for some plans due to data system limitations, it is usually possible to combine a complete tabulation of all out-of-plan claims costs (hospital, referrals, and so on) with a reasonable estimate of in-plan costs for each group (using data from a broad sample of visits and other encounters). Various administrative and marketing expenses can be allocated on a per member, per premium, per claim, or per group basis. In addition, similar data should be constructed for the total enrolled membership population for comparison purposes.

Using the assembled data, a variety of statistics can be computed for each group, including loss ratio (benefit costs to premiums), operating margin (premiums less benefit costs), profit/loss (premiums less all group costs), and profit rate (profit as a percent of premiums). The claims can be aggregated for each of the preceding two years for each group (assuming that sufficient time has elapsed since the end of the most recent year for a complete tabulation of claims). The costs can also be aggregated, across all groups, according to the following categories: age of member, sex of member, relationship to sponsor (subscriber/spouse/dependent), and industry (with appropriate subcategories and subtotals).

It is recommended that three issues be investigated using this data base: (1) analyze the overall cost experience of the plan, (2) conduct a review of major employers, and (3) conduct feasibility studies for adjusted community rating and for more detailed forms of group-specific rating. The objectives of the first task are to conduct an in-depth investigation of the HMO cost structure and to determine how the plan costs are distributed across population subgroups. This is accomplished using the tabulation of costs, across all members, with breakdowns by age, sex, family composition, and industry. The detailed data are analyzed on a per member per month basis to determine the logical breakpoints (i.e., appropriate age categories) and subcategories (i.e., individual contracts, two-person contracts, families of three or more) that explain the largest degree of variation in the PMPM costs. This is very similar to the process used to determine appropriate rating factors to be used in community rating by class. In fact, this analysis should produce a set of relative cost factors that explain major variations in health costs according to an appropriate stratification of the enrolled membership population.

In addition, if the plan has multiple product lines (commercial groups, individual members, group conversions, Medicare, Medicaid, long-term care), then an analysis should be conducted of plan profitability by line of business. This is essential if the plan is to accurately price a variety of products. Acceptable plan financial results on an aggregate basis can mask serious problems for individual lines of business. The basic principle is that each line of business should be self-supporting. This principle should only be violated when (1) there are solid reasons to do so (e.g., development of a new product requires front-end investment, but it is anticipated that the product will result in an adequate return on investment within a defined period of time), and (2) the HMO is cognizant of the inherent risks and has a detailed plan for this line of business, with contingency options for unforeseen problems.

Further, this analysis should be done by type of service. A plan should know not only how much in total its members cost, but also which services they are using. This is very important in pricing more flexible product designs for specific employer groups.

The second task is to conduct a review of the experience of major employers. The tabulation of costs for groups with 100 or more members could be used. The objectives of the task are to determine the surplus and deficit accounts. Knowledge of the size and direction of the plan's current internal cross-subsidies is essential to an evaluation of the exposure of the plan to competition and to evaluate alternative strategies to protect the plan's enrollment, especially for the largest commercial accounts.

The first step in the evaluation is to prepare a summary that lists employers in major size groups in descending order, according to the total surplus or loss from the account during the previous two years, along with such quantitative characteristics as total employees, total enrollment at end of period, industry, initial date of contract, total premiums, dollar profit or loss (year 1, year 2, and total), loss ratio (by year and total), credibility factor, and actual-to-expected cost ratio. A second summary should be prepared according to decreasing loss ratio. These two reports should be used to determine a subgroup of employers for further examination. Criteria for selection of this subgroup could include any group in the top 5 percent or bottom 5 percent of total surplus/loss, any group of size 100–250 (over 250) whose loss ratio exceeded 150 percent (120 percent), and any group of size 100–250 (over 250) whose loss ratio was lower than 25 percent (50 percent).

After selection of this subgroup of employers, the data should be analyzed to determine potential reasons for the results. For example, each group should be examined to determine if there is a consistent pattern across both years, or if one year is average and one year is exceedingly high or low. To assist in this analysis, we assume that a tabulation has been prepared of all claims costs in each calendar year (on an individual member basis within each group) that exceed the following thresholds: $5,000, $10,000, $15,000, $20,000 and $25,000. They are tabulated together with the primary diagnosis and whether or not the member is still alive, still sick, and still enrolled. This tabulation should be examined to determine if high costs for the group in one or both years are due to catastrophic cases.

Further analysis should focus on determining the reasons for the good and poor performances of the groups. Reasons could include (1) certain industries have consistently good (poor) experience,

(2) employers' indemnity rates are substantially higher or lower than the HMO's community rates, and (3) the HMO experienced either very favorable selection or adverse selection due to the competitive situation or other factors. Another consideration is whether the situation can be expected to persist or is likely to prove temporary.

A much more precise analysis of gains and losses can be made through use of the actual-to-expected technique (see Section 7.5). These ratios are formed from the relative cost factors that were developed in the first task described above. First, the expected costs for each group would be determined by multiplying the number of enrollees in each stratified cell (age, sex, family composition, industry) by the appropriate relative cost factor (i.e., the factor that would be used if the HMO followed community rating by class). Second, the actual cost for each group would be divided by the expected cost for that group to obtain the actual-to-expected ratio. Groups with actual-to-expected ratios below unity are contributing a surplus of income to the HMO, compared to a community rating by class, and those groups with ratios above unity are receiving a cross-subsidy. Third, an analysis similar to that described above would be conducted to determine which groups are contributing a surplus and which groups are being subsidized. Again, it is important to determine the probable cause of the results for each group.

The results of the above analyses should provide a considerable amount of information concerning the dynamics that are occurring within the plan with respect to cost experience. For example, the "winners and losers" analyses should identify those groups where the plan has consistently had surpluses and those for which there are persistent losses. It is to be expected that there will be a substantial amount of "noise" (random variation in a statistical sense) in the results, especially if all groups with 100 or more members are included in the analysis. For this reason, considerable judgment must be exercised in using the information. At least at first, it may be desirable to focus only on the largest groups in the plan, where the results have the highest credibility.

It is important to distinguish between knowledge of the sources of gains and losses (relative to both income and a class rating system) and the use of such knowledge. The policy of an HMO may quite properly be to use gains from the fortunate (healthy persons or low-risk groups) to subsidize those whose costs are higher than expected. This policy may originate in the charter of the plan or simply reflect the goals of a consumer board. It may also be based on a belief that, over a period of time, gains and losses from any group are likely to even out.

However, an increasingly competitive environment will likely reduce the surpluses many HMOs now obtain, forcing them to reduce internal cross-subsidies to offset this loss. In other words, when survival is at stake, tight competitive conditions may force HMOs to modify their policy with regard to cross-subsidies between groups. Further, at a time of rapid change and unreasonable employer demands, an HMO's financial managers and underwriters must be in a position to determine where they stand with regard to aggregate expected surpluses and subsidies if they are to make prudent rating decisions.

Finally, feasibility studies can be conducted for implementing methods that would permit group-specific rating (either adjusted community rating or a more detailed form of group-specific rating). The analyses recommended above would provide the basic data needed for this task. The primary objectives would include (1) developing criteria necessary to implement ACR (group selection criteria, credibility formulas, and formulas for determining prospective rates for future time periods that take into account historical and projected utilization and cost experience), and (2) analyzing each major group to evaluate the impact of ACR on the projected rates for all major groups, the competitive position of the plan, and how other strategic planning would be affected (modification of benefit package, low-option plans, and so on). For example, with the passage of the amendments permitting ACR, it is expected that large employers will pressure HMOs to implement some form of experience-rated premiums. However, the wisest course of action would be to consider a move to implement ACR in the broader context of the HMO's strategic plans for handling all of its large groups—not just for rating purposes but also for benefit design and increased flexibility to improve the plan's overall competitive position.

In addition to the choice of alternative rating methods, there are a variety of other factors and considerations that affect an HMO's approach to rating, the feasibility of alternative rating methods, and the key decisions that must be made for development and implementation of the most appropriate rating system for a given plan, notably underwriting considerations and HMO data system considerations.

Underwriting Considerations

Although rating and underwriting are closely related in practice, they are separate functions. A premium rating system is defined as the process and methods for determination of premium rates to be charged to policyholders for a specific insurance product, or, more generally, the pricing methods applicable to a particular line of business in an insurance-type organization. Objectives of rating systems include (1) ensuring the adequacy of the rate structure, (2) ensuring the competitiveness of rates, (3) equity among policyholders, (4) simplicity and ease of understanding and implementation, (5) flexibility and adaptability (minimizing the degree of difficulty in making changes or adapting to new conditions), and (6) ensuring the consistency of the rating process and methods.

Although this book has focused on alternative rating methods for HMOs, it should be recognized that the rating process relies on an associated underwriting process. In addition, it is necessary for the two functions to be properly integrated and coordinated. The underwriting process involves evaluating a risk, determining the conditions of its acceptability, and establishing an appropriate rating basis. The objectives of group underwriting are (1) to determine which customers who have applied for insurance coverage (or been marketed to) should be accepted, (2) to identify which potential customers should be rejected, (3) to determine which customers present a level of risk that requires a unique (higher) rate, and (4) to specify and approve the financial terms and conditions for the insurance contract.

The standard of performance for a group underwriter is the financial performance of the portfolio of business (i.e., all group contracts combined). This is measured by the profitability of the insurance product, or line of business, that is being underwritten. Thus, a primary goal of group underwriting is to minimize the possibility of adverse financial experience for the insurer (HMO) based on the entire portfolio of business (i.e., to maximize profitability and to minimize losses that may be incurred). In other terms, the job of the underwriter is to reduce the probability of loss resulting from premiums that are, in aggregate, less than the costs of incurred claims, administrative costs, and other expenses for all insurance contracts written within a defined line of business.

In essence, this means that the underwriting function has the responsibility for making the multitude of specific decisions that are required to maintain a profitable insurance product, or line of business. This requires implementation of the insurer's pricing guidelines and principles, evaluation of the risks presented by potential customers, and determination of the appropriate basis for renewal (or termination) of current contracts that will expire in the near future. An additional task for a group underwriter is to protect the insurer from antiselection (e.g., to ensure that the members in each risk class represent an average selection of risks, with the average for each risk class corresponding to the assumptions built into the pricing structure).

In the past, many HMOs have used community-rating methods, with the built-in simplicity and ease of administration that community rating affords. In addition, compared to private insurance companies and Blue Cross plans, most HMOs have not employed rigorous group underwriting standards and practices. In order to respond to the demands of employers and other competitive pressures, many HMOs are now exploring more flexible rating alternatives such as group-specific pricing methods. However, HMO underwriting practices also require attention, especially when rating methods are changed.

HMO Data System Considerations

The degree of sophistication in HMO data systems varies greatly. Many of the traditional prepaid group practice plans do not collect outpatient encounter data in an automated format. Some plans have separate data systems for different categories of data (e.g., membership, billing, claims, encounter, pharmacy, and laboratory) that are not integrated and that are difficult to use for tasks required by group-specific rating. In general, IPA-model plans with claims-based systems have the highest level of detailed data available for analysis and rating purposes. However, plans with good data systems in general may not capture selected components of utilization or cost data due to capitation arrangements or other factors. In addition, data may not be sufficiently complete, reliable, or consistent to permit rating on a group-specific basis.

The capabilities of an HMO's data system and the requirements of an alternative rating method are key issues that must be examined by HMO management. As discussed above, in order to implement a more sophisticated rating system, it is necessary that the HMO's management information system (MIS) be fully capable of supporting the data requirements of the rating system. The feasibility of a rating option is constrained by the data elements that are captured by the MIS system. In addition, it is likely that a new rating system will require substantial MIS development work to produce new reports and data tabulations from existing data files. However, even an HMO with an extremely limited data system can employ a less detailed form of group-specific rating, such as the adjusted community-rating option (see Section 7.2).

Other Relevant Factors and Considerations

Other factors that should be considered as part of the decision process for a new rating system include (1) the need for pricing flexibility, (2) the HMO's capacity for financial analysis, and (3) desirable by-products from group-specific rating. Most HMO's have traditionally offered few benefit packages and options. With increasing competition, however, there is a need for greater pricing flexibility on the part of most plans. In addition to consideration of more flexible rating methods, many HMOs would find it profitable to broaden the range of benefit plans that they offer or, at least, to evaluate the design of their products compared to what is offered in their marketplace. If the HMO is constrained, or at a competitive disadvantage, due to limited offerings, then there may be a need to develop an ability to price out a larger variety of options (e.g., benefit packages, cost-sharing options, riders, limits on services, and low-option plans) as part of the analysis of different rating alternatives.

Currently, many HMOs do not have the types of financial analysis and underwriting capacities that are normally found in insurance companies and that are necessary for implementation of more complex rating systems. A prerequisite for use of any of the more complex rating methods is the ability to acquire and analyze utilization and cost data on a group-specific basis. For example, to develop group-specific premium rates, it is necessary to obtain historical utilization and cost data for individual employer groups and to have the capacity to analyze the resulting cost and utilization patterns. Therefore, for some HMOs, adoption of a new rating method may also require hiring additional specialized personnel or otherwise upgrading internal capabilities for financial analysis.

The development of a group-specific rating capability may result in desirable by-products or other benefits. For example, exploration of alternative rating methods focuses attention on the organization's financial goals and objectives, in general, and on many aspects of an HMO's financial performance, in particular. In addition, analysis of group-specific utilization and cost data permits evaluation of a plan's profit/loss experience for individual groups. All of these activities are desirable and sound business practices for any insurance-type organization. However, many HMOs do not currently perform these types of analysis on a systematic basis.

From a broader perspective, all of the features discussed above (rating methods, underwriting practices, financial analysis capabilities, and MIS and data systems) can be viewed as tools that an HMO can utilize to (1) improve bottom-line financial results by raising plan profitability and reducing potential losses, and (2) increase the effectiveness of a plan's approach to pricing and financial management. A greater understanding of the dynamics underlying the profitability of a plan's portfolio of business is also essential to the future success of an HMO in an increasingly competitive health care environment.

Notes

1. Little attention is devoted in this book to flexible benefit plans such as cafeteria plans and flexible spending accounts. However, these plans have become increasingly popular and can affect the enrollment in HMOs, especially in regards to selection effects. Federal law and Internal Revenue Service regulations concerning the requirements and tax status of flexible benefit plans have continued to evolve in recent years, and future changes should be monitored.
2. Again, other observers (and many personnel in the HMO industry) do not believe that the current competitive pressures make it imperative for HMOs to change from community rating. They argue that (1) the advantages of community rating outweigh the potential advantages of switching to adjusted community rating or experience rating, (2) the arguments against community rating are speculative and cannot be proven, and (3) there is a long-standing philosophical belief held by many HMO personnel (especially among prepaid group practice personnel) that community rating is the best pricing method.
3. The topic of Medicare payment rates is outside the scope of this book. However, the term "adjusted community rate" is used by Medicare for HMO and CMP risk contractors. In this context, an adjusted community rate is defined as "the equivalent of the premium that a risk organization would have charged to Medicare enrollees independently of Medicare payments, for Medicare covered services using, as a basis, the same rates it charges to its non-Medicare enrollees, and adjusting for Medicare enrollees' utilization." See Chapter 3 of Part 5 in *Medicare Manual: Health Maintenance Organizations and Competitive Medical Plans,* HCFA Pub. No. 75, Department of Health and Human Services (Washington, DC: U.S. Government Printing Office, 1985).
4. Richard V. Anderson, "Designing New Options II—Putting Flexibility into Rating Systems," Presentation at the 1987 Group Health Institute, Seattle, Washington, June 1987.
5. The regulations are currently under development at the Office of Prepaid Health Care, Health Care Financing Administration, U.S. Department of Health and Human Services, 200 Independence Avenue, SW, Washington, DC 20201.

6. Kaiser's ACR system was initiated and developed jointly by Kaiser's largest West Coast regions and the central office's Department of Medical Economics under the direction of Richard V. Anderson, Vice President for Medical Economics. Ann E. Evans, Manager of Pricing and Benefits Design, was responsible for supervising and coordinating the ACR effort. Corporate staff play a major role in disseminating information about ACR methods to the Kaiser regions and provide technical assistance in the development and implementation of the regional systems.

7. While the proposed group-specific rating methods are generally consistent with the 1988 amendments and the congressional intent, some modifications may be necessary to the methods discussed in this section, in order to conform to the final regulations. It is also expected that the Office of Personnel Management will issue requirements for ACR for HMOs that participate in the Federal Employees Health Benefits Program.

8. This surplus-back guarantee practice should really be called "participating" rather than experience rating, although the rates are normally set following experience-rating techniques. Participating arrangements have been popular with employers because the employee benefits manager can demonstrate that the employer pays for its own costs and no more.

9. Stephen H. Long, Russell F. Settle, and Charles W. Wrightson, "Employee Premiums, Availability of Alternative Plans, and HMO Disenrollment," *Medical Care* 26, no. 10(1988): 927–38.

Suggested Readings

Ammeter, H. "A Rational Experience Rating Technique for Group Insurance on the Risk Premium Basis." In *Transactions of the Fifteenth International Congress of Actuaries* (International Congress of Actuaries, 1957) 507–21.

Barnhart, E. P. "A New Approach to Premium, Policy and Claim Reserves for Health Insurance." *Transactions, Society of Actuaries* 37(1985): 13.

Bragg, J. M., and Green, E. A. "Health Insurance Claim Reserves and Liabilities." *Transactions, Society of Actuaries* 16, no. 3 (1964): 17.

Dobson, Robert H., and Doran, Phyllis A., moderators. "Managing the Group Health Line: Technical Approaches to Analyzing, Monitoring and Projecting Group Health Experience." *Record, Society of Actuaries* 8, no. 4 (October 1982): 1717.

Gal, Samuel, and Landsberger, Michael. "On Small Sample Properties of Experience Rating Insurance Contracts." *Quarterly Journal of Economics* 103, no. 1 (February 1988): 233.

Halvorson, W. A. "Expense Analysis and Allocation." *Transactions, Society of Actuaries* 20, no. 4 (1968): D554.

Jackson, P. H. "Experience Rating." *Transactions, Society of Actuaries* (1953): 239.

Jones, Donald A., and Gerber, Hans U. "Credibility Formulas of the Updating Type." *Transactions, Society of Actuaries* 27 (1975): 31.

_____. "Dividend Formulas in Group Insurance." *Transactions, Society of Actuaries* 26, no. 4 (1974): 77.

Maguire, Ralph D. "An Empirical Approach to the Determination of Credibility Factors." *Transactions, Society of Actuaries* 21, no. 1 (1969): 1.

Margolin, Myron H. "On the Credibility of Group Insurance Claim Experience." *Transactions, Society of Actuaries* 23, no. 1 (1971): 229.

Panjer, Harry H., and Mereu, John A. "Analysis of the Deficit Risk in Group Insurance." *Transactions, Society of Actuaries* 32 (1980): 305.

Pike, Bertram N. "Gain and Loss Analysis and Related Concepts for Group Insurance." *Transactions, Society of Actuaries* 13, no. 2 (1961): 412.

_____. "Some Considerations in Determining Incurred Claims Used in the Computation of Dividends under Group Accident and Health Insurance." *Transactions, Society of Actuaries* 10 (1958): 630.

Spellman, Lewis J.; Witt, Robert C.; and Rentz, William F. "Investment Income and Non-Life Insurance Pricing." *Journal of Risk and Insurance* 42, no. 4 (1975): 567.

Chapter 8

Selection Bias and Premium Rate Setting

One of the most controversial—and most misunderstood—topics in health care cost containment today is "risk skimming." Also known as "anti-selection," "negative selection," "risk creaming," and "risk pool manipulation," no other topic has generated more energy and less data. . . . You (the employer) do deserve to know if your employees who enrolled in an HMO are very low users of health care services. From your perspective as the buyer of health services, you deserve to know what level of care and service is being provided to your employees by both your HMO and insurance plans. Keep in mind that HMOs are truly more efficient than almost every insurance based cost containment approach. If your HMO enrollees are being hospitalized at one-half the rate of your insurance plan people, you can attribute the majority of that hospitalization difference to the HMO's efficiency. Part of that saving could also be due to risk selection, however, and you need to investigate to see if that might be the case for your group.

G. C. Halvorson, *How to Cut Your Company's Health Care Costs*

8.1   Introduction

One of the objectives of increased competition in health care markets is to contain costs by encouraging enrollment in cost-effective health plans.[1] Competitive efforts, however, can place a higher premium on enrolling healthy persons or low-cost groups than on developing delivery networks and providing services in an efficient manner. Thus, the impact of biased selection can be to raise total health costs, because not only would fewer persons be enrolled in the more efficient plans, but the most costly persons with the most to gain from a cost-effective plan would remain in the fee-for-service system.[2] Clearly, this is not the result intended from increased competition. In addition, if biased selection is severe and persistent over time, it could lead to instability in health insurance markets, as plans compete for the healthiest lives rather than the most efficient delivery of services. This, in turn, might lead to a breakdown in health insurance markets as we know them today.

Some health plans offer premiums that are lower than average because they have highly efficient health care delivery systems. However, selection effects can overwhelm differences in efficiency or cost effectiveness between health plans. Thus, selection bias could limit the success of the most efficient plans.[3]

Identification and analysis of selection bias among alternative health plans is a complex task. It is an important problem for HMO premium rate setting because adverse selection can lead to premiums being underpriced and adverse financial experience for the HMO. On the other hand, favorable selection (without appropriate adjustments to premiums charged to contract holders) can result in justifiable claims of "skimming." Selection bias can also result in an individual employer experiencing significantly higher health care costs in the aggregate. However, analysis of selection effects in multiple-option health benefits programs sponsored by employers is a complicated task. In addition, the interactions among the health plans chosen by individual subscribers, the enrollment patterns across alternative health plans, premium rate–setting practices, and the resulting costs to employers are very complex.

From one perspective, selection bias occurs because people are not randomly assigned to HMOs and other health plans. If a group of persons has only one choice of health plan, then selection bias is not a problem. In most cases, however, HMOs enroll their members from populations that have at least two options, and multiple-option health benefits programs are common. In highly competitive areas with many alternative plans, the selection bias problem is usually more severe.

Without random assignment, there will be some type of selection bias in HMO enrollment patterns, either favorable or adverse in any particular case. There is a debate among employers, HMOs, health benefit managers, consultants, academics, and others regarding the type of selection effects that HMOs receive. As discussed in Chapter 4, there is considerable concern on the part of employers that HMOs usually receive favorable selection, to the detriment of employers' indemnity plans. Representatives of HMOs counter that the selection issue is more complicated and that they do not receive favorable selection in all, or most, cases.

This chapter examines the topic of selection bias, first defining the issue and then discussing its implications for HMO premium rate setting. The appendix to this chapter contains a brief review of the literature on this topic. In addition, the current state of knowledge regarding selection bias in multiple-option health benefit programs is described.

8.2 What Is Selection Bias?

One way to understand selection bias is to consider a situation where it does *not* exist. This would arise from a random distribution of persons among a set of health plans from which they can choose, where each plan expects to enroll a distribution of individuals representative of the whole group. Selection bias, then, results from a systematic correlation (i.e., a nonrandom pattern) between the choice of plan and the characteristics of employees related to their health needs, health condition, preferences for providers, and general tendency to use health services. Consequently, from the perspective of a participating plan, if selection is biased, then the plan does not obtain a random sample from the population of those persons eligible to make a choice. If subscribers representing higher than average risk choose the plan, then that plan is said to have experienced "adverse selection" from the group in question (the health plan has more than its "fair share" of high-cost enrollees).

There are many different definitions of selection bias. Focusing on employers that offer more than one health plan, one definition of biased selection is "where employees with different levels of health-related financial risk systematically choose one health plan over another."[4] Thus, in the context of an employer's health program, selection bias refers to an unequal distribution of health risks across participating health plans.[5] In this case, selection bias occurs because of systematic differences in choices made by persons with different levels of health risk. Usually, the subscriber has more information regarding personal health status, dependents' health status, and the probability of serious illness than the insurer. This information and other factors (e.g., degree of being risk-adverse and level of out-of-pocket premiums) can be viewed as inputs into the decision-making process concerning choice of health plan.

From the perspective of a participating health plan, selection bias may be either "favorable" or "adverse." It is favorable when lower than average expected risks enroll and adverse when higher than average expected risks enroll.[6] In other words, selection bias is adverse, from a health plan's standpoint, when the enrollees are higher risk (i.e., higher cost) than anticipated when premiums were set (e.g., the pool of enrollees requires more than the anticipated amount of health care).

Similarly, an employer with a self-insured plan (or basic indemnity plan) suffers adverse selection when lower-risk employees choose alternative health plans (e.g., HMOs and PPOs), leaving a higher-risk enrollment in the employer's traditional plan. This results in the employer's basic plan having a disproportionate share of persons with high medical costs.

From a slightly different viewpoint, the pattern of selection effects results from the choices made by employees within the context of the overall health benefits program of the employer. Key characteristics of an employer's health program include the number and type of plans offered, and the benefit packages, cost-sharing requirements, provider panels, and premiums of alternative plans.[7]

Selection bias also involves the choice of different levels of insurance. For example, suppose that the alternative health plans represent a range of high-option and low-option plans (if the plans differ significantly with respect to degree of cost-sharing and comprehensiveness of benefits) with premium differentials reflecting the differences in the actuarial values of the benefits offered by each plan. Overall, there will be a tendency for persons who expect to use health services to choose the higher-option (more expensive) plans. Alternatively, healthy persons who do not expect to use services will have a tendency to choose the low-option (less expensive) plans.[8]

This phenomenon also applies to selected health services. For example, if alternative health plans differ with respect to coverage of specific services (maternity care, mental health, vision care, prescription drugs, and substance abuse services), then it is to be expected that persons with a tendency to use these services will choose the health plan with the best coverage.[9]

These tendencies, however, can be overcome by other factors that also affect selection bias.[10] For example, the level of out-of-pocket premiums that employees must pay is a key factor.[11] If the employer pays the entire premium, then employees will be encouraged to enroll in the high-option plans. In contrast, if there are substantial out-of-pocket premium differentials between the plans, this will tend to exacerbate the favorable selection for the low-option plans and adverse selection for the high-option plans. Moreover, this pattern of selection bias over time can force the premiums higher and higher on the high-option plans, and the low-option plans may reap windfall profits, purely through favorable selection effects.

Selection Bias and Premium Rate Setting

In order to set premium rates, a thorough evaluation of selection bias is required.[12] Groups are often classified by risk and different premiums are determined for each risk classification. It is important to estimate the effect of antiselection for each risk classification, in order to determine the appropriate premium. Thus, selection bias must be examined relative to risk class (i.e., within a rate cell or rating category, adverse selection occurs when enrollees represent higher than average expected risk for that rate cell or risk class). As discussed by Shepherd and Webster,

> A more complete term for the process is "Selection and Classification of Risks." . . . The selection process is necessary if we accept the principle that every insured should contribute his fair share toward the risk involved—that only applicants who are exposed to comparable degrees of risk should be placed in the same premium class. . . . The insurer will determine how many classes or gradations of risk he will recognize in his premium rates on the basis of practical considerations.[13]

This issue is also discussed by Wilensky and Rossiter: "Patient self-selection is said to be biased when premium payments for health care do not equal actual costs because some, perhaps unknown, factor about the insured population influencing service use and costs is not factored into the calculation of the payment."[14] Thus, evaluation of selection bias must take into account both the enrollment patterns among alternative health plans and their premium rate–setting methods. According to Welch: "Biased selection per se is not a problem if the premium compensates for differences in expected expenditure. A problem exists only if selection is biased even after adjusting for premium differences."[15]

With respect to premium rate setting, the most important aspect of selection bias concerns the health care cost patterns of the population subgroups that are in different risk classifications. For example, it is likely that premiums will be experience rated or that a set of rate categories will be used to determine the rates. In either case, the rates assume an underlying enrolled population distribution according to significant characteristics for historical and projected cost experience of the group covered by a particular health plan.

In order to rate accurately, the potential for selection bias must be evaluated when estimating the expected experience of the group and in setting the premium. If the actual enrollment pattern deviates from the expected distribution with respect to "cost-important" variables, then biased selection is said to exist (with specific implications for premium rate setting among the alternative health plans). If the enrollment pattern is biased, then each health plan will receive either adverse or favorable selection, depending on which persons actually enroll with that plan. Again, with dual or multiple options available in a particular employer group, it is extremely unlikely that any plan will receive "neutral" selection (i.e., that there will be an absence of selection bias).

HMO Underwriting and Adverse Selection

The selection of risks represented in an HMO's enrollment patterns is determined in part by the underwriting practices used by the HMO. Federal laws and regulations place restrictions on underwriting practices for federally qualified HMOs. Similarly, state-licensed HMOs, including federally qualified HMOs, must abide by state laws and regulations.

As discussed in Chapter 5, the costs incurred by a health plan depend in part on the plan's underwriting guidelines and implementation practices. Strictly controlled underwriting practices can lead to a more uniform, lower-cost enrolled population. In contrast, less well defined (or looser) underwriting practices usually result in higher costs and a less predictable population (from the standpoint of health status and medical risks).

In addition to the federal government, HMOs are regulated by state insurance and health departments. In general, HMOs have less flexibility with respect to underwriting practices than do Blue Cross plans or private insurance carriers.

For group enrollment, federally qualified HMOs are prohibited from any form of selective enrollment (i.e., medical underwriting via questionnaires or other forms of screening, use of preexisting conditions or waiting periods, or exclusions for persons with poor health status). In addition, federally qualified HMOs must provide all mandated basic health services to all members of a group, regardless of the health status of any member(s) of the group.

Depending on state law, state-licensed HMOs that are not federally qualified may have more flexibility concerning the use of selective enrollment techniques. For example, in some states, HMOs are allowed to medically underwrite individual members of a group or to establish waiting periods or limitations of coverage for preexisting conditions.

For small groups (e.g., fewer than 25 employees), private insurers typically use medical underwriting for premium rate setting and possibly for excluding or limiting coverage for individual members of the group (or imposing substandard rates for these members). Federally qualified HMOs are prohibited from using medical underwriting for small groups. If a group is accepted, the group must be given community rates, and all members who enroll with the HMO must be given the basic benefit package. As discussed above, state-licensed HMOs have greater freedom in setting underwriting requirements for small groups.

All HMOs are permitted to medically underwrite applicants for individual coverage. However, if the individual is accepted for enrollment, federally qualified HMOs must provide all basic health services mandated by the HMO Act. State-licensed HMOs may impose preexisting condition requirements or limit the benefit package due to health status or other conditions, depending on the HMO laws of the state.

On the other hand, private insurers generally impose higher restrictions on individual enrollment, and medical underwriting standards are usually higher than HMO standards. While federally qualified HMOs are forced to community rate, private insurers may employ a variety of premium rate–setting practices for individual contracts (e.g., age/sex rates, standard/substandard). In addition, for individual applicants, private insurers virtually always exclude preexisting conditions and may restrict coverage for specified services (e.g., maternity) or impose high deductibles for selected services. In contrast, federal and state HMO laws require coverage of all basic services.

In general, HMOs have less flexibility in underwriting methods than do their competitors due to federal and state laws and regulations. Most HMOs have been quite unsophisticated with respect to both the use and the potential impact of underwriting practices. In the past, although a small number of HMOs (mostly nonfederally qualified plans) may have ignored applicable regulations on permissible HMO underwriting methods, many more HMOs have ignored the potential benefits to be gained from development and implementation of well-defined underwriting guidelines.

Analysis of Selection Bias:
Prospective Versus Retrospective Approaches

Analysis of selection bias can focus on a variety of characteristics of the population under observation. The analysis usually attempts to find those characteristics that are significantly related to health care expenditure patterns and to give some insight into which plan an individual is likely to prefer (e.g., demographic characteristics, socioeconomic characteristics, health status, and prior utilization rates). For example, we can ask if the persons who enroll in Plan A are younger than the persons who enroll in Plan B. Similarly, differences can be examined for characteristics such as income, marital status, family size, overall health status, chronic conditions, and inpatient or outpatient utilization.

Selection bias can be studied from both a "prospective" and a "retrospective" perspective. After persons have chosen their health plans, but before actual cost experience is available, it is possible to analyze whether any particular plan has received favorable or adverse selection by looking at factors such as (1) health status at the time of choice, (2) prior health services utilization patterns, (3) demographic or socioeconomic variables related to cost experience, or (4) the historical cost experience of selected population subgroups. These prospective studies are not always accurate, however, because future health care utilization and costs can differ from prior (prechoice) patterns due to the random nature of health service use, the differences in practice patterns among alternative providers and health plans (if persons switch from one plan to another), the "regression to the mean" phenomenon, and other factors.

Some of these limitations are solved by the retrospective approach to analysis of selection bias. With this approach, the actual cost experience of different population subgroups is evaluated after the health plan decision has been made (i.e., during a postchoice period), usually in conjunction with demographic and socioeconomic characteristics and prior utilization or cost experience. However, retrospective studies must still consider the effects of random (year-to-year) variations, practice pattern differences, and regression to the mean patterns.

8.3 HMOs and "Skimming"

The topic of selection bias is quite complicated, and it is difficult to find generalizable results that are applicable to every type of situation where biased selection may occur. Additional information on selection bias is presented in the appendix to this chapter.

Many persons in the worlds of business, health benefits consulting, academia, and health insurance believe that HMOs receive favorable selection in most dual- or multiple-choice situations. In addition, they believe that the extent of favorable selection is significant and that premium formulas should compensate for this bias, so that HMOs do not reap windfall profits while employers are charged community rates. In addition, if HMOs "skim" the better risks (healthier employees), the less healthy employees are left in the employer's traditional plan. Over time, this can lead to an increasing concentration of higher-cost, higher-risk persons in the traditional plan. As a result, the premiums for the employer's traditional plan will rise substantially, and eventually the enrollees in the traditional plan will not be able to afford the premiums.

It is important that HMOs directly confront the charge of "skimming." Confronting the issue means answering questions such as these:

- Do HMOs consciously try to "skim"?
- Even if not attempted consciously, do HMOs receive favorable selection, in general?
- Given that selection bias will always occur in dual- or multiple-choice situations, what are fair and equitable methods for compensating for this phenomenon in premium formulas?

As a summary of the material presented in this chapter, these questions and their implications for concerned HMOs are addressed in the following pages.

Do HMOs Consciously Try to "Skim"?

Health maintenance organizations can consciously attempt to "skim" by developing and implementing explicit strategies: (1) to target low-risk persons and selectively enroll them, (2) to identify high-risk persons and prevent them from enrolling (or encourage them not to enroll), or (3) to avoid providing needed care to high-risk persons or to encourage them to disenroll from the HMO. To exacerbate the perceived problem, some HMOs have used strategies (including benefit design, cost sharing, and premium contribution policies) that tend to encourage lower-risk persons to enroll. Some non-federally qualified HMOs, similar to private insurers, have used waiting periods and exclusions on preexisting conditions to discourage some high-risk persons from enrolling.

In general, it is difficult to distinguish policies that attempt to enhance a plan's competitive position (and attract enrollees) from those designed with favorable selection as their objective.[16] The great majority of HMOs, especially those that developed in the 1970s and earlier, use standard community-rating methods and do not use techniques that are predatory in nature to obtain a low-risk enrollment. However, a few plans have been very aggressive and have obtained low-cost membership populations through favorable selection.

Most plans have not employed specific strategies to target healthy enrollees or to discourage sick enrollees for several reasons. First, it is difficult to identify and selectively enroll low-risk employees (and their dependents) and explicitly discourage potential high-risk enrollees. Second, large employers are keenly aware of this issue, and HMOs would have to be quite sophisticated to successfully employ predatory methods in the current environment. (As discussed earlier, the vast majority of HMOs do not have the underwriting expertise and analytical capacity required to mount strategies of this type on a large scale.) Third, it is difficult to withhold needed care from high-risk persons or provide incentives for them to choose alternate carriers (e.g., "dumping the queen of spades" strategy). Some enrollees will not be satisfied with either the available physicians or the medical advice provided by the HMO, and they will disenroll from the HMO at their next opportunity. This dissatisfaction, however, does not necessarily mean that the HMO consciously withheld needed care or encouraged these persons to disenroll.

Favorable Selection without Skimming

Even if HMOs do not consciously attempt to "skim," do they still receive favorable selection in general? There are many cases and situations in which HMOs can be expected to receive favorable selection. These cases, discussed more fully in the appendix to this chapter, include the following:

- Persons with established ties to particular physicians may be unwilling to break these ties to join an HMO, especially a staff-model or group-model plan. These persons usually have higher-cost medical profiles than persons without a regular physician. Once enrolled in a staff- or group-model plan, the opposite phenomenon appears to be applicable to HMOs (if enrolled in an HMO, persons with health problems tend to remain with their HMO physician).

- If HMOs are offered for the first time to an employer group, it is likely that the HMO will receive favorable selection compared to the employer's basic health plan (the "Jackson-Beeck" phenomenon). [17] With the growth in the number of HMOs and HMO enrollment over the past ten years, this has been a frequent phenomenon. However, with the virtual halt in formation of new HMOs and with the growth of alternatives such as PPOs and new managed care indemnity plans, HMOs may be victims (rather than beneficiaries) of this phenomenon over the next five to ten years.

- Some persons who expect to need medical care in the near future may not be familiar with the HMO concept or may be reluctant to try a new provider. In contrast, persons who are new to an area or who are not concerned about their health may be more willing to try a new health plan. Again, HMOs should receive favorable selection from this group.

- Under the ''equal contribution'' requirement of the federal HMO Act, many employers have contributed as much to HMOs as to their basic indemnity plan. For employers with high indemnity rates, this has created a situation where low-risk employees have had incentives to join HMOs. However, the ''equal contribution'' requirement is not applicable for nonmandated employers. In addition, the new HMO Act amendments provide for much greater flexibility in determining employer contributions. Therefore, HMOs should benefit less in the future from this aspect of favorable selection.

On the other hand, there are cases where HMOs can be expected to receive adverse selection:

- Some persons who anticipate needing medical care may find the comprehensiveness of HMO benefits and low cost sharing to be attractive.

- The premium rates determined under community-rating methods may be attractive to high-risk, high-cost groups or subscribers.

- The redesign of some employers' health plans, with higher cost sharing and more limited benefits, will likely encourage some employees who expect to need medical care to choose HMO coverage.

- In most cases, HMOs experience adverse selection from persons who disenroll, compared to continuing HMO members.

- There is some evidence that, for employer groups that have been with an HMO for several years, the HMO experiences adverse selection from the new enrollees in these groups who choose the HMO.

In many cases in the past, HMOs have received favorable selection at the expense of an employer's indemnity program. In other cases, HMOs have suffered adverse selection when competing in multiple-option health benefits programs sponsored by employers. Most HMOs can point to specific cases where biased selection has occurred in both directions.

Although it is impossible to determine precisely, it is likely that HMOs, as a group, have received favorable selection over the past five to ten years, and that employers' indemnity plans, in the aggregate, have experienced adverse selection as a result. Most of the favorable selection for HMOs probably occurred when they were offered to employer groups for the first time. It is likely that new HMOs received the best selection, in general, and that established HMOs received more neutral selection, especially for groups where they had long-standing contractual relationships. Again, selection results are very complicated, and it is difficult to generalize for any particular group.

Given the halt in development of new HMOs since approximately 1987, many of the forces that result in favorable HMO selection are likely to stop. Other developments that will tend to reverse the trend are (1) actions by many employers to reduce the number of HMOs they offer, (2) restructuring of benefit, cost-sharing, and contribution levels to reduce the attractiveness of HMOs compared to indemnity plans, and (3) the aging of HMO members over time and the regression toward the mean phenomenon, which will tend to moderate the effects of prior favorable selection for employees who remain in HMOs.

Compensation for Favorable Selection

Given that selection bias will always occur in dual- or multiple-choice situations, what are fair and equitable methods for compensating for this phenomenon in premium formulas? A variety of group-specific rate-setting formulas are discussed in Chapter 7. Many of these options are applicable to HMOs now that the 1988 HMO amendments have been signed into law. Of most concern to employers, however, are the required employer contributions for health insurance coverage. Many employers believe that their contributions should reflect the relative risk of persons enrolled in alternative health plans. For example, if younger employees choose HMO coverage, then employer contributions should not be fixed but should be adjusted to reflect the costs represented by that subgroup of enrollees.

Basically, the objective is to correct for biased selection through risk-adjusted employer contribution rates. One method of achieving this objective is to develop "classes" of employees, using age/sex groups or other methods. Rather than a single, fixed contribution rate, the employer can establish a higher contribution rate for a class with higher-risk persons (and lower rates for lower-risk classes). Examples of this technique are discussed in Chapter 4. The advantages of this approach are that (1) lower-risk employees have less incentive to choose HMO coverage, (2) the employer's total health care costs are more directly controlled, (3) health benefits are made more affordable for all employees, and (4) the effects of biased selection are neutralized. It is important, however, for HMOs to negotiate with employers so that HMO premiums can be recomposited into the same "classes" as employer contributions and so that the selection effects are not aggravated, especially from the HMO's perspective.

Fair and equitable premium rates and employer contribution rates, along with other issues, are part of an ongoing debate between HMOs and the business community. It is extremely important for HMOs to be viewed by the business community as (1) "good business partners," (2) effective agents in containing medical costs while increasing employee satisfaction with health benefits, and (3) progressive and flexible in negotiating on issues of concern to employers, including premium rate setting and contribution formulas. In many geographic areas, the relationship between employers and health plans is both fragile and competitive, and HMOs have a lot to lose by not taking advantage of current opportunities to improve relations with their biggest customers. This does not preclude the fact that many HMOs will continue to believe that community rating is the best premium rate–setting method for their plan. It will be important, though, for these plans to convince their major clients that community rates are fair and equitable, possibly in conjunction with constructive negotiations on risk-adjusted employer contribution rates.

Appendix
Selection Bias: An Overview

This appendix provides additional information related to the topic of selection bias and the effects on premium rate setting. It begins with an overview of the literature, which is followed by an examination of selection bias in multiple-option health benefits programs.

Literature Review

The phenomenon of antiselection has been well known in the insurance business for many decades.[18] Selection is also a major topic in the fields of econometrics, demography, biostatistics, actuarial science, and epidemiology.[19] For example, numerous econometric methods have been developed to correct for selection bias.[20] Also, the effects of antiselection in health insurance programs have been studied extensively by actuaries.[21] This review, however, will focus primarily on the health services research and HMO literature.[22]

The literature review has been divided into time periods. Even before the term "health maintenance organization" came into being (prior to 1973), there were a number of studies that examined the demographic characteristics and utilization rates of persons enrolled in prepaid group practices. Many of these studies were conducted by Donabedian at the University of Michigan, Roemer at UCLA, Shapiro at Johns Hopkins University, and Densen at Harvard University.[23]

During the mid- to late 1970s, the focus shifted to comparisons between HMOs and indemnity plans, enrollment patterns within selected employer groups, and selection effects as represented by utilization differences. Studies were conducted by Berki et al.; Bice; Scitovsky, McCall, and Benham; Mechanic; Wollstadt, Shapiro, and Bice; and others.[24]

Out of these studies came a number of theories and hypotheses about enrollment patterns and the resulting selection effects on HMOs. One of these was the "risk/vulnerability" hypothesis that persons who are at greater risk or who are vulnerable to high health care costs would be attracted by the comprehensive benefits offered by HMOs. In addition, if HMO premium rates were higher than competitors' rates, this would exacerbate the adverse selection experienced by plans.

The concept of "self-selection" for persons choosing among alternative health plans was also examined. In 1981, Luft published *Health*

Maintenance Organizations: Dimensions of Performance, which contains a detailed discussion of what was known about selection and HMOs at that point in time.[25]

From 1980 to 1985, the volume of selection studies increased, and many of them took different forms. Many studies continued to analyze enrollment patterns in individual plans and individual employers. However, new types of studies were also conducted:

1. HMO *disenrollment* patterns were studied, led by efforts by Wintringham, Gold, and others.[26]

2. Eggers looked at *Medicare* eligibles who joined HMOs and their prior experience in the fee-for-service sector.[27]

3. Price and Mays conducted a series of studies on selection effects in the Federal Employees Health Benefits Program.[28]

4. Other studies analyzed the prior fee-for-service experience of persons from commercial groups who joined HMOs the *first time* they were offered in a group (Jackson-Beeck and Kleinman).[29]

In 1985 Scheffler and Rossiter published an interesting collection of articles on selection issues.[30] In addition, a summary and review of existing literature on patient self-selection in HMOs was published by Wilensky and Rossiter in 1986.[31]

Between 1985 and 1988, there were some new developments in the literature. First, the concept of "regression to the mean" appeared. Although this concept was not new in the actuarial science literature, it had not been used extensively in health services research studies. In its first application to HMOs, Welch published results of "Regression toward the Mean in Medical Care Costs: Implications for Biased Selection in HMOs" in 1985.[32] Lubitz et al. considered this concept in relation to improving the Medicare payment formula for HMOs.[33] Beebe also published an interesting article on this topic in 1988.[34]

Second, multi-HMO studies have attempted to determine generalizable results that are applicable to broad categories of HMOs. For example, as part of the National Evaluation of the Medicare Competition Demonstrations, Mathematica Policy Research conducted a study of this type on Medicare selection and HMOs. Other studies of this type include Wrightson, Genuardi, and Stephens on HMO disenrollment patterns.[35]

Third, there have been more studies on Medicare and Medicaid. The National Evaluation of the Medicare Competition Demonstration was a very large study of HMO experience with Medicare.[36] For Medicaid, Freund has published interesting results from the Medicaid Capitation Demonstration Evaluation.[37] Also, Wintringham and Bice have conducted a comprehensive study of the Medicaid experience of Group Health Cooperative of Puget Sound.[38]

Fourth, there have been a variety of other studies on specific topics. Feldman and Dowd completed a study that distinguished between "biased selection" and "selectivity bias," using econometric methods. Luft has examined methods for compensating for biased selection in health insurance.[39] Enthoven has called for a "managed competition" approach to help solve the selection bias problem, among other objectives.[40]

Finally, Hellinger and Luft and Miller have published the most recent review articles.[41] Hellinger reaches the following conclusion:

> Review of the available literature leads one to conclude that prepaid group practice HMOs do experience favorable selection. Numerous studies demonstrate that prior use of health services for HMO enrollees is less than prior use of health services for those who remain in the fee-for-service sector. There is considerable evidence that shows a statistically significant positive relationship between prior use and current use. These findings reflect the experience of HMOs with both the elderly and non-elderly populations.[42]

Although it is natural to attempt to determine whether or not HMOs receive favorable selection in all cases, the topic of selection for HMOs (or, more generally, selection in multiple-option health programs) is a very complex topic. It is important to be very careful about how we measure selection and also how we define different types of situations where we look at selection effects.

Luft and Miller have discussed many factors that are relevant to analysis of HMO selection bias, including risk-adjusted HMO premiums:

> The evidence from the literature suggest that HMOs are subject to some favorable selection of new enrollees according to prior health care use and cost measures, although no selection bias at all is also a common result in many studies. The prepaid group practice model and the Medicare demonstrations account for much of the favorable selection findings according to these measures. No such favorable selection exists according to health status measures. . . . Health status for people already enrolled is also generally favorable to HMOs. The preponderance of evidence from disenrollment studies suggests HMOs are subject to unfavorable disenrollment.[43]

In summary, there is an extensive body of literature on HMOs and selection bias. We have progressed from the 1960s, when selection for HMOs (prepaid group practices) was perceived as neutral or not considered at all; through the 1970s, when many observers believed that HMOs received adverse selection (risk/vulnerability); to the early 1980s, which might be viewed as a transition period; to the present, when many employers and other observers believe that HMOs receive favorable selection, unless it is proven otherwise.

What Is Known about HMO Selection Bias?

Although the topic of selection bias has not been completely analyzed to the satisfaction of all observers, some general conclusions have been established. These conclusions appear to hold in the majority of cases, but not in every case:

1. Selection bias exists when HMOs and other health plans compete (or, more generally, in multiple-option health benefits programs). This fact has been confirmed by many studies.

2. From work by Jackson-Beeck[44] and related articles, it appears that HMOs receive *favorable* selection when they are offered for the first time to an employer group. This also appears to be true for PPOs and other plans. In fact, any new plan is likely to get a favorable selection of risks because people with health problems or established physician relationships are less likely to change from their current health plan. This is especially true for persons in the midst of a serious health condition or problem. Thus, an indemnity plan is also likely to receive favorable selection when it is offered for the first time to an employer group that previously had only HMO coverage.

3. Based on HMO disenrollment studies, it appears that HMOs receive *adverse* selection from voluntary disenrollees. Compared to continuing members, the disenrollees are younger, use less services, and are less costly. This result is not surprising given the second conclusion. If individuals who switch plans tend to be less costly than average, then the plan they enroll in will experience favorable selection, while the plan they leave will experience adverse selection.

4. Based on studies of Medicare enrollees in HMOs, it appears that group and staff models get *favorable* initial selection, while

IPAs get neutral or *adverse* initial selection. These findings have been confirmed by the study conducted by Mathematica Policy Research as part of the Medicare demonstration evaluation.[45] Note that the second, third, and fourth conclusions are based on studies that used the "prospective" approach to analyzing selection effects (e.g., comparing the prior utilization and cost patterns of "switchers" vs. "stayers"). There is some evidence that, in some cases, future (postchoice) experience may differ from prior (prechoice) experience.

5. A study by Group Health Inc. in Minneapolis shows that established HMOs receive *adverse* selection from new enrollees from established employer groups (i.e., groups that have had contracts with the plan for several years and that have large numbers of employees enrolled with the plan).[46] However, more studies are necessary to explore this type of phenomenon in more detail.

6. It appears that regression to the mean should be considered in studies that examine selection effects. Selection effects result from an individual's desire to enroll in the plan most favorable to his or her current situation. For example, if the individual is healthy and does not expect to use any medical services in the foreseeable future, he or she may enroll in the plan with the lowest premium, or a plan with good catastrophic coverage and little first-dollar coverage. Conversely, an individual who expects to use extensive medical services soon may enroll in the plan with the most comprehensive coverage, with little regard to the levels of out-of-pocket premiums among available plans. Other factors related to choice of health plan are discussed below.

   These initial effects, whether favorable or adverse, are likely to diminish over time so that the experience of each plan converges toward some "average" experience that would be expected for the enrollees of each plan (i.e., the initial selection effects moderate, or die out, over time). However, the average may be specific to the subgroup and may not be the same as the planwide average. For example, in the Jackson-Beeck case, if new HMO enrollees from new groups are healthier than average, their first-year experience in the HMO will likely be lower than the HMO's planwide average experience, but it may not be as low as their previous fee-for-service experience. Over the first few years in the HMO, the experience of this cohort can be expected to regress higher towards its mean experience. However, this mean is likely to be lower than the planwide mean because the selected cohort represents a group of persons who are healthier than average.

7. In addition to the results from the studies cited above, there have been numerous studies that have examined the selection effects for particular cases (i.e., one employer, or one HMO, or one indemnity plan, or a group of employers, or one market area). The various studies have often shown conflicting results because of differences in methodology, data collection methods, competitive market conditions, or other factors. However, a variety of specific variables have been identified that play a significant role in this process. Examples of important variables include the following:

- Differences in benefit packages and cost-sharing features of alternative health plans
- Differences in premium rates, especially out-of-pocket premiums
- Other factors that affect an individual's choice of health plan, such as personal utility functions, risk/vulnerability theory, demographic and socioeconomic characteristics, prior patterns of use of health services, and expectations about future use of health services and changing needs
- Characteristics of the employer group setting that affect employee choice of health plan, such as the number and type of health plan options offered, the number of years offered (each plan), and the penetration rate of each plan
- Characteristics of the local health care marketplace and the competitive environment that affect individual choice of health plan *within the employer group setting*

What Is Not Known about HMO Selection Bias?

Although much is known about HMO selection bias in terms of what normally happens in some generic situations, there is still much to learn about the total picture of HMO selection bias. Little is understood about the relationship between HMOs and selection effects in the following areas:

1. Few studies have distinguished between the selection effects for new plans (less than three to five years old) and those for older, more established plans. Since new plans are naturally going to deal with a higher proportion of new groups (first time offerings), new plans should expect to obtain a favorable selection of risks (in most but not all cases). On the other hand, older HMOs have an established membership population, where regression to the mean has already taken place for most members. For example, the utilization and cost pattern of a member who has been enrolled for ten years will depend more on personal characteristics and health status than on the initial (transient) selection effects from when he or she first became a member of the HMO. If new health plans (HMOs and PPOs) receive favorable initial selection in a given marketplace, then the established health plans in that marketplace (older HMOs, indemnity plans, self-insured plans) will necessarily receive adverse or less favorable selection.

   No studies have been conducted on the selection effects experienced by both existing HMOs and indemnity plans when a new health plan emerges on the scene and is successful in obtaining a large enrollment in its first two to three years of operation. However, in addition to the Jackson-Beeck phenomenon, many other factors can lead to adverse selection against established HMOs: their comprehensive benefits, community rating, and increasing risk levels in their population over time due to the aging, or "graying," of the enrolled membership. Many observers feel that, when new entrants come into the marketplace, they often get favorable selection, and the established plans (both HMO and indemnity) suffer adverse selection as a result.[47]

2. The picture for Medicare and Medicaid eligibles who are enrolled in HMOs is not clear. The early Eggers studies showed that, when measured using a prospective approach based on the prior fee-for-service experience, group-model and staff-model plans were likely to receive favorable selection.[48] However, in recent years, many HMOs (of all model types) have suffered significant losses from Medicare enrollees. It has not been determined whether the losses are coming from new enrollees, old enrollees, or certain adjusted average per capita costs (AAPCC) rate categories, or whether the HCFA payment rates are uniformly low compared to the HMO's actual costs.

   Similarly, most HMOs have had poor financial experience

with Medicaid. This is supported by a study by Wintringham and Bice which showed that the costs experienced by Group Health Cooperative of Puget Sound for Medicaid enrollees were significantly higher than the state's payment rates.[49]

More comprehensive studies of Medicare and Medicaid, across numbers of HMOs, would be desirable. In addition, identification and analysis of adverse selection patterns for Medicare and Medicaid enrollees would provide very useful information for many HMOs.

3. In terms of patterns of selection effects over time, the phenomenon of an "adverse selection spiral" has been documented and is well known for indemnity plans. Briefly, an adverse selection spiral occurs in a multiple-option health benefits program when the indemnity plan's premiums are higher than the other choices. This leads to healthier subscribers leaving the indemnity plan, but higher-risk subscribers remain in the plan and the indemnity rates are forced higher and higher over time.

Although this phenomenon is well known, there has not been any attention paid to the opposite type of phenomenon. For simplicity, it will be termed a "favorable selection spiral." For example, consider an employer with an indemnity plan and one HMO, with the indemnity rates significantly lower than the HMO's rates. Under the favorable selection spiral hypothesis, the HMO experiences adverse selection initially and, over time, it gets worse. The indemnity plan, however, gets favorable selection initially, and it gets better over time. As a result, the indemnity rates stay constant or even decline, or they go up by less than inflation (or other comparable rate increases or trend factors).[50]

4. Little attention has been devoted to analysis of the selection effects for individual contract holders (nongroup enrollees, direct pay, and group conversion). Although few health plans get good experience from these groups, the issue of whether HMOs receive worse selection effects from these groups, compared to the experience of private insurers, has not been examined. Do HMOs get adverse selection from these groups, in relative terms?

5. Some studies have indicated that the postchoice utilization experience of persons who switch health plans can be significantly different from their prechoice patterns. For example, it is likely

that any type of "selective enrollment" or switching (plan hopping) behavior would involve (1) known conditions (e.g., non-emergency, high-cost surgery), (2) planned conditions (e.g., obstetrics/maternity), or (3) specialized services such as mental health, substance abuse, vision care, and dental care, which are only available on a limited number of health plans offered.

Since subscribers are much more knowledgeable about their health status and needs, changing conditions, and future expectations about use of health services, it is to be expected that they will make intelligent decisions concerning the choice of health plans. (Consumers have much better information about their short-term needs and intentions than do insurers, and this knowledge will be used to choose between the health plan options available to them.) Their choice will likely involve an assessment of features of the alternative health plan options, such as benefits and limits on covered services, cost-sharing requirements, access to selected providers, and expected out-of-pocket costs (including both employee premiums and expected deductibles and copayments). Thus, consumers who face changing needs or conditions will be more likely to switch health plans, and these "switchers" will be likely to have postchoice use patterns that are significantly different from their prechoice health services utilization patterns. Since "persistence" is the norm in decisions relating to the individual choice of health plan, persons switching health plans are likely to be responding to changing needs, expectations, or other motives.[51]

Many studies have relied on prior utilization in the fee-for-service sector to determine HMO selection bias effects using a prospective perspective. The potential for changing patterns in prechoice versus postchoice behavior has not been adequately investigated. This would apply equally to persons switching from indemnity plans to HMOs, as well as to persons switching from HMOs to indemnity plans.

6. Recently, many indemnity plans have instituted significantly higher cost-sharing provisions or introduced a very low-option plan (sometimes in conjunction with flexible benefits). Although the actual selection effects of such changes are a function of many factors, plans with comprehensive benefits and low cost sharing (like HMOs) are likely to suffer adverse selection as a result. This topic, however, has not been analyzed in detail.

7. The regression to the mean phenomenon has been recognized for some time in different disciplines. In insurance programs, differences in incidence rates and cost patterns by duration since enrollment have been studied extensively by actuaries. With individual life insurance, for example, rigorous underwriting of new applicants usually results in initial mortality rates that are significantly below the expected rates for a given type of policy and a group of policyholders with specified characteristics. This initial selection effect is referred to as "select" mortality, as compared to the "ultimate" mortality rates that will result from the group as the initial selection effects wear off over time.

In health services research, however, regression to the mean has only recently been applied to analysis of health services utilization and expenditure patterns.[52] The concept is applicable to many situations involving analysis of how health services utilization and expenditure patterns can be expected to change over time. However, we do not yet know the expected magnitude of changes in different population subgroups or how the effects of the concept change in different situations. Welch has attempted to estimate the magnitude of the effects of regression to the mean under certain assumptions in a first attempt at this problem, and he has provided a set of interesting results.[53]

Much work still needs to be done to understand this problem in its entirety. In particular, the concept of regression to the mean has not been adequately explored in relation to analysis of health care expenditure patterns. The topic is important because it appears to be applicable to a range of current issues of interest, including the following:

1. Reimbursement to HMOs under TEFRA risk contracts for Medicare eligibles

2. Analysis of selection effects in multiple-option health benefits programs

3. Evaluation of results of HMO choice studies[54]

There are many methodological issues to be considered in analyzing this phenomenon. Clear distinctions must be made between results using (1) individual-level (person-based) data, (2) family-level data, (3) data for population subgroups, and (4) aggregated data for the total population being considered. The statistical properties and nature of trends over time will differ significantly for different levels of data aggregation. Two studies using aggregated, multiyear data demonstrated regression to the mean over time.[55] However, this statistical behavior would be expected due to the method of defining population subgroups in these studies (each population was stratified into subgroups according to the level of expenditures in the base year).

The applicability of these types of results to the general case is not clear. In the general case, although the average expenditure level can be calculated for any subgroup of a larger population, in most cases the subgroup will not be defined according to the expenditure level of its members (e.g., Medicare eligibles choosing an HMO, employees choosing alternative health plans in a multiple-choice environment).

Key Unresolved Issues

Although many studies on HMO selection effects have been completed, there are still many topics and particular situations that have not been adequately analyzed. One of the key unresolved issues is the appropriate "unit of analysis" to be used in these selection studies. Many studies have used individual members as the basic unit of analysis. Some studies have used individual employer groups. Other studies have identified a number of groups and then used all of the members of those groups as the study population. Some studies have used a plan (HMO) as the unit of analysis. Different units of analysis have advantages and disadvantages, and some may be more appropriate for analysis of some issues than others.[56]

A second unresolved issue concerns the measurement of selection bias, especially with respect to the impact on HMO premium rate setting. For example, it is relatively easy to determine if HMO enrollees are younger than indemnity plan enrollees (or to calculate the average number of chronic conditions or prior use rates). Other factors, however, may have a much greater impact than age.[57]

Analysis of selection effects in multiple-option health benefits programs is a very difficult and complicated problem. There are many different types of situations that need to be considered. In addition, it may be impossible to find completely generalizable results that hold in all possible situations for all types of HMOs. Rather, it may be necessary to determine generalizable results for pieces of the problem (particular types of situations and types of HMOs) in order to understand the total picture.

Does favorable selection occur for HMOs? Yes, it has been demonstrated to occur in many situations. In addition, results for new enrollees from groups in a first-time HMO offering (like the Jackson-Beeck case) appear to be generalizable (for most but not all cases).

Does adverse selection exist for HMOs? Again, yes—especially in HMO disenrollment situations and possibly for new enrollees from established groups (e.g., the Group Health case), although further evidence is required to prove that this is a generalizable result.

Much research and many practical studies are still required to develop a complete picture of HMO selection bias. Of course, it would be desirable to have a comprehensive theoretical structure that ties together all of the results with an appealing conceptual framework. In addition, it would be desirable to have a more complete theoretical framework that explains a greater number of cases that actually occur in practice. More thorough documentation of specific types of situations would also be desirable, so that generalizable results would be available across entire "classes" of situations that would be applicable to broad categories of HMOs.

Selection bias for HMOs and other health plans can interact with premium rate–setting practices to produce undesirable situations. For example, an employer's total costs for health care may increase when alternative, supposedly lower-cost plans are offered. However, to determine the true effect of biased selection involving HMOs, it is necessary to evaluate the total picture (postchoice as well as prechoice experience), including all of the possible scenarios in which significant interactions could take place. Identification, measurement, and analysis of selection effects in multiple-option health benefits programs are not simple or straightforward tasks.

Changing Perspectives on Medicare Risk Contracts

An interesting example of how the approach to selection changes over time is the case of Medicare risk contracts.[58] During the 1970s, there were a number of proposals to reimburse HMOs on a risk/capitation basis for services provided to Medicare eligibles who were enrolled in HMOs. Since the payment basis for most of these proposals was 95 percent of fee-for-service Medicare costs for comparable beneficiaries, most policy analysts assumed that there would be cost savings to Medicare resulting from implementation of the risk contracts.

During this time period, the Office of the Actuary in the Health Care Financing Administration was quite concerned about the potential for antiselection for the Medicare program as a result of the HMO risk contracts. From the perspective of the actuaries who were charged with estimating the cost impact of the various proposals, there was a very real potential danger that relatively healthy Medicare eligibles would enroll with the HMOs and that the Medicare program would realize negative savings as a result. For example, if the HMO enrollees represented an average cost of 80 percent of the fee-for-service equivalent costs, rather than the 95 percent that was the basis for the HCFA payment rate, then Medicare total costs would increase as a result.

A second form of biased selection was from the HMOs that chose to participate in risk contracts. For HMOs with a large number of enrollees over the age of 65, some plans would have per capita costs for Medicare eligibles that were less than 95 percent of the AAPCC, while other plans would have costs that exceeded 95 percent of the AAPCC. The Medicare actuaries believed that the HMOs with lower costs would have a significantly greater incentive to participate in risk contracts than plans with higher costs. If only the low-cost HMOs went "at-risk" (i.e., entered into risk contracts), then Medicare's aggregate expenditures would increase as a result.

A third factor was the approach and detailed provisions embodied in most of the legislative proposals for Medicare HMO risk contracts. There were no marketing constraints associated with many of the proposals, which increased the level of concern on the part of the actuaries that some prepaid plans could develop marketing approaches that would exacerbate the antiselection from Medicare's standpoint.

Thus, the Medicare actuaries predicted (or at least planned for) favorable selection for HMOs with risk contracts as early as 1970.[59] During the period from 1970 to 1980, there were many conflicts and differences of opinion between the Office of the Actuary and HCFA policy analysts. During this same time period, most of the academic literature indicated that HMOs usually experienced adverse selection or, at most, neutral selection.

How have the perspectives changed during the 1980s? The health services research and HMO literature has evolved with the numerous studies identified in the first section of this appendix. The late 1970s and early 1980s were a transition period, and by the mid-1980s, there was a modest trend in studies that concluded that HMOs received favorable selection.[60]

The first few years of experience under the risk contracts have provided critical "operating" data from which actuaries have revised their initial assessment of the selection effects of Medicare risk contracts. Factors related to evaluation of the selection effects of the risk contracts, from an actuarial perspective, include the following:

- The process used to determine the HCFA reimbursement rates (AAPCC) and the adequacy of the HCFA payment rates
- The actual enrollment patterns and selection experienced by different types of HMOs
- Effects of regression to the mean
- The financial experience of participating HMOs (losses experienced by many plans)
- The financial effects on consumers and providers

Many HMOs have fared well with risk contracts. During the past three to four years, they have established solid bases of enrollment (in addition to delivery systems and other requirements for Medicare enrollees), and they have had financial experience ranging from satisfactory to good to excellent. In some cases, HMOs have made profits that were substantially better than projected.

On the other hand, there have been many HMOs that have suffered adverse financial experience from their Medicare risk contracts. The financial problems incurred by these plans result from many factors:

- Underestimates of the actuarial value of the benefit package that they offered to Medicare eligibles, in relation to the HCFA payment rate
- Offering benefits that were too "rich," and attracting substantial adverse selection
- Responding to competitive pressures and underpricing premiums to consumers
- Underestimating the difference between Medicare reimbursement rates to physicians and what the plan paid to its participating physicians, as well as the impact of higher payments on biased selection

- Underestimating the value of Medicare cost sharing that was included in the plan's benefit package
- Perceptions of inadequate HCFA payment rates (AAPCC) by some HMOs
- Inadequate control over utilization of health services by Medicare beneficiaries

There have been many different outcomes, viewed on a plan-by-plan basis, and evaluation of the resulting selection effects is a complicated endeavor.

What are actuaries' current views regarding Medicare risk contracts with HMOs? Most actuaries believe that risk contracts have to be examined very carefully to determine whether a plan should enter into such a contract (or renew a current contract). For example, since Medicare eligibles are a relatively high-risk population (compared to the normal HMO enrollment population), and the HMO is assuming full risk under the contract, it is incumbent upon the plan's management to evaluate all aspects of the arrangement—including the financial, delivery system, and other implications.

The attitudes of the actuarial community to Medicare risk contracts, in general, and to the selection effects for HMOs, in particular, are represented by the general advice and recommendations that actuaries offer to HMOs in these situations. First, there should be a careful assessment of the adequacy of the HCFA payment rates for the area served by the HMO. This involves evaluation of (1) benefit package design, including cost sharing and limitations on services, (2) careful estimation of expected costs, (3) provider reimbursement policies, (4) competitive market conditions, (5) marketing approach and enrollment projections (including the number of roll-over versus new Medicare enrollees), (6) adequacy of utilization control mechanisms for Medicare patients, (7) accurate determination of premiums to be charged to consumers, (8) concern regarding the future level of HCFA payments, and (9) a realistic comparison of the expected costs with the amount of the reimbursement from HCFA for the projected enrollees. In general, IPAs have to be especially careful with Medicare risk contracts. Due to the potential for antiselection and the other risks involved, many actuaries recommend against IPAs entering into risk contracts, unless the conditions are very favorable (e.g., high level of the AAPCC in the area, the HMO has strong relations with its physician providers, participating hospitals are willing to accept risk on a capitation basis for Medicare patients, favorable competitive market conditions).

The attitudes of actuaries concerning the selection effects of HMOs with Medicare risk contracts has evolved substantially during the past five years. Initially, the actuaries in the Office of the Actuary were very concerned about the possibility that antiselection would increase Medicare costs while HMOs received favorable selection when enrolling Medicare eligibles. Based on the actual experience of the past few years, many actuaries have changed their perspective. Each case must be assessed according to a variety of factors and plan-specific conditions. The financial experience for the HMO can be favorable or unfavorable, depending on how the contract is implemented and the selection of risks that actually enroll with the HMO.

Notes

1. See A. C. Enthoven and R. Knonick, "A Consumer-Choice Health Plan for the 1990s," *New England Journal of Medicine* 320 no. 1(1989): 29–37; A. Enthoven, "Managed Competition of Alternative Delivery Systems," *Journal of Health Politics, Policy and Law* 13, no. 2 (1988): 305–21; A. C. Enthoven, "Managed Competition: An Agenda for Action," *Health Affairs* 7, no. 2 (1988): 25–47; A. C. Enthoven, "Managed Competition in Health Care and the Unfinished Agenda," *Health Care Financing Review* 1986 Annual Supplement: 105–20; and A. C. Enthoven, *Health Plan: The Only Practical Solution to the Soaring Cost of Medical Care* (Reading, MA: Addison-Wesley, 1980).
2. If selection bias is severe, the low-cost plans will be those that obtain the most favorable selection of risks (i.e., select expertly), rather than the plans that are most effective in containing costs. These low-cost plans, rather than those plans that provide services efficiently, will attract the most members. In this case, the average cost for those remaining will be increased.
3. See A. Enthoven, *Theory and Practice of Managed Competition in Health Care Finance* (Amsterdam: North Holland, 1988); and J. P. Newhouse, "Is Competition the Answer?" *Journal of Health Economics* 1, no. 1 (1982): 109–15.
4. B. Dowd and R. Feldman, "Biased Selection in Twin Cities Health Plans," in *Advances in Health Economics and Health Services Research: Biased Selection in Health Care Markets,* ed. R.M. Scheffler and L.F. Rossiter (Greenwich, CT: JAI Press, 1985), 253.
5. This is often referred to as "risk segmentation." If an employer offers multiple health plans, it is likely that the formation of groups of employees who choose alternative plans will result in biased selection (i.e., an unequal segmentation of health risks among the plans).
6. This basis of comparison is established from the health plan's perspective. For example, for a community-rated HMO, the experience of a subgroup

of enrollees from a particular group would be compared to the HMO's planwide experience to determine if favorable or adverse selection had occurred. For experience-rated plans or plans that use group-specific premiums (e.g., community rating by class), the subgroup experience would be compared to the basis used for determination of the group-specific premium.

7. According to Luft, "[a]dverse selection arises from two decision-making processes: the enrollment decision made by the individual employee, and the overall design of a health benefits program by an employer. On the employee side, there are three factors which influence the choice of health plan: (1) economic factors, primarily income, as defining the ability to pay for services; (2) health risk factors, including family size, sex and age, current health status, and prior use of services; and (3) individual attitudes and values related to use of health services and to preferred type of care and preferred setting to receive treatment." See H. S. Luft, J. B. Trauner, and S.C. Maerki, "Adverse Selection in a Large, Multi-Option Health Benefits Program: A Case Study of the California Public Employees' Retirement System," in *Biased Selection in Health Care Markets,* ed. R.B. Scheffler and L. F. Rossiter (Greenwich, CT: JAI Press, 1985), 198.

8. Another factor affecting selection patterns is the length of time that each health plan has been offered by the employer. For example, if an employer has offered a single health plan for many years, and a new plan is offered to the group for the first time in conjunction with the old plan, then employees will have to make a conscious choice to change to the new plan. The resulting selection effects for the new plan and the old plan will depend on (1) the relative incentives offered by the two plans in terms of benefit levels, cost-sharing requirements, provider panels, and premium rates, and (2) the characteristics of the group of "switchers" to the new plan. See J. Neipp and R. Zeckhauser, "Persistence in the Choice of Health Plans," in *Biased Selection in Health Care Markets,* ed. R.M. Scheffler and L.F. Rossiter (Greenwich, CT: JAI Press, 1985).

9. For example, some indemnity policies have limited coverage of maternity care, and well-baby services are excluded. In contrast, most HMOs cover maternity care and well-baby services in full, with minimal cost sharing, if any.

10. The composition of provider panels of alternative health plans also affects selection bias. Indemnity plans with freedom of choice of physician will be more likely to suffer adverse selection in a multiple choice situation. In contrast, closed-panel HMOs offering a limited set of physician providers will be more likely to enroll low-risk persons without an established physician relationship.

11. See S. H. Long, R. F. Settle, and C. W. Wrightson, "Employee Premiums, Availability of Alternative Plans, and HMO Disenrollment," *Medical Care* 26 (1988): 927–38.

12. The discussion in this section takes the perspective of a health plan that

must set premium rates. In contrast, the perspective of an employer may be very different. For example, if the employer is self-insured or has an experience-rated indemnity plan, the main concern is whether HMOs, PPOs, or alternative health plans are enrolling the healthiest employees and forcing the employer's indemnity plan into an adverse selection "death spiral" (i.e., the premiums of the indemnity plan are forced higher and higher as lower-risk persons leave the plan over time and only high-risk persons remain).

13. P. Shepherd and A. C. Webster, *Selection of Risks* (Chicago, IL: Society of Actuaries, 1957), 2–3.

14. G. R. Wilensky and L. F. Rossiter, "Patient Self-Selection in HMOs," *Health Affairs* 5, no. 1 (1986): 67.

15. W. P. Welch, "Medicare Capitation Payments to HMOs in Light of Regression toward the Mean in Health Care Costs," in *Biased Selection in Health Care Markets,* ed. R. M. Scheffler and L. F. Rossiter (Greenwich, CT: JAI Press, 1985), 76.

16. With respect to explicit strategies to "skim," the author's opinion, based on consulting experience and first-hand knowledge of several major plans in the industry, is that few HMOs "play the selection game" consciously and with a primary goal of obtaining low-risk enrollees.

17. The utilization experience of persons choosing HMOs is analyzed in M. Jackson-Beck and J. Kleinman, "Evidence for Self-Selection Among Health Maintenance Organization Enrollees," *The Journal of the American Medical Association* 250, no. 20 (1983): 2826–29. The analysis is limited to employer groups that offered HMOs for the first time. The authors found that the persons who joined the HMOs had significantly lower prior utilization than the persons who continued in the employers' indemnity plans. This result is referred to as the "Jackson-Beck phenomenon" in this book.

18. See P. Shepherd and A. C. Webster, "Introduction to Selection," Chapter 1 in *Selection of Risks* (Chicago, IL: Society of Actuaries, 1957).

19. See A. M. Lilienfeld and D. E. Lilienfeld, *Foundations of Epidemiology* (New York: Oxford University Press, 1980), 199–205.

20. See G.S. Maddala, "Models with Self-Selectivity," Chapter 9 in *Limited-Dependent and Qualitative Variables in Econometrics* (New York: Cambridge University Press, 1983); L. F. Lee, "Some Approaches to the Correction of Selectivity Bias," *Review of Economic Studies* 49 (1982): 355–72; L. F. Lee, "Generalized Econometric Models with Selectivity," *Econometrica* 51 (1983): 507–12; and G. S. Maddala, "A Survey of the Literature on Selectivity Bias as It Pertains to Health Care Markets," in *Biased Selection in Health Care Markets,* ed. R. M. Scheffler and L. F. Rossiter (Greenwich, CT: JAI Press, 1985).

21. See F. T. O'Grady, ed., *Individual Health Insurance* (Chicago, IL: Society of Actuaries, 1988); and E. L. Bartleson, *Health Insurance* (Chicago, IL: Society of Actuaries, 1968).

22. This literature review is more of an overview than an in-depth evaluation

of the comprehensive literature that exists on this topic. For other reviews of the literature, see R. M. Scheffler and L. F. Rossiter, eds., *Biased Selection in Health Care Markets* (Greenwich, CT: JAI Press, 1985); H. S. Luft, *Health Maintenance Organizations: Dimensions of Performance* (New York: John Wiley, 1981); and H. S. Luft and R. H. Miller, "Patient Selection in a Competitive Health Care System," *Health Affairs* 7, no. 3 (1988): 97–119.

23. See P. M. Densen, E. Balamuth, and S. Shapiro, *Prepaid Medical Care and Hospital Utilization* (Chicago: American Hospital Association, 1958); P. M. Densen, N. Deardorff, and E. Balamuth, "Longitudinal Analyses of Four Years of Experience of a Prepaid Comprehensive Medical Care Plan," *Milbank Memorial Fund Quarterly* 36, no. 1 (1958): 5–45; P. M. Densen, S. Shapiro, and M. Einhorn, "Concerning High and Low Utilizers of Service in a Medical Care Plan, and the Persistence of Utilization Levels Over a Three Year Period," *Milbank Memorial Fund Quarterly* 37, no. 3 (1959): 217–50; A. Donabedian, "An Evaluation of Prepaid Group Practice," *Inquiry* 6, no. 3 (1969): 3–27; M. I. Roemer and W. Shonick, "HMO Performance: The Recent Evidence," *Milbank Memorial Fund Quarterly* 51, no. 3 (1973): 271–317; M. I. Roemer et al., *Health Insurance Effects: Services, Expenditures, and Attitudes under Three Types of Plans* (Ann Arbor, MI: University of Michigan School of Public Health, 1972); S. Shapiro, L. Weiner, and P. Densen, "Comparison of Prematurity and Perinatal Mortality in a General Population and in the Population of a Prepaid Group Practice Medical Care Plan," *American Journal of Public Health* 48, no. 2 (1958): 170–85; and S. Shapiro et al., "Further Observations on Prematurity and Perinatal Mortality in a General Population and in the Population of a Prepaid Group Practice Medical Care Plan," *American Journal of Public Health* 50, no. 9 (1960): 1304–17.

24. See S. E. Berki et al., "Enrollment Choice in a Multi-HMO Setting: The Roles of Health Risk, Financial Vulnerability, and Access to Care," *Medical Care* 15, no. 2 (1977): 95–114; S. E. Berki et al., "Enrollment Choice in Different Types of HMOs: A Multivariate Analysis," *Medical Care* 16, no. 8 (1978): 682–97; S. E. Berki et al., "Health Concern, HMO Enrollment, and Preventive Care Use," *Journal of Community Health* 3, no. 1 (1977): 3–31; T. W. Bice, "Risk Vulnerability and Enrollment in a Prepaid Group Practice," *Medical Care* 13, no. 8 (1975): 698–703; D. Mechanic, "The Organization of Medical Practice and Practice Orientation Among Physicians in Prepaid and Nonprepaid Primary Care Settings," *Medical Care* 13, no. 3 (1975): 189–204; D. Mechanic, N. Weiss, and P. D. Cleary, "The Growth of HMOs: Issues of Enrollment and Disenrollment," *Medical Care* 21, no. 3 (1983): 338; A. Scitovsky, N. McCall, and L. Benham, "Factors Affecting the Choice between Two Prepaid Plans," *Medical Care* 16, no. 8 (1978): 660–81; L. J. Wollstadt, S. Shapiro, and T. W. Bice, "Disenrollment from a Prepaid Group Practice: An Actuarial and Demographic Description," *Inquiry* 15, no. 2 (1978): 142–50. Addi-

tional references are listed at the end of this chapter. A comprehensive review of the literature prior to 1981 can be found in H. S. Luft, *Health Maintenance Organizations: Dimensions of Performance* (New York: John Wiley and Sons, 1981).

25. Luft, *Health Maintenance Organizations,* Chapter 3.

26. K. Wintringham, "Impact of Step-Rating and Price Sensitivity on Disenrollment and Risk Selection: The Experience of a Group Practice HMO," *The Group Health Journal,* Summer 1982; and W. E. Gold, "Predicting HMO Disenrollment Behavior: Results of a Study of Demographic and Behavioral Characteristics of HMO Members," *Proceedings of the 1981 Group Health Institute* (Washington, DC: Group Health Association of America, 1982).

27. P. Eggers, "Risk Differential between Medicare Beneficiaries Enrolled and Not Enrolled in an HMO," *Health Care Financing Review* 1, no. 3 (1980): 91; P. Eggers and R. Prihoda, "Pre-Enrollment Reimbursement Patterns of Medicare Beneficiaries Enrolled in 'At-Risk' HMOs," *Health Care Financing Review* 4, no. 1 (1982): 55.

28. J. R. Price, J. W. Mays, and G. R. Trapnell, "Stability in the Federal Employees Health Benefits Program," *Journal of Health Economics* 2, no. 3 (1983): 207–23; J. R. Price and J. W. Mays, "Biased Selection in the Federal Employees Health Benefits Program," *Inquiry* 22, no. 1 (1985): 67–77; J. R. Price, and J. W. Mays, "Selection and the Competitive Standing of Health Plans in a Multiple-Choice, Multiple-Insurer Market," in *Biased Selection in Health Care Markets,* ed. R. M. Scheffler and L. F. Rossiter (Greenwich, CT: JAI Press, 1985).

29. M. Jackson-Beeck and J. H. Kleinman, "Evidence for Self-Selection among Health Maintenance Organization Enrollees," *Journal of the American Medical Association* 250, no. 20 (1983): 2826–29.

30. Scheffler and Rossiter, eds., *Biased Selection in Health Care Markets.*

31. Wilensky and Rossiter, "Patient Self-Selection in HMOs."

32. W. P. Welch, "Regression toward the Mean in Medical Care Costs: Implications for Biased Selection in HMOs," *Medical Care* 23, no. 11 (1985): 1234.

33. J. Lubitz, J. Beebe, and G. Riley, "Improving the Medicare HMO Payment Formula to Deal with Biased Selection," in *Biased Selection in Health Care Markets,* ed. R.M. Scheffler and L.F. Rossiter (Greenwich, CT: JAI Press, 1985).

34. J. C. Beebe, "Medicare Reimbursement and Regression to the Mean," *Health Care Financing Review* 9, no. 3 (1988): 9–22.

35. W. Wrightson, J. Gennardi, and S. Stephens, "Demographic and Utilization Characteristics of HMO Disenrollees," *GHAA Journal* 8 (1987): 23.

36. K. M. Langwell and J. P. Hadley, *National Evaluation of the Medicare Competition Demonstrations: Summary Report,* prepared under Contract No. 500-83-0047 for the Health Care Financing Administration, Mathematica Policy Research, Princeton, NJ, 31 January 1989.

37. D. A. Freund and F. Neuschler, "Overview of Medicaid Capitation and Case-Management Initiatives," *Health Care Financing Review,* 1986 Annual Supplement: 21–30; D. A. Freund, "Competitive Health Plans and Alternative Payment Arrangements for Physicians in the United States: Public Sector Examples," *Health Policy* 7 (1987): 163.
38. K. Wintringham and T. W. Bice, "Effects of Turnover on Use of Services by Medicaid Beneficiaries in a Health Maintenance Organization," in *Proceedings of the 1985 Group Health Institute* (Washington, DC: Group Health Association of America, June 1985).
39. H. S. Luft, "Compensating for Biased Selection in Health Insurance," *Milbank Memorial Fund Quarterly/Health and Society* 60, no. 2(1982): 268.
40. A. C. Enthoven, "Managed Competition: An Agenda for Action," *Health Affairs* 7, no. 3 (1988): 25–47.
41. F. J. Hellinger, "Selection Bias in Health Maintenance Organizations: Analysis of Recent Evidence," *Health Care Financing Review* 9, no. 2(1987): 55; and H. S. Luft and R. H. Miller, "Patient Selection in a Competitive Health Care System," *Health Affairs* 7, no. 3(1988): 97–119.
42. Hellinger, "Selection Bias in Health Maintenance Organizations."
43. H. S. Luft and R. H. Miller, "Patient Selection in a Competitive Health Care System," *Health Affairs* 7, no. 3(1988): 97–119.
44. M. Jackson-Beeck and J. H. Kleinman, "Evidence for Self-Selection among Health Maintenance Organization Enrollees," *Journal of the American Medical Association* 250, no. 20(1983): 2826.
45. R. Brown, "Biased Selection in the Medicare Competition Demonstration," prepared under Contract No. 500-83-0047 from the Health Care Financing Administration, Mathematica Policy Research, Princeton, NJ, February 1987.
46. G. C. Halvorson, and P. Stix, "Hospital Use by New and Continuing HMO Enrollees," *HMO Practice* 2, no. 3(1988): 97–100.
47. This phenomenon has been termed "selection deterioration" and has been explored in depth by Price and Mays in their studies of the Federal Employees Health Benefits Program (see in note 28 above).
48. P. Eggers, "Risk Differential between Medicare Beneficiaries Enrolled and Not Enrolled in an HMO," *Health Care Financing Review* 1, no. 3(1980): 91; and P. Eggers and R. Prihoda, "Pre-Enrollment Reimbursement Patterns of Medicare Beneficiaries Enrolled in 'At Risk' HMOs," *Health Care Financing Review* 4, no. 1(1982): 55.
49. Wintringham and Bice, "Effects of Turnover on Use of Service."
50. As reported in J. Gabel et al., "Employer-Sponsored Health Insurance in America: Preliminary Results from the 1988 Survey," (Washington, DC: Health Insurance Association of America, January 1989), approximately 30 percent of employers had no increase in health premiums from spring 1987 to spring 1988. This occurred during a period of relatively strong increases in health premiums in general.

51. They may also be reacting to changing prices, especially out-of-pocket premiums.
52. See Welch, "Medicare Capitation Payments to HMOs in Light of Regression toward the Mean"; J. C. Beebe, "Medicare Reimbursement and Regression to the Mean," *Health Care Financing Review* 9, no. 3 (1988): 9; G. Anderson and J. Knickman, "Patterns of Expenditures among High Utilizers of Medical Care Services," *Medical Care* 22, no. 2(1984): 143; G. Anderson and J. Knickman, "Adverse Selection under a Voucher System: Grouping Medicare Recipients by Level of Expenditure," *Inquiry* 21, no. 2(1984): 135; U.S. Congressional Budget Office, *Catastrophic Medical Expenses: Patterns on the Non-Elderly, Non-Poor Population* (Washington, DC: Congressional Budget Office, December 1982); and G. Riley, E. Rabey, and J. Kasper, "Biased Selection and Regression toward the Mean in Three Medicare HMO Demonstrations: A Survival Analysis of Enrollees and Disenrollees," *Medical Care* 27, no. 4(1989): 337.
53. Welch, "Medicare Capitation Payments to HMOs in Light of Regression toward the Mean."
54. See Eggers and Prihoda, "Pre-Enrollment Reimbursement Patterns"; and Jackson-Beeck and Kleinman, "Evidence for Self-Selection."
55. See Anderson and Knickman, "Patterns of Expenditures among High Utilizers of Medical Care Services"; and U.S. Congressional Budget Office, *Catastrophic Medical Expenses.*
56. In general, my preference is for the individual employer group to serve as the basic unit of analysis (or other appropriately defined subgroup for non-commercial group cases like Medicare and Medicaid). In essence, the individual employer group is where all of the important variables converge. For example, it is the setting where an individual's choice of health plan is made. It is also a unique point of confluence of "macro" variables, such as the group-specific variables (number of options, premium rates, benefits, penetration), plan-specific variables (model type, age, size, providers), and competitive market area variables. Thus, the dynamics and history of each group are unique, and the outcome of every open enrollment competition is a function of both the "micro" individual-level variables and the "macro" variables. In order to have a complete understanding of selection effects for HMOs (or, more generally, in multiple-option health benefits programs), it is necessary to understand the dynamics at the group-specific level. Therefore, the individual employer group appears to be the most appropriate "unit of analysis."
57. For example, if a group has a two-tier premium rate structure (separate rates for singles and families), then it may be more difficult to determine the selection bias and cost implications of different enrollment patterns. Consider a 25-year-old married male subscriber (with spouse but no children) who switches from the indemnity plan to the HMO (assume that both adults are healthy and have no chronic conditions). For comparison, consider a

40-year-old male subscriber in the indemnity plan, who has a 39-year-old spouse (with a minor chronic condition) and an 18-year-old daughter living at home.

In the year prior to choice, there are no costs (fee-for-service claims) for the family unit with the 25-year-old male subscriber, but the expenses for the 40-year-old male are equal to the indemnity plan's average cost per family subscriber. According to the methods of analysis used in many selection studies, the HMO would be judged to have received favorable selection by statistical analysis of all prechoice variables of interest.

Now consider the following scenario for the postchoice experience of both family units. In the year after the choice of health plan (postchoice period), the daughter leaves home and the expenses for the older subscriber's family is slightly below the average for the indemnity plan. In addition, the indemnity plan's cost experience for this family unit of two adults would be expected to remain fairly stable during the next five years.

In contrast, suppose that the 25-year-old subscriber and his wife have a baby during the next year (postchoice). This would result in (1) prenatal, obstetric, inpatient hospital, and postnatal services for the mother, (2) hospital nursery, well-baby, immunization, and sick-child services for the baby, and (3) possibly a few other office visits for both adults during the year. Under reasonable assumptions, the HMO's expenses for these services result in a loss ratio of 2.5 (the HMO's medical expenses are 2.5 times higher than the premium received for this family unit during the postchoice year), compared to a desired loss ratio of .90. If the newborn is premature or there are complications, then the costs to the HMO could increase significantly. In addition, the family size of this subscribing unit is now three instead of two, and this family unit represents increased risk/costs for the HMO for the next five years (expected costs that are significantly higher than the HMO's average), especially if the family has more children.

Although this example is hypothetical, it does illustrate the differences between the prospective and retrospective perspectives regarding biased selection for HMOs (and other health plans).

58. This section is based on discussions with Gordon Trapnell and David McKusick who were the head Medicare actuaries during the 1970s.
59. The initial proposals were in connection with the development of the 1972 amendments to Medicare.
60. See, for example, "HMOs Experience Favorable Selection," *Research Activities,* no. 104, Rockville, MD: National Center for Health Services Research, 1988), 1. Also, see Suggested Readings at the end of this chapter.

Suggested Readings

Beebe, James C. "Medicare Reimbursement and Regression to the Mean." *Health Care Financing Review* 9, no. 3(1988): 9.

Berki, S. E., and Ashcraft, Marie L. F. "HMO Enrollment: Who Joins What and Why: A Review of the Literature." *Milbank Memorial Fund Quarterly/ Health and Society* 58, no. 4(1980): 588.

Eggers, Paul, and Prihoda, Ronald. "Pre-Enrollment Reimbursement Patterns of Medicare Beneficiaries Enrolled in 'At Risk' HMOs." *Health Care Financing Review* 4, no. 1(1982): 55.

Enthoven, Alain C. "Managed Competition: An Agenda for Action." *Health Affairs* 7, no. 3(1988): 25.

Halvorson, George C. *How to Control Your Company's Health Costs.* Englewood Cliffs, NJ: Prentice-Hall, 1988.

Halvorson, George C., and Stix, Peter. "HMO Use by New and Continuing HMO Enrollees." *HMO Practice* 2, no. 3(1988): 58.

Hellinger, Fred J. "Selection Bias in Health Maintenance Organizations: Analysis of Recent Evidence." *Health Care Financing Review* 9, no. 2(1987): 55.

Jackson-Beeck, Marilyn, and Kleinman, John H. "Evidence for Self-Selection among Health Maintenance Organization Enrollees." *Journal of the American Medical Association* 250, no. 20(1983): 2826.

Long, Stephen H.; Settle, Russell F.; and Wrightson, Charles W. "Employee Premiums, Availability of Alternative Plans, and HMO Disenrollment." *Medical Care* no. 10(1988): 927.

Luft, Harold S. *Health Maintenance Organizations: Dimensions of Performance.* New York: John Wiley & Sons, 1981.

Welch, W. P. "Regression towards the Mean in Medical Care Costs, Implications for Biased Selection in Health Maintenance Organizations." *Medical Care* 23, no. 11(1985): 1234.

Wrightson, William; Genuardi, James; and Stephens, Sharman. "Demographic and Utilization Characteristics of HMO Disenrollees." *GHAA Journal* 8, no. 1(1987): 23.

Additional Readings

Selection Articles

Anderson, Gerard and Knickman, James. "Adverse Selection under a Voucher System: Grouping Medicare Recipients by Level of Expenditure." *Inquiry* 21, no. 2(1984): 135.

————. "Patterns of Expenditures among High Utilizers of Medical Care Services." *Medical Care* 22, no. 2(1984): 143.

Angermeier, Ingo. "Impact of Community Rating and Open Enrollment on a Prepaid Group Practice." *Inquiry* 13, no. 1(1976): 48.

Ashcraft, Marie; Penchansky, Roy; Berki, S. E.; Fortus, Robert; and Gray, John. "Expectations and Experience of HMO Enrollees after One Year: An

Analysis of Satisfaction, Utilization, and Costs." *Medical Care* 16, no. 1(1978): 14.

Blumberg, Mark S. "Health Status and Health Care Use by Type of Private Health Coverage." *Milbank Memorial Fund Quarterly/Health and Society* 58, no. 4(1980): 663.

————. "Risk Adjusting Health Care Outcomes: A Methodologic Review." *Medical Care Review* 43, no. 2(1986): 351.

Brown, R., et al. *Biased Selection in the Medicare Competition Demonstration.* Prepared by Mathematica Policy Research for the Health Care Financing Administration. Contract no. 500–83–0047. Department of Health and Human Services. February 1987.

Buchanan, Joan L., and Cretin, Shan. "Risk Selection of Families Electing HMO Membership." *Medical Care* 24, no. 1(1986): 39.

Dahlby, B. G. "Monopoly Versus Competition in an Insurance Market with Adverse Selection." *Journal of Risk and Insurance* 54, no. 2(1987): 325.

Densen, Paul M.; Deardorff, Neva R.; and Balamuth, Eve. "Longitudinal Analyses of Four Years of Experience of a Prepaid Comprehensive Medical Care Plan." *The Milbank Memorial Fund Quarterly* 36, no. 1(1958): 5.

Densen, Paul M.; Shapiro, Sam; and Einhorn, Marilyn. "Concerning High and Low Utilizers of Service in a Medical Care Plan, and the Persistence of Utilization Levels over a Three Year Period." *The Milbank Memorial Fund Quarterly* 37, no. 3(1959): 217.

Diehr, Paula; Martin, Diane P.; Price, Kurt F.; Friedlander, Lindy J.; Richardson, William C.; and Riedel, Donald C. "Use of Ambulatory Care Services in Three Provider Plans: Interactions between Patient Characteristics and Plans." *American Journal of Public Health* 74, no. 1(1984): 47.

Dowd, Bryan, and Feldman, Roger. "Biased Selection in Twin Cities Health Plans." In *Advances in Health Economics and Health Services Research,* edited by Richard M. Scheffler and Louis F. Rossiter, vol. 6. Greenwich, CT: JAI Press, 1985.

Eggers, Paul. "Risk Differential between Medicare Beneficiaries Enrolled and Not Enrolled in an HMO." *Health Care Financing Review* 1, no. 3(1980): 91.

Eggers, Paul, and Prihoda, Ronald. "Pre-Enrollment Reimbursement Patterns of Medicare Beneficiaries Enrolled in 'At Risk' HMOs." *Health Care Financing Review* 4, no. 1(1982): 55.

Ellis, Randall P. "The Effect of Prior Year Health Expenditures on Health Coverage Plan Choice." In *Advances in Health Economics and Health Services Research,* edited by Richard M. Scheffler and Louis F. Rossiter, vol. 6. Greenwich, CT: JAI Press, 1985.

Farley, Pamela J., and Monheit, Alan C. "Selectivity in the Demand for Health Insurance and Health Care." In *Advances in Health Economics and Health Services Research,* edited by Richard M. Scheffler and Louis F. Rossiter, vol. 6. Greenwich, CT: JAI Press, 1985.

Feldman, Roger D., and Dowd, Bryan E. "Simulation of a Health Insurance

Market with Adverse Selection." *Operations Research* 30, no. 6(1982): 1027.

Fuller, Norman; Patera, Margaret; and Koziol, Krista. "Medicaid Utilization of Services in a Prepaid Group Practice Health Plan." *Medical Care* 15, no. 9(1977): 705.

Gaus, Clifton R.; Cooper, Barbara S.; and Hirschman, Constance G. "Contrast in HMO and Fee-For-Service Performance." *Social Security Bulletin* 39, no. 3(1976): 3.

Gold, Marsha. "Competition within the Federal Employees Health Benefits Program: Analysis of the Empirical Evidence." Office of the Assistant Secretary for Planning and Evaluation. U.S. Department of Health and Human Services, November 1981.

Greenlick, Merwyn R. "An Investigation of Selection Bias in an HMO Enrollment Experiment." *The Group Health Journal* 5, no. 1(1984): 22.

Jensen, Gail; Feldman, Roger; and Dowd, Bryan. "Corporate Benefit Policies and Health Insurance Costs." *Journal of Health Economics* 3, no. 3(1984): 275.

Lairson, David R., and Herd, J. Alan. "The Role of Health Practices, Health Status, and Prior Health Care Claims in HMO Selection Bias." *Inquiry* 24, no. 3(Fall 1987): 276.

Langwell, Kathryn M., and Hadley, James P. *National Evaluation of the Medicare Competition Demonstrations: Summary Report.* Prepared by Mathematica Policy Research for the Health Care Financing Administration. Contract No. 500-83-0047. Department of Health and Human Services, 31 January 1989.

Lubitz, James; Beebe, James; and Riley, Gerald. "Improving the Medicare HMO Payment Formula to Deal with Biased Selection." In *Advances in Health Economics and Health Services Research,* edited by Richard M. Scheffler and Louis F. Rossiter, vol. 6. Greenwich, CT: JAI Press, 1985.

Luft, Harold S. "Compensating for Biased Selection in Health Insurance." *Milbank Memorial Fund Quarterly* 64, no. 4(1986): 566.

————. "Health Maintenance Organizations and the Rationing of Medical Care." *Milbank Memorial Fund Quarterly/Health and Society* 60, no. 2(1982): 268.

Luft, Harold S., and Miller, Robert H. "Patient Selection in a Competitive Health Care System." *Health Affairs* 7, no. 3(1988): 97.

Luft, Harold S.; Trauner, Joan B.; and Maerki, Susan C. "Adverse Selection in a Large, Multiple-Option Health Benefits Program: A Case Study of the California Public Employees' Retirement System." In *Advances in Health Economics and Health Services Research,* edited by Richard M. Scheffler and Louis F. Rossiter, vol. 6. Greenwich, CT: JAI Press, 1985.

Maddala, G. S., "A Survey of the Literature on Selectivity Bias as It Pertains to Health Care Markets." In *Advances in Health Economics and Health Services Research,* edited by Richard M. Scheffler and Louis F. Rossiter, vol. 6. Greenwich, CT: JAI Press, 1985.

Manning, Willard G.; Leibowitz, Arleen; Goldberg, George A.; Rogers, William H.; and Newhouse, Joseph P. "A Controlled Trial of the Effect of a Prepaid Group Practice on Use of Services." *New England Journal of Medicine* 310, no. 23(1984): 1505.

Marcus, Alfred C. "Mode of Payment as a Predictor of Health Status, Use of Health Services and Preventive Health Behavior: A Report from the Los Angeles Health Survey." *Medical Care* 19, no. 10(1981): 995.

McCall, Nelda, and Wai, Hoi. "An Analysis of the Use of Medicare Services by the Continuously Enrolled Aged." *Medical Care* 21, no. 6(1983): 567.

McClure, Walter. "On the Research Status of Risk-Adjusted Capitation Rates." *Inquiry* 21, no. 3(1984): 205.

McFarland, Bentson H.; Freeborn, Donald K.; Mullooly, John P.; and Pope, Clyde R. "Utilization Patterns and Mortality of HMO Enrollees." *Medical Care* 24, no. 3(1986): 200.

Newhouse, Joseph P. "Cream Skimming, Asymmetric Information, and a Competitive Insurance Market." *Journal of Health Economics* 3, no. 1(1984): 97.

Nycz, Gregory R.; Wenzel, Frederick J.; Lohrenz, Francis N.; and Mitchell, John H. "Composition of the Subscribers in a Rural Prepaid Group Practice Plan." *Public Health Reports* 91, no. 6(1976): 504.

Pauly, Mark V. "Is Cream-Skimming a Problem for the Competitive Medical Market?" *Journal of Health Economics* 3, no. 1(1984): 87.

Perkoff, Gerald T.; Kahn, Lawrence; and Haas, Phillip J. "The Effects of an Experimental Prepaid Group Practice on Medical Care Utilization and Cost." *Medical Care* 14, no. 5(1976): 432.

Price, James R., and Mays, James W. "Biased Selection in the Federal Employees Health Benefits Program." *Inquiry* 22, no. 1(1985): 67.

———. "Selection and the Competitive Standing of Health Plans in a Multiple-Choice, Multiple-Insurer Market." In *Advances in Health Economics and Health Services Research,* edited by Richard M. Scheffler and Louis F. Rossiter, vol. 6. Greenwich, CT: JAI Press, 1985.

Price, James R.; Mays, James W.; and Trapnell, Gordon R. "Stability in the Federal Employees Health Benefits Program." *Journal of Health Economics* 2, no. 3(1983): 207.

Roemer, Milton I. "Sickness Absenteeism in Members of Health Maintenance Organizations and Open-Market Health Insurance Plans." *Medical Care* 20, no. 11(1982): 1140.

Roghmann, Klaus J.; Sorensen, Andrew A.; and Wells, Sandra M. "Hospitalizations in Three Competing HMOs during Their First Two Years, A Cohort Study of the Rochester Experience." *Group Health Journal* 1, no. 1(1980): 26.

Rossiter, Louis F., and Freund, Deborah A. "Adverse Selection in the Market for Health Insurance: A Simultaneous Logit Model." Paper presented at the annual meeting of the American Public Health Association, November 1979.

Rossiter, Louis F.; Nelson, Lyle M.; and Adamache, Killard W. "Service Use and Costs for Medicare Beneficiaries in Risk-Based HMOs and CMPs." *American Journal of Public Health* 78, no. 8(1988): 937.

Schuttinga, James A.; Falik, Marilyn; and Steinwald, Bruce. "Health Plan Selection in the Federal Employees Health Benefits Program." *Journal of Health Politics, Policy and Law* 10, no. 1(1985): 119.

Sorensen, Andrew A.; Saward, Ernest W.; and Wersinger, Richard P. "The Demise of an Individual Practice Association: A Case Study of Health Watch." *Inquiry* 17, no. 3(1980): 244.

Sorensen, Andrew A.; Wersinger, Richard; Saward, Ernest; and Katz, Phillip. "Health Status, Medical Care Utilization, and Cost Experience of Prepaid Group Practice and Fee-For-Service Populations. An Analysis of the Rochester, New York Market." *Group Health Journal* 2, no. 1(1981): 4.

Thomas, J. William, and Lichtenstein, Richard. "Including Health Status in Medicare's Adjusted Average Per Capita Cost Capitation Formula." *Medical Care* 24, no. 3(1986): 259.

Thomas, J. William; Lichtenstein, Richard; Wyszewianski, Leon; and Berki, S. E. "Increasing Medicare Enrollment in HMOs: The Need for Capitation Rates Adjusted for Health Status." *Inquiry* 20, no. 3(1983): 227.

Unger, Walter. "Largest Competitive Health Program Faces a Crisis." *Hospital Financial Management Journal* 12, no. 3(1982): 18–30.

Welch, W. P. "Health Care Utilization in HMOs, Results from Two National Samples." *Journal of Health Economics* 4, no. 4(1985): 293.

————. "HMO Enrollment: A Study of Market Forces and Regulations." *Journal of Health Politics, Policy and Law* 8, no. 4(1984): 743.

————. "Medicare Capitation Payments to HMOs in Light of Regression Towards the Mean in Health Care Costs." In *Advances in Health Economics and Health Services Research*, edited by Richard M. Scheffler and Louis F. Rossiter, vol. 6. Greenwich, CT: JAI Press, 1985.

Welch, W. P.; Frank, Richard G.; and Diehr, Paula. "Health Care Costs in Health Maintenance Organizations." In *Advances in Health Economics and Health Services Research*, edited by Richard M. Scheffler and Louis F. Rossiter, vol. 6. Greenwich, CT: JAI Press, 1985.

Wersinger, Richard; Roghmann, Klaus J.; Gavett, J. William; and Wells, Sandra M. "Inpatient Hospital Utilization in Three Prepaid Comprehensive Health Care Plans Compared with a Regular Blue Cross Plan." *Medical Care* 14, no. 9(1976): 721.

Wilensky, Gail R., and Rossiter, Louis F. "Patient Self-Selection in HMOs." *Health Affairs* 5, no. 1(1986): 66.

HMO Enrollment/Choice

Acito, Franklin. "Consumer Decision Making and Health Maintenance Organizations: A Review." *Medical Care* 16, no. 1(1978): 1.

Barr, Judith K.; Schachter, Mark; and Visnyey, Noemi. "Expectations and Experience in an HMO: Consumer Perspectives." Paper presented at the annual meeting of the American Public Health Association, 13–17 November 1983.

Bashshur, Rashid L., and Metzner, Charles A. "Vulnerability to Risk and Awareness of Dual Choice of Health Insurance Plan." *Health Services Research* 5, no. 2(1970): 106.

Benjamini, Yael, and Benjamini, Yoav. "The Choice among Medical Insurance Plans." *American Economic Review* 76, no. 1(1986): 221.

Berki, S. E.; Ashcraft, Marie; Penchansky, Roy; and Fortus, Robert. "Enrollment Choice in a Multi-HMO Setting: The Roles of Health Risk, Financial Vulnerability, and Access to Care." *Medical Care* 15, no. 2(1977): 95.

Berki, S. E.; Penchansky, Roy; Fortus, Robert; and Ashcraft, Marie. "Enrollment Choices in Different Types of HMOs." *Medical Care* 16, no. 8(1978): 682.

Bice, Thomas W. "Risk Vulnerability and Enrollment in a Prepaid Group Practice." *Medical Care* 13, no. 8(1975): 698.

Bonanno, James Bautz, and Wetle, Terrie. "HMO Enrollment of Medicare Recipients: An Analysis of Incentives and Barriers." *Journal of Health Politics, Policy and Law* 9, no. 1(1984): 41.

Brown, R., and Langwell, K. "Enrollment Patterns in Medicare HMOs: Implications for Access to Care." In *Advances in Health Economics and Health Services Research,* edited by Richard M. Scheffler and Louis F. Rossiter, vol. 9. Greenwich, CT: JAI Press, 1988.

Budenstein, Mary Jane, and Hennelly, Virginia D. "Deterrents to Family Enrollment in a Prepaid Group Practice." *Medical Care* 18, no. 6(1980): 649.

Ellis, Randall P. "The Effect of Prior-Year Health Expenditures on Health Coverage Plan Choice." In *Advances in Health Economics and Health Services Research,* edited by Richard M. Scheffler and Louis F. Rossiter, vol. 6 Greenwich, CT: JAI Press, 1985.

Friedman, Bernard. "Risk Aversion and the Consumer Choice of Health Insurance Option." *The Review of Economics and Statistics* (1973): 209–214.

Galiher, Claudia B., and Costa, Marjorie A. "Consumer Acceptance of HMOs." *Public Health Reports* 90, no. 2(1975): 106.

Gaus, C. "Who Enrolls in a Prepaid Group Practice: The Columbia Experience." *Johns Hopkins Medicine* 128(1971): 9.

Hershey, John C.; Kunreuther, Howard; Schwartz, J. Sanford; and Williams, Sankey V. "Health Insurance under Competition: Would People Choose What Is Expected?" *Inquiry* 21, no. 4(1984): 349.

Homan, Rick K.; Glandon, Gerald L.; and Counte, Michael A. "Perceived Risk: The Link to Plan Selection and Future Utilization." *The Journal of Risk and Insurance* 56, no. 1(1989): 67.

Juba, David A.; Lave, Judity R.; and Shaddy, Jonathan. "An Analysis of the Choice of Health Benefits Plans." *Inquiry* 17, no. 1(1980): 62.

McGuire, Thomas G. "Price and Membership in a Prepaid Group Medical Practice." *Medical Care* 19, no. 2(1981): 172.

Mechanic, David. "Consumer Choice among Health Insurance Options." *Health Affairs* 8, no. 1(1989): 138–48.

Merrill, Jeffrey; Jackson, Catherine; and Reuter, James. "Factors That Affect the HMO Enrollment Decision: A Tale of Two Cities." *Inquiry* 22, no. 4(1985):388.

Metzner, Charles A., and Bashshur, Rashid L. "Factors Associated with Choice of Health Care Plans." *Journal of Health and Social Behavior* 8, no. 4(1967):291.

Moustafa, A. Taher; Hopkins, Carl E.; and Klein, Bonnie. "Determinants of Choice and Change of Health Insurance Plan." *Medical Care* 9, no. 1(1971): 32.

Neipp, Joachim, and Zeckhauser, Richard. "Persistence in the Choice of Health Plans." In *Advances in Health Economics and Health Services Research,* edited by Richard M. Scheffler and Louis F. Rossiter, vol. 6. Greenwich, CT: JAI Press, 1985.

Nelson, Lyle M.; Langwell, Kathryn M.; and Brown, Randall S. "Comparison of 'Rollovers' and 'Switchers' among Enrollees of Medicare HMOs." *GHAA Journal* 8, no. 2(1987/1988): 63.

Piontkowski, Dyan, and Butler, Lewis H. "Selection of Health Insurance by an Employee Group in Northern California." *American Journal of Public Health* 70, no. 3(1980: 274.

Roghmann, Klaus J.; Gavett, J. William; Sorensen, Andrew A.; Wells, Sandra; and Wersinger, Richard. "Who Chooses Prepaid Medical Care: Survey Results from Two Marketings of Three New Prepayment Plans." *Public Health Reports* 90, no. 6(1975): 516.

Rossiter, L., et al. *Analysis Report of Patient Satisfaction for Enrollees and Disenrollees in Medicare Risk-Based Plans.* Prepared by Mathematica Policy Research for the Health Care Financing Administration. Contract No. 500–83–0047. Department of Health and Human Services, May 1988.

Scitovsky, Anne A.; McCall, Nelda; and Benham, Lee. "Factors Affecting the Choice between Two Prepaid Plans." *Medical Care* 16, no. 8(1978): 660.

Tessler, Richard, and Mechanic, David. "Factors Affecting the Choice between Prepaid Group Practice and Alternative Insurance Programs." *Milbank Memorial Fund Quarterly/Health and Society* 53, no. 2(1975): 149.

Ullman, Ralph. "The HMO Enrollment Decision: A Transactions Analysis and Literature Review." Discussion Paper No. 1, University of Pennsylvania National Health Care Management Center, January 1979.

Walsh, Deborah J., and Lewis, Kenneth M. "Premium Costs and Employer Contributions as Factors in HMO Penetration." In *Proceedings of the 1982 Group Health Institute.* Washington, DC: Group Health Association of America, 1982.

Welch, W. P., and Frank, Richard G. "The Predictors of HMO Enrollee Populations: Results from a National Sample." *Inquiry* 23, no. 1(1986): 16.

Wolfson, Daniel B.; Bell, Christy W.; and Newbery, Denyse A. "Fallon's Senior Plan: A Summary of the Three Year Marketing Experience." *The Group Health Journal* 5, no. 1(1984): 4.

HMO Disenrollment

Baloff, Nicholas, and Griffith, Mary Jane. "Start-Up Utilization by Disenrollees: A Reply." *Medical Care* 20, no. 12(1982): 1243.

Boxerman, Stuart B., and Hennelly, Virgina D. "Determinants of Disenrollment: Implications for HMO Managers." *The Journal of Ambulatory Care Management* 6, no. 2(1983): 12–23.

Brown, R., et al. *Enrollment and Disenrollment in Medicare Competition Demonstration Plans: A Descriptive Analysis.* Prepared by Mathematica Policy Research for the Health Care Financing Administration. Contract No. 500–83–0047. Department of Health and Human Services, September 1986.

DesHarnais, Susan I. "Enrollment in and Disenrollment from Health Maintenance Organizations by Medicaid Recipients." *Health Care Financing Review* 6, no. 3(1985) 39.

Donaldson, Molla S.; Keith, Karla J.; Ott, John E.; and Pawlson, L. Gregory. "Linking Disenrollment with Dissatisfaction." In *Proceedings of the 1981 Group Health Institute.* Washington, DC: Group Health Association of America, 1981.

Dowd, Bryan E., and Kralewski, John. "Disenrollment Effects in Insurer-Based Utilization Studies: A Comment on Griffith and Baloff." *Medical Care* 20, no. 12(1982): 1241.

Forthofer, Ron N.; Glasser, Jay H.; and Light, Nancy. "Life Table Analysis of Membership Retention in an HMO." *Journal of Community Health* 5, no. 1(1979): 46.

Gold, William E. "Predicting HMO Disenrollment Behavior: Results of a Study of Demographic and Behavioral Characteristics of HMO Members." In *Proceedings of the 1981 Group Health Institute,* Washington, DC: Group Health Association of America, 1981.

Grazier, Kyle L.; Richardson, William C.; Martin, Diane P.; and Diehr, Paula. "Factors Affecting Choice of Health Care Plans." *Health Services Research* 20, no. 6, pt. 1(1986): 659.

Griffith, Mary Jane; Baloff, Nicholas; and Spitznagel, Edward L. "Utilization Patterns of Health Maintenance Organization Disenrollees." *Medical Care* 22, no. 9(1984): 827.

Hennelly, Virginia D., and Boxerman, Stuart B. "Disenrollment from a Prepaid Group Plan: A Multivariate Analysis." *Medical Care* 21, no. 12(1983): 1154.

————. "Managing Disenrollment in HMOs." In *Proceedings of the 1983 Group Health Institute.* Washington, DC: Group Health Association of America, 1983.

————. "Out-of-Plan Use and Disenrollment: Outgrowths of Dissatisfaction with a Prepaid Group Plan." *Medical Care* 21, no. 3(1983): 348.

Lewis, Kathleen. "Comparison of Use by Enrolled and Recently Disenrolled Populations in a Health Maintenance Organization." *Health Services Research* 19, no. 1(1984): 1.

Mechanic, David; Weiss, Norma; and Cleary, Paul D. "The Growth of HMOs: Issues of Enrollment and Disenrollment." *Medical Care* 21, no. 3(1983): 338.

Sorensen, Andrew A., and Wersinger, Richard P. "Factors Influencing Disenrollment from an HMO." *Medical Care* 19, no. 7(1981):766.

Stiefel, Matthew C.; Gardelius, David A.; and Hayami, Dawn E. "Selection Bias: A Comparison of Inpatient Utilization, Demographics, and Premiums for HMO 'Leavers', 'Stayers', and 'Joiners'." In *Proceedings of the 1984 Group Health Institute.* Washington, DC: Group Health Association of America, 1984.

Tucker, Anthony M., and Langwell, Kathryn. "Disenrollment Patterns in Medicare HMOs: A Preliminary Analysis." *GHAA Journal* 9, no. 1(1988): 22.

Welch, W. P. "HMO Enrollment and Medicaid: Survival Analysis with a Weibull Function." *Medical Care* 26, no. 1(1988): 45.

Wersinger, Richard P., and Sorensen, Andrew A. "Demographic Characteristics and Prior Utilization Experience of HMO Disenrollees Compared with Total Membership." *Medical Care* 20, no. 12(1982): 1188.

Wintringham, Karen. "Impact of Step-Rating and Price Sensitivity on Disenrollment and Risk Selection: The Experience of a Group Practice HMO." *The Group Health Journal* 3, no. 2(1982).

Wintringham, Karen, and Bice, Thomas W. "Effects of Turnover on Use of Services by Medicaid Beneficiaries in a Health Maintenance Organization." In *Proceedings of the 1985 Group Health Institute.* Washington, DC: Group Health Association of America, 1985.

Wollstadt, Loyd J.; Shapiro, Sam; and Bice, Thomas W. "Disenrollment from a Prepaid Group Practice: An Actuarial and Demographic Description." *Inquiry* 15, no. 2(1978): 142.

Medicare

Adamache, K., and Rossiter, L. "The Entry of HMOs into the Medicare Market: Implications for TEFRA's Mandate." *Inquiry* 23, no. 4(1986): 349.

Anderson, Gerard; Cantor, Joel; Steinberg, Earl P.; and Holloway, James. "Capitation Pricing: Adjusting for Prior Utilization and Physician Discretion." *Health Care Financing Review* 8, no. 2(1986): 27.

Anderson, Gerard, and Knickman, James. "Adverse Selection under a Voucher System: Grouping Medicare Recipients by Level of Expenditure." *Inquiry* 21, no. 2(1984): 135.

Ash, Arlene, and Ellis, Randall P. *Refining the Diagnostic Cost Group Model: A Proposed Modification to the AAPCC for HMO Reimbursement.* Prepared for the Health Care Financing Administration. HCFA Cooperative Agreement No. 18–C–98526/1–03. Department of Health and Human Services, February 1988.

Beebe, James; Lubitz, James; and Eggers, Paul. "Using Prior Utilization to

Determine Payments for Medicare Enrollees in Health Maintenance Organizations." *Health Care Financing Review* 6, no. 3(1985): 27.

Bonanno, James Bautz, and Wetle, Terrie. "HMO Enrollment of Medicare Recipients: An Analysis of Incentives and Barriers." *Journal of Health Politics, Policy and Law* 9, no. 1(1984): 41.

Brown, R., and Langwell, K. "Enrollment Patterns in Medicare HMOs: Implications for Access to Care." In *Advances in Health Economics and Health Services Research,* edited by Richard M. Scheffler and Louis F. Rossiter, vol. 9. Greenwich, CT: JAI Press, 1988.

Brown, R., et al. *Enrollment and Disenrollment in Medicare Competition Demonstration Plans: A Descriptive Analysis.* Prepared by Mathematica Policy Research for the Health Care Financing Administration. Contract No. 500–83–0047. Department of Health and Human Services, September 1986.

Brown, R., et al. *Biased Selection in the Medicare Competition Demonstration.* Prepared by Mathematica Policy Research for the Health Care Financing Administration. Contract No. 500–83–0047. Department of Health and Human Services, February 1987.

Eggers, Paul. "Risk Differential between Medicare Beneficiaries Enrolled and Not Enrolled in an HMO." *Health Care Financing Review* 1, no. 3 (1980): 91.

Ginsburg, P. B. "A New Payment System for Risk-Based Programs under Medicare." Paper presented at HCFA Conference, Risk-Based Payments for Public Programs, October 1987, Williamsburg, Virginia.

Greenberg, Jay; Leutz, Walter; Greenlick, Merwyn; Malone, Joelyn; Ervin, Sam; and Kodner, Dennis. "The Social HMO Demonstration: Early Experience." *Health Affairs* 7, no. 3(1988): 66.

Greenlick, Merwyn P. "Comments on Medicare Capitation Payments to HMOs." In *Advances in Health Economics and Health Services Research,* edited by Richard M. Scheffler and Louis F. Rossiter, vol. 6. Greenwich, CT: JAI Press, 1985.

Greenlick, M.; Lamb, S.; Carpenter, T.; Fischer, T.; Marks, S.; and Cooper, W. "Kaiser-Permanente's Medicare Plus Project: A Successful Medicare Prospective Payment Demonstration." *Health Care Financing Review* 4, no. 4(1983): 85.

Harrington, Charlene; Newcomer, Robert J.; and Friedlob, Alan. *Social Health Maintenance Organization Demonstration Evaluation—Report on the First Thirty Months.* Institute for Health and Aging, University of California, San Francisco, September 1987.

Langwell, Kathryn M., and Hadley, James P. "Marketing Strategies for Medicare HMOs: Experience from 20 Demonstration Plans." In *New Health Care Systems: HMOs and Beyond.* Washington, DC: Group Health Association of America, 1986.

————. *National Evaluation of the Medicare Competition Demonstrations: Summary Report.* Prepared by Mathematica Policy Research for the Health Care Financing Administration. Contract No. 500–83–0047. Department of Health and Human Services, 31 January 1989.

Langwell, Kathryn M.; Rossiter, Louis; Brown, Randall; Nelson, Lyle; Nelson, Shelly; and Berman, Katherine. "Early Experience of Health Maintenance Organizations under Medicare Competition Demonstrations." *Health Care Financing Review* 8, no. 3(1987): 37–55.

Lichtenstein, Richard, and Thomas, J. William. "Including a Measure of Health Status in Medicare's Health Maintenance Organization Capitation Formula: Reliability Issues." *Medical Care* 25, no. 2(1987): 100.

Lubitz, James. "Health Status Adjustments for Medicare Capitation." *Inquiry* 24, no. 4(1987): 362.

Lubitz, James; Beebe, James; and Riley, Gerald. "Improving the Medicare HMO Payment Formula to Deal with Biased Selection." In *Advances in Health Economics and Health Services Research*, edited by Richard M. Scheffler and Louis F. Rossiter, vol. 6, Greenwich, CT: JAI Press, 1985.

McCall, Nelda, and Wai, Hoi. "An Analysis of the Use of Medicare Services by the Continuously Enrolled Aged." *Medical Care* 21, no. 6(1983):567.

Milliman and Robertson, Inc. *Actuarial Review of the AAPCC Methodology.* Prepared for the Department of Health and Human Services. Contract No. 500–86–0036. Task Order 004. July 1987.

―――. *Review of AAPCC Methodology for Implementing Prospective Contracts with HMOs.* Prepared for the Health Care Financing Administration. Contract No. 500–83–0018. Department of Health and Human Services, November 1983.

Nelson, Lyle M.; Langwell, Kathryn M.; and Brown, Randall S. "Comparison of 'Rollovers' and 'Switchers' among Enrollees of Medicare HMOs." *GHAA Journal* 8, no. 2(1987/1988): 63.

Newhouse, Joseph P. "Rate Adjusters for Medicare under Capitation." *Health Care Financing Review,* 1986 Annual Supplement: 45–56.

Palsbo, Susan J. "The AAPCC Explained." Research Brief No. 8. Washington, DC: Group Health Association of America, February 1989.

―――. "Analysis of the 1988 AAPCCs in Metropolitan Statistical Areas," Research Brief No. 3. Washington, DC: Group Health Association of America, December 1987.

―――. "Analysis of 1989 USPCCs and AAPCCs." Research Brief No. 6. Washington, DC: Group Health Association of America, 1988.

―――. "The USPCC Explained." Research Brief No. 5. Washington, DC: Group Health Association of America, June 1988.

Porell, F.; Tompkins, C.; and Turner, W. "An Empirical Analysis of Alternative Geographic Configurations for Basing Medicare Payments to HMOs." Bigel Institute for Health Policy, Brandeis University, August 1988.

Riley, Gerald; Rabey, Evelyne; and Kasper, Judith. "Biased Selection and Regression toward the Mean in Three Medicare HMO Demonstrations: A Survival Analysis of Enrollees and Disenrollees." *Medical Care* 27, no. 4(1989): 337.

Rossiter, Louis F. *An Analysis of Long-Run Rate Setting Strategies for Risk-Based Contracting under Medicare.* Prepared for the Health Care Financing Administration. HCFA Cooperative Agreement No. 18–C–98737/3–02.

Department of Health and Human Services, 1989.

Rossiter, L.; Friedlob, A.; and Langwell, K. "Exploring Benefits of Risk-Based Contracting under Medicare." *Healthcare Financial Management* 39, no. 5(1985) 42–58.

Rossiter, Louis F., and Langwell, Kathryn. "Medicare's Two Systems for Paying Providers." *Health Affairs* 7, no. 3(1988): 120.

Rossiter, L.; Langwell, K.; Brown, R.; and Adamache, K. "Medicare's Expanded Choices Program: Issues and Evidence from the HMO Experience." Paper presented at HCFA Conference, Risk-Based Payments for Health Care Under Public Programs, October 1987, Williamsburg, Virginia.

Rossiter, Louis F.; Nelson, Lyle M.; and Adamache, Killard W. "Service Use and Costs for Medicare Beneficiaries in Risk-Based HMOs and CMPs." *American Journal of Public Health* 78, no. 8(1988): 937.

Rossiter, L., et al. "Operational Issues for HMOs and CMPs Entering the Medicare Market." In *New Health Care Systems: HMOs and Beyond.* Washington, DC: Group Health Association of America, 1986.

Rossiter, L., et al. *Analysis Report of Patient Satisfaction for Enrollees and Disenrollees in Medicare Risk-Based Plans.* Prepared by Mathematica Policy Research for the Health Care Financing Administration. Contract No. 500–83–0047. Department of Health and Human Services, May 1988.

Thomas, J. William, and Lichtenstein, Richard. "Including Health Status in Medicare's Adjusted Average Per Capita Cost Capitation Formula." *Medical Care* 24, no. 3(March 1986): 259.

Thomas, J. William; Lichtenstein, Richard; Wyszewianski, Leon; and Berki, S. E. "Increasing Medicare Enrollment in HMOs: The Need for Capitation Rates Adjusted for Health Status." *Inquiry* 20, no. 3(1983): 227.

Trapnell, Gordon R.; McKusick, David; and Genuardi, James. *An Evaluation of the Adjusted Average Per Capita Cost (AAPCC) Used in Reimbursing Risk-Based HMOs Under Medicare.* Prepared for the Health Care Financing Administration. Contract No. HCFA–80–ORDS–87, Department of Health and Human Services, April 1982.

Tucker, Anthony M., and Langwell, Kathryn. "Disenrollment Patterns in Medicare HMOs: A Preliminary Analysis." *GHAA Journal* 9, no. 1(1988): 22.

U.S. General Accounting Office. *Medicare: Health Maintenance Organization Rate-Setting Issues.* Report No. GAO/HRD–89–46, January 1989.

Wallack, Stanley S.; Tompkins, Christopher P.; and Gruenberg, Leonard. "A Plan for Rewarding Efficient HMOs." *Health Affairs* 7, no. 3(1988): 80.

Welch, W. P. "Improving Medicare Payments to HMOs: Urban Core Versus Suburban Ring." *Inquiry* 26, no. 1(1989): 62.

————. "Regression towards the Mean in Medical Care Costs, Implications for Biased Selection in Health Maintenance Organizations." *Medical Care* 23, no. 11(1985): 1234.

Yordi, Cathleen L. "Case Management in the Social Health Maintenance Organization Demonstrations." *Health Care Financing Review,* 1988 Annual Supplement: 83–88.

Part III

HMO Competitive Strategy

Chapter 9

Issues, Trends, and Goals Affecting HMO Competitive Strategy

Health care inflation, intense competition and increasingly demanding purchasers are just a few ingredients in the bitter pill health maintenance organizations now are swallowing. Add to these the specter of the huge financial losses of companies once considered wunderkinds of this young industry and new federal regulations that will affect the ways HMOs price and design their products. As a result of these pressures, HMOs are being forced to rethink their business strategies, HMO executives and consultants say. Only a year ago, most HMOs were concentrating on expanding into as many cities as possible, in search of creating mighty "national HMO networks" that would attract national employer accounts and big premium revenues. But, today, in an era of hemorrhaging balance sheets, the issue for many HMOs is survival, the experts say.

D. DiBlase, "Growing Pains: HMOs Rethink Plans to Build Large Networks"

9.1 Introduction

The health care marketplace is currently in a state of flux. Health costs again threaten to spiral out of control, leading to continued and increasing emphasis on cost containment. Technological advances, medical breakthroughs, and malpractice premiums fuel cost increases. Buyers face a daunting array of problems, including government mandates, retiree health costs, COBRA extensions, Section 89 requirements,[1] looming Federal Accounting Standards Board (FASB) requirements,[2] and subtle cost shifting with concomitant cost pressures on premiums.[3] In the past year, many employers have felt the shock of health insurance premium increases of 30 percent or more.[4]

When viewed in this context, the HMO industry's future appears uncertain, indeed. While HMOs are generally recognized as efficient providers of medical services, and while they appear to be among the most effective agents for containing increases in health care costs, the HMO environment has become increasingly competitive, with most plans facing difficult future negotiations with their health care providers and also with their major customers (employers).

With predictions (and evidence) of HMO industry consolidation and restructuring, individual plans face a demanding set of conditions when planning for the future. To compete effectively, HMOs must fend off threats to their financial stability (including market share and profitability concerns), while at the same time finding improved ways to contract effectively with providers and establishing a stronger relationship with employer clients.

With respect to increased competition in health care, some observers believe that we are in the middle of a 15- to 20-year cycle, one that began with an acceleration of competition around 1980. The growth of the HMO industry has been a key component of this cycle. The final outcomes, however, will not be fully evident for some years to come. In addition, it is likely that the pluralistic nature of the U.S. health care delivery system will have a significant effect on the outcomes. Competition, for example, will yield different results across different geographic markets. And, outcomes in areas affected earliest by increased competition are likely to affect results in other areas. Overall, it is very difficult to predict the exact contours of the HMO industry by the year 2000, although substantial changes will undoubtedly take place in the composition and characteristics of plans.

This final chapter explores various aspects of HMO competitive strategy. At the present time, many plans are maintaining the basic approach and strategy that has been successful for them in the past. However, others are experimenting with a variety of new and different strategies in attempts to respond to competitive pressures and to improve the competitive position of their plans for the future. Notable among these efforts are strategies for product line diversification, expansion of provider networks/geographic service areas, and joint ventures with insurance companies for development of PPOs, triple-option plans, and other products.

Overall, it is accurate to say that every plan faces a unique set of conditions resulting from factors such as the competitive environment, the history and current status of the plan, the opportunities that are available in the marketplace, the commitments and capabilities of the plan, pressures from employers and other purchasers, and the strategy used by each of the plan's major competitors. With these caveats in mind, the remainder of this chapter addresses (1) current issues that affect HMO competitive strategy, (2) forecast of future trends, (3) realistic goals for HMOs during the next five years, (4) financial strategies, (5) relations with major constituencies, and (6) other competitive strategy issues.

9.2 Current Issues Affecting HMO Competitive Strategy*

With the growth in the number of HMOs and the proportion of employers offering a broad choice of different HMOs and other health insurance options, competition for enrollees has reached a new stage. The introduction of PPOs and captive HMOs that are jointly rated with indemnity options in double- or triple-option offerings have compounded the impact of multiple HMO offerings. The competition is especially keen among plans that offer open panels with a broad selection of primary care physicians and specialists.

The price pressures produced by competing (group by group, category by category) with other multiple options has seriously eroded HMO profit margins, leading to large financial losses experienced by many plans. For many, fear of enrollment decreases and antiselection prevent adequate rate increases.[5]

Despite inadequate premiums, many HMOs are under increasing pressure from employers for further rate concessions. Underlying this pressure is a perception by many employee benefit managers that HMOs are selecting against them by taking the lower-cost employees, thus driving up the cost for the remainder, especially those who stay in a residual indemnity plan. This has led in turn to demands by employers for further rate cuts. The capacity and willingness of some plans with "deep pocket" financial backers to buy market share has further exacerbated the general situation.

Another important trend arises from the nature of the relationships that open-panel (IPA-type) HMOs and PPOs have established with phy-

---

*Portions of Sections 9.2, 9.3, and 9.4 were adapted from Gordon R. Trapnell and Charles W. Wrightson, "HMO Pricing Issues from an Actuarial Perspective," in *Proceedings of the 1988 Group Health Institute* (Washington, DC: Group Health Association of America, 1989). Reprinted with the permission of Group Health Association of America, Inc., 1129 20th Street, NW, Washington, DC 20036.

sicians. In most areas in which multiple open-panel HMOs have been introduced, there are overlapping physician panels. A majority of physicians in these areas seem to have decided either to participate in most of the HMOs or to participate in none. Relatively few appear to have examined the nature of the HMO and its risk and other financial arrangements in deciding whether to join. This has led to a situation in some market areas in which the physicians believe that they can dictate terms to the HMOs regarding such essential elements of the contract as the level of fees, withholds, and physician responsibility for losses through risk pools. In some cases, the most intense competition has been competition among the HMOs (for enrollees and physicians to offer on their panels) rather than between physicians (to offer more favorable financial terms in order to gain the patients enrolling in the HMOs). Physicians in some areas appear to believe that they can persuade their patients to change to another open-panel HMO with more favorable terms for the physicians at the next open enrollment. This impression of control also undermines the willingness of physicians to cooperate with the utilization controls of the HMO or to report the nature of services performed consistently over time (i.e., the phenomenon known as "CPT creep" or "diagnosis creep").

A similar restiveness may also occur between a multispeciality physician group and the management corporation operating an HMO that offers their services. For some groups, seemingly inseparable links between the HMO and the physician group have been severed as the management group pursued other goals, such as the formation of holding companies, public stock offerings, expansion to other areas, or entering new businesses. In addition, many medical groups have been approached by other HMOs or HMO management companies wishing to offer their services, permitting them to force the HMOs to compete for their services.

Some of these pressures stem from the maturation of the HMO industry. In a number of service areas, there does not seem to be enough room for the number of plans that have entered, especially among IPA models with largely overlapping physician panels. Many employers have indicated a desire to rationalize the number of HMOs offered, and to use the opportunity to choose those providing the best value.

On the other hand, an abrupt halt has occurred in the development of new HMOs. Now that the stock prices of HMOs have fallen dramatically, risk capital for new HMO ventures has disappeared and those already in place find it difficult to raise additional capital. This is especially the case for the management companies that have attempted to expand beyond their initial marketing area. In addition, insurers that paid large premiums for existing HMOs as recently as 1987 are now reducing their exposure or leaving the field altogether (e.g., Travelers, Aetna, Lincoln National and Hancock). Much greater circumspection may be expected from other insurers interested in obtaining a position in the HMO industry.

9.3 Forecast of Trends

The process of sorting out the strongest competitors among existing HMOs has already begun and will probably continue through the early 1990s. Some HMOs may be forced to close or to merge with stronger plans. This is particularly true of HMOs that are either not yet established with an adequate enrollment, lacking in adequate sources of capital, financially overextended, plagued with high-cost enrollments, unable to cope effectively with design flaws in their organization or risk arrangements, or suffering from weak management, including consumer boards that refuse to recognize economic realities. A consolidation of HMO staffs and reduced opportunities for managers may be expected as a result. For value-conscious buyers, however, there should be a unique opportunity to acquire HMOs with sound fundamentals at bargain prices.

The insurance industry, in particular, is likely to continue to attempt to protect their remaining market share by following strategies to regain lost enrollees (through expanded offerings of PPOs and improved capacity to manage care in existing indemnity plans), thereby narrowing the differences between their coverages and IPA-model HMOs. Some of the insurers may be expected to provide extensive capital resources, if necessary, to back up strategies to preserve market shares, including HMO affiliates.[6]

Relations between open-panel HMOs and participating physicians are likely to become more difficult, as physicians become conscious of their power to force the HMOs to compete for their participation and as they become more sophisticated (and better advised) concerning the impact of different risk and capitation arrangements.[7] Word of any perceived success of physicians in any area of coping with HMOs will spread quickly to other market areas.

Perhaps the greatest obstacle to HMO success will come from employers. The next few years will be marked by increasing demands by employers regarding nearly every facet of HMO operation. In particular, employers are likely to demand documented proof that HMOs enrolling their employees provide care at a lower cost than available elsewhere. Those HMOs that cannot provide the data needed to determine the actual cost for the enrollees of a specific employer may be forced to reduce their premium rate arbitrarily or to be dropped. In addition, employers will come to negotiations armed with consultants' reports purporting to show how efficiently the HMO's provider panels and hospitals practice medicine and how much the employer should be paying the HMO (normally less than the HMO is asking). Increasingly, employers can be expected to deny access to their employees for HMOs not meeting their demands.

A related obstacle is that employee benefit managers tend to have a poor understanding of how to use HMOs in health care cost-containment efforts. It is difficult for employee benefit managers to understand how offering HMOs under different conditions affects their costs. Some HMOs have profited from this situation by enrolling lower-cost groups and driving up the cost of the remaining employees. Although employers are now well aware of this relationship, they still do not understand the mechanics of how it happened and how HMOs can be harnessed to reduce their overall costs. As a result, they are subject to incorrect premises that may lead to actions that hurt those HMOs that could help them most in providing high-quality care at the most economical cost. In this vacuum of knowledge, employee benefit managers may become prey to consultants who advise them to follow strategies that may not be in their best interests.[8]

It is incumbent upon HMOs to adopt a financial viewpoint for their relationships with employers. They must be ready to leave groups rather than accept the likelihood of losses (or they must have a well-defined strategy for dealing with losses). This requires identifying all cases in which the HMO is being required to underwrite a group at an inadequate rate for the circumstances. Since HMOs are not only providers but also insurers, they must subject themselves to the same disciplines that have guided insurers. The skills required are those needed to identify likely losses and to react to the probabilities as insurers would. In addition, HMOs must develop and implement underwriting practices that lead to sound and profitable portfolios.

9.4 Immediate Goals for HMOs

From 1973 to the early 1980s, the HMO industry was in its formative stages; the plans started during this period had to concentrate on issues such as capital financing, organizational development (including development of their health care delivery system), and enrollment growth. More recently, however, the HMO industry has entered a transition period in which HMOs have faced increased competition and more pressures on plan profitability. The HMO industry has matured in many areas of the country, and some areas are now oversaturated with new and established plans. Most observers predict a continuing period of consolidation, with increasing pressures on financial solvency. Thus, many HMO chief executive officers (CEOs) and other industry participants believe that HMOs will need to change past patterns of behavior (if they have not already done so) in response to current trends. In fact, many HMOs have already redirected their goals and objectives in recent years.

The goals that HMOs must meet to survive and prosper in the difficult times ahead are presented below, in the order of their importance.

Survival

The primary goal for any HMO during the next five years is financial survival. All other objectives must be subordinated to this. Only when survival is assured can attention be given to other corporate goals such as expansion, fairness among enrollment groups, or service to members. As obvious as it may sound, the owners (or consumer boards) of many HMOs have been unable to recognize survival as a priority or to direct their management efforts accordingly. Recognizing survival explicitly as a primary goal can help to focus attention on the actions needed to obtain it, while educating both management and ownership that survival is not guaranteed in the current environment.

Financial Strength

Since there are a number of backers of HMOs and PPOs who are willing to commit substantial capital in the form of sustaining major losses to obtain market share, even the most efficient and well-managed HMOs are likely to need substantial reserves to get through the next five years. Independent HMOs that have made provisions for building and maintaining adequate reserves, and that have avoided committing their surplus to rapid expansion or other diversification, will be in far better shape to withstand the period of mergers and consolidation. Reserves will be needed to cover losses incurred when plans are forced to operate with inadequate profit margins as a result of competition or to cover inadvertent, unplanned losses. It is, unfortunately, the very nature of the insurance business (in which HMOs are participants) to be forced to sustain unanticipated losses from time to time as a result of unforeseen events.

An important prerequisite for financial strength is to have an accounting and management information system that provides the information that management and owners need to ascertain the real financial position of the HMO. Those HMOs that have paid careful attention to development of sound accounting and financial planning systems will benefit over the next few years. There will be a premium on competence in such mundane and frequently neglected matters as maintaining a complete enumeration of cost elements, preparing realistic projections of claims incurred but not reported, accounting for all claims in process and other contractual liabilities, and what an insurance company would call a "premium deficiency reserve" (the liability from a commitment to provide insurance for less than its projected cost).

In order to know that reserves are adequate, it is necessary that the HMO know its financial position. The most rigorous standard for judging the financial position at any time is the "going out of business" standard, which measures the surplus that would exist at the end of an accounting period if the entity were to be liquidated. The consolidation of the industry will reward those HMOs that can meet this standard.

Adequate Profit Margins

The necessity of building and maintaining a strong financial position requires close attention to actual profit margins. Only a few HMOs, however, are in a position to assess their margins for individual groups.

Determining the actual profit margins requires precise information concerning the cost structure of the HMO. This is much easier for an open-panel HMO, since payment of providers normally requires maintaining the data needed to determine costs. An HMO based on a multispeciality group may also maintain charge information that is close enough to actual costs to provide realistic cost information.

Competitive Cost Structure

The rigors of competing for enrollees in open enrollments places an unusual premium on the level of rates. It is crucial for the HMO to be in a position to offer competitive rates in each rating category (which includes family type, age/sex, and any other separate category). Adequate and competitive rates can only be offered if the HMO has a cost structure no higher than its principal competitors (including PPOs) in their service area. And this may not be enough over the next few years. Independent HMOs will probably have to maintain significantly lower costs than competitors that are willing to absorb losses to gain market share.

The most important goal is to be a low-cost provider/health plan. This goal has three essential components:

- An enrollment with health care needs no greater than that of principal competitors
- Providers with operating costs and practice styles no more expensive than those of competitors, and negotiated rates that reflect these determinants of cost
- Capacity of the HMO to manage utilization, especially for the most expensive conditions and for mental health

The sum total of all these factors is what matters. HMOs have traditionally taken the view that their management capacity and negotiating flexibility could overcome any problems posed by the cost of a group. But only if the HMO breaks even on selection, or close enough that other efficiencies can overcome the cost differential, can the HMO offer competitive rates that will not lead to antiselection in open enrollments. The cost of treating any group is relative to the health of that group. Even HMOs offering the most efficient providers can be overwhelmed by the service needs of an unhealthy group of enrollees. Although HMOs can reduce the level or cost of services needed by a particular group of enrollees, the change is relative to the underlying level of health needs.

Another way to look at this is that the returns from efficiency can be overwhelmed by the returns from selection. In other words, of the two strategies for achieving a low-cost structure (i.e., selecting a healthy group of enrollees or providing only needed services at relatively low cost), the easiest or most effective strategy is to have a very healthy group that needs few services.

In determining provider cost levels, it is crucial to distinguish between low cost and low prices. A number of HMOs have found that they can negotiate deals with providers, especially hospitals, at rates far below the nominal price level and frequently below cost. But such deals cannot be sustained over time. As insurers representing more and more of the patient loads of providers demand the same rates, the providers will eventually be forced to raise their rates to cover their full average costs, or go out of business. Similarly, after failure to pay withholds once or twice, the actual payment rate becomes the price, as far as physicians are concerned. Other payers will demand the same fee. As the providers become more sophisticated in dealing with HMOs, we can expect a gradual erosion in the terms available from providers. Thus, only where low prices are the result of low costs can they be sustained in the long run.

A Close Relationship of Service to Employers

The difficulties HMOs are now experiencing with employers are largely attributable to the types of relationships that have typically been established. The perspective that HMOs need to adopt is similar to that developed and honed by the insurance industry over decades of providing group insurance to employers. The insurers function much more as advisers and consultants than as insurers—for example, as administrators for self-insured plans. Similarly, HMOs should seek to work as consultants and suppliers to employers rather than as adversaries in negotiating favorable prices. They need to be able to explain, from the employer's perspective, why it is in the employer's interest to enroll a substantial portion of the work force in the HMO. This must include evidence that the HMO is not charging more for the employees in question than would be the employer's experience in other modes of insurance. It must also include assistance with the details of providing employee benefit programs, such as administering the residual indemnity plan and providing a funding mechanism that encompasses both HMO and non-HMO employees and documents the savings that the HMO can produce for the specific HMO enrollees employed by that employer.

The principal need is to educate employers concerning what HMOs can and cannot do for them. Employers want an HMO to take over a portion of the employment group and provide health care to that group at the same or a lower cost than their competitors, with the employees in question fully satisfied with the arrangement. It is not enough for an HMO to fulfill this mission through the care they offer. The HMO should also provide the same kind of consulting and educational support that insurers provide as a basic component of their service. This requires a high level of communication with employers, in order to ascertain their needs, and sufficient flexibility to fulfill their needs without overextending the HMO or incurring losses.

Maintaining Market Share

An HMO must maintain a certain level of market share to remain financially viable. At lower levels of enrollment, fixed overhead costs are spread over fewer enrollees, leading to higher average costs. All financial calculations must take into consideration the impact of lower enrollments on average costs.

The perception of many in the industry is that the critical level is at least as high as the current level and usually somewhat larger. The notion that large size is a prerequisite to success has its foundation in the early theoretical writings about HMOs, in which it was assumed that HMOs have a very high overhead component which had to be spread over a critical level of minimum enrollment to produce economical operation. It is evident, however, that HMOs have wide latitude to adjust their fixed costs to meet their actual enrollment and financial situation. For example, there are both open-panel and closed-panel plans that are operating successfully in the Arizona Health Care Cost Containment System (AHCCCS) program with only small fractions of the enrollments that have traditionally been regarded as essential for economical average operating costs. Recent studies of rural HMOs have also found that plans are viable even with relatively small enrollments.[9]

Maintaining market share must be viewed as a means to survival and not as a goal in itself. The problem of fixed costs requires informed calculations by the HMO of the joint effect of any decision to withdraw from a group (or loss of enrollment in a group) and the likely impact on the profit margin if the opposite decision is reached (maintaining the contractual relationship). Better information concerning the degree to which overhead costs are really fixed will be needed over the next few years so that these calculations can be made.

Growth

The perception of growth as an objective in itself may have begun with the theoretical HMO model in which there is a certain level of fixed costs and, the higher the enrollment, the lower would be the average of these fixed costs per enrollee. This view has been reinforced by the practical experience of most existing HMOs, who have found that profit margins (positive or negative) tend to be a constant percentage of the capitation rate. Until recently, there has also been an implicit assumption in investment circles that HMO profits would be proportionate to enrollment.

If the projections concerning the competitive environment are correct, the HMO industry will be entering a phase in which growth is no longer a desirable objective, in and of itself, unless it can be demonstrated that the growth will result in increased profitability. Thus, it would appear that one component of an HMO's strategy should be to identify and cull unprofitable groups, regardless of the impact on enrollment, to preserve an adequate profit margin and surplus (e.g., for a group with significant losses that are expected to persist into the future, it will be necessary to terminate the contract with this group, or to redefine the financial terms of the contract so that the expected losses are eliminated). Here, it is merely argued that profitable growth is a desirable goal, but one that can be given high priority only by HMOs that are assured survival as viable independent entities.[10]

Summary

The combination of pressures outlined above may require HMOs to adopt a totally different operating philosophy, especially with regard to growth and rating. Perhaps the most important element of the recommended approach is the adoption of a revised perspective on rating that attempts to respond to the concerns expressed by major employers. Other crucial elements include (1) the adoption of realistic goals for the next five years, and (2) the implementation of disciplined measures to accomplish those goals.

Overall, then, to be successful during the next five years, a plan will require astute management with the flexibility and foresight to identify and adapt to rapidly changing competitive conditions. Efforts to improve the competitive position of an HMO will require increased attention to the following factors:

- Marketing approaches
- New product development
- Rating and underwriting practices
- Provider relations and contract negotiations
- Cost-containment procedures
- Data systems and MIS reporting

- Utilization review and quality of care protocols
- Accounting, actuarial, and financial planning methods
- Provider reimbursement and risk-sharing arrangements

With the changes taking place in health care delivery, organization, and financing, achieving success during the next five years will be a difficult, though not impossible, task for most HMOs.[11] An important part of the recipe for success will be found in more specific financial strategies.

9.5 Financial Strategies

How does an HMO gain a competitive edge over competing health plans? There are many alternative financial strategies that can be considered. To be successful, a strategy should reflect the unique characteristics and competitive position of the HMO. Strategies that are appropriate for one plan may be disastrous for another. This section considers financial strategies related to a plan's cost-containment methods and risk-sharing techniques, alternative benefit design options, and rating and data analysis capabilities.

Cost-Containment Methods and Risk-Sharing Techniques

To maintain a plan's profitability, the plan's management must continually monitor the cost structure of the plan and attempt to find ways to reduce costs without harming quality of care or patient satisfaction. The three primary avenues for reducing costs are (1) internal cost control, (2) provider reimbursement, and (3) risk management. (See Chapter 3 for a detailed discussion of these topics.)

In a highly competitive environment, it is sometimes difficult to focus on the mundane "nuts and bolts" activities related to internal cost control, provider contracting, and other ongoing tasks. However, savings resulting from diligent efforts at these activities might spell the difference between a profitable and an unprofitable year, or they might provide the difference in cash flow that permits an important expansion or restructuring project.

Benefit Design Options

Flexibility in benefit design should be given strong consideration by most plans. Some HMOs still have one basic benefit package with a limited number of riders for optional services such as pharmacy, eye care, and dental care. All HMOs, however, should evaluate the feasibility of offering multiple benefit options with additional cost sharing and possibly limitations on some services. Some form of limited open-ended plan where enrollees could obtain reimbursement for services received from nonplan providers, subject to appropriate limitations and cost sharing, should also be considered (e.g., a self-referral option to obtain care from non-HMO providers at the point of service). The point is that increased flexibility in benefit design will make a plan much more competitive, especially among employers that only offer limited indemnity programs with rates substantially below the HMO's community rates and where it has been impossible for the plan to be competitive previously. It might also be advisable to consider development of a number of lower options, at least some with markedly lower premiums. This can be achieved through reduced benefit coverage, higher cost sharing, and the use of riders between the lowest and highest benefit plan options offered, in order to permit more price flexibility and to improve the competitive position of the plan in the marketplace.

Increased cost sharing. The combination of comprehensive benefits and low cost sharing offered by most HMOs provides, basically, first-dollar coverage for a wide range of health services. Most HMOs should seriously consider offering options with much higher cost sharing in their benefit plans. Higher cost sharing offers the following advantages:

- Increased level of direct revenue (or offsets to expenses)
- Lower utilization rates, as demonstrated by the RAND studies[12]
- A selection advantage in dual- or multiple-choice situations (there will be a tendency for persons expecting to use health services to choose plans with low cost sharing, and a tendency for infrequent users to select plans with lower premiums and higher cost sharing, all other things being equal)

For a given value of increased cost sharing (e.g., the actuarial value of higher copays), the HMO can expect to reduce its costs by as much as twice that amount for the impact on utilization and may find selection advantages of a greater amount, depending on the specific circumstances of the case. The amount for any particular subgroup of enrollees will vary, of course, depending on their age, sex, prior utilization rates, characteristics of the employer's health benefits program, posture of competing health plans, and level of out-of-pocket premium rates.

It would be difficult for many HMOs to approach the level of cost sharing that is part of many indemnity plans. However, HMOs should consider visit copays of $8, $10, or $12, rather than common values such as $2, $3, or $5. Higher levels of inpatient cost sharing should be considered to correspond to the levels of deductibles found in indemnity programs. Where an indemnity plan may have a $200 per year deductible per individual, an HMO could institute a hospital benefit copayment of $500 per year, $50 per day for up to ten inpatient days, or 20 percent coinsurance up to out-of-pocket limits of $1,000 per individual or $2,000 per family. Other sources of cost sharing could include 50 percent copays for outpatient mental health, emergency room visits, and selected elective procedures; and instituting copays for x-rays, laboratory tests, other ancillary services, and other outpatient services or procedures (outpatient surgery, comprehensive physicals, allergy testing and injections). Copayments are most effective on those services over which the patient has most control. The most important point is that most HMOs have minimal cost sharing compared to indemnity plans, and there is substantial ''competitive space'' for HMOs to develop benefit options with increased cost-sharing provisions.

Multiple benefit options.   If they do not already do so, most HMOs should explore the feasibility of offering a wide range of benefit packages, extending from first-dollar coverage plans to very low option plans with limited benefit packages and high cost sharing. The advantages of multiple benefit options include the following:

- The HMO is better able to respond to employer desires.
- The HMO is better able to adapt to changes in competitive conditions for different employers.
- The HMO has greater flexibility—instead of increasing premiums, the HMO can offer the employer a reduced benefit package or guaranteed, multiyear rates (as long as the HMO has the flexibility to modify benefits marginally).

With a combination of benefit options and cost-sharing options, HMOs should be able to offer custom-tailored benefit packages that are responsive to competitive conditions.

Integrated products and open-ended HMOs.   There is a great need for integrated products in the changing marketplace. For HMOs, this usually means adding some form of choice plan (i.e., enrollees can receive some services from non-HMO providers and be reimbursed for these services).[13] These plans are proliferating and numerous alternatives have been implemented. Many plans simply have two levels of benefits— a more comprehensive benefit package for members who use HMO providers and a lower level of benefits for members who use non-HMO providers. In many cases, HMO members are not locked in and can choose desired providers at the point of service.

Historically, a major drawback to HMOs has been the limited provider network (especially for staff and group models, but also for IPAs and networks). "Freedom of choice" is a very important factor for many potential enrollees. During the past few years, many alternatives have been designed and tested in the marketplace. To date, no design has become predominant. Emphasis on development of a variety of open-ended options and integrated products is likely to continue. To maintain or improve a plan's competitive position, the feasibility of alternative product designs should be considered.

It is not possible to identify all of the options that have been put forth in the last few years. Examples of alternatives for closed-panel (staff and group) plans include primary care swing plans and opt-out or "wrap around" plans:

- *Primary care swing plans.* To prevent members from being locked in to the closed panel of HMO providers, some plans have permitted members to go to their own primary care physician (out-of-panel) with higher copays or other cost sharing imposed. However, members are required to use the HMO's specialists for referrals. Also, hospital admissions and selected procedures (e.g., greater than a specified dollar value) must be approved by the HMO.

- *Opt-out or "wrap around" plans.* Some closed-panel plans have granted virtually unlimited access to out-of-plan primary care and specialist physicians with an indemnity-like "wrap around" plan. These plans usually have moderate to high deductibles ($200 or more per individual) and coinsurance (20 percent or higher) for out-of-plan services, and they usually have a more restricted benefit package. Some closed-panel plans have entered into joint ventures with insurance companies or third-party administrators to implement these types of programs.

For network and IPA-model plans, the following are examples of alternatives for open-ended or integrated products.

- *Triple-option plans.* Typically, these alternatives use "lock-in" features whereby employees must choose to enroll in one of three alternative options: (1) an option with a selected group of preferred providers that corresponds to the most cost-effective group of primary care and specialist physicians available in the open panel (this option may be covered with minimal or no cost sharing), (2) an intermediate option that contains the full set of providers in the HMO's panel (this option may be covered with the HMO's regular cost sharing, similar to a low-option plan), and (3) total access to all providers (in or out of the HMO's panel), usually with increased cost sharing similar to indemnity deductibles and coinsurance.

- *Point-of-service plans.* Typically, these "multi-option" or "instant choice" plans do not lock employees into one of the options. Rather, a covered member is able to select a provider when he or she receives service. In these plans, there is usually minimal or no cost sharing if the core group of preferred providers is used. If other in-panel providers are used, the cost sharing may be 20 percent or higher. If out-of-panel providers are used, patients are subject to deductibles and coinsurance and may be responsible for balance billing (e.g., the HMO will reimburse out-of-panel providers up to 80 percent of the maximum fee schedule, with patients being responsible for the balance of the provider's bill). If out-of-panel providers are used, it may be the patient's contractual responsibility to obtain preadmission certification, second surgical opinion, and so on (or bills may not be reimbursed for nonemergency services).

- *Exclusive provider organizations (EPOs).* Some broad-based IPAs have established PPOs or EPOs to offer indemnity-type plans under administrative services only (ASO) arrangements with utilization review and managed care services billed separately as unbundled services.

The dangers associated with these plan designs include (1) the HMO loses control over utilization of services delivered by non-HMO physicians, (2) HMO physicians resent the loss of income resulting from the out-of-plan services, and (3) the cost-containment potential of the HMO is diminished. To make these plans work, there must be an adequate penalty for opting out (e.g. reduced benefits or much higher cost sharing for non-HMO providers). In addition, the requirements for effective utilization control are increased.

Since many of these open-ended plans are quite new, there is little documented evidence on the level of utilization and costs resulting from use of non-HMO providers. Preliminary evidence from several plans, however, appears to indicate that out-of-panel utilization/costs can be held to minimal levels with well-designed benefit packages that provide appropriate financial incentives for using the HMO providers.

Rating and Data Analysis Strategies

The following financial strategies related to rating methods and data analysis capabilities are among those discussed in Section 7.6:

1. Strategy for rate increase
2. Feasibility study for adjusted community rating or other form of group-specific rating
3. Review of financial experience of major employer clients
4. Analyze ''portfolio'' of group business
5. Study of profitability by line of business
6. Analyze cost structure and cost experience of plan

It is evident that HMOs should carefully assess and use all relevant financial-based strategies that would improve the competitive positions of their plans.

Creative Cost Containment and Financing Arrangements

Three topics mentioned frequently as employer objectives in dealing with HMOs are (1) group-specific premiums, (2) risk-adjusted employer contributions, and (3) multiyear rate guarantees. However, perhaps the most pressing problem for many employers is the spiraling cost of their basic indemnity plan. Premium increases of 20 to 50 percent or more have been commonplace in the past few years for many employers. Whether due to risk selection, cost shifting, inadequate cost controls, or other factors, the indemnity rate increases have caused widespread employer concern that their indemnity plans are locked in a cost spiral.

It would benefit both employers and HMOs to find ways for managed care plans to contribute to solving this problem. It is likely that several options will need to be explored, including (1) taking a comprehensive cost-containment approach to the employer's entire health benefits program, (2) developing group-specific premium rates and risk-adjusted employer contribution methods so that employers do not suffer financial penalties for offering HMOs, (3) redesigning both indemnity and HMO benefit levels and cost-sharing requirements so that an appropriate proportion of an employer's work force is directed to managed care options, and (4) developing creative financing arrangements whereby HMOs share the risk for containing an employer's aggregate costs.[14]

9.6 Other HMO Competitive Strategy Issues

Although financial issues are expected to continue to occupy the attention of those involved in HMO strategic planning during the next five years, the subject of HMO competitive strategy is much broader than financial planning alone. The most important nonfinancial, competitive strategy issues for HMOs include the problem of relating effectively to key constituencies and the more general problems affecting management of HMOs in the increasingly competitive environment.

Relations with Key Constituencies

There appears to be a changing emphasis on the part of employers regarding what they want most from HMOs. Concerns raised more and more often are (1) value, (2) administrative simplicity, (3) retiree medical costs, (4) "skimming," and (5) "fair" premium rates.

Employers want value for their health care dollar. In the past, a major problem for employers was their perception that HMOs could not demonstrate either the quantity or quality of the health care services that were delivered to their employees who were enrolled in the HMO. This led to a feeling on the part of employers that they were not obtaining a "good value" for their premium dollar. Many employers who have been enthusiastic supporters of HMOs still believe that HMOs are cost-effective and provide a tightly controlled managed care system that results in lower overall costs to the employer. Other employers, however, want demonstrated proof of these assertions in a format that they can understand (e.g., data on HMO utilization and costs). If HMOs can explain how they provide value to employers in terms of lower overall costs (and equal or higher quality and satisfaction) for a given group of employees, then it will contribute significantly to an improved HMO/employer relationship.

A second topic that has been emphasized is "administrative simplicity.'' Most employers (especially national employers) are burdened by the administrative requirements of maintaining multiple health plan offerings. In addition, the Section 89 antidiscrimination requirements of the 1986 Tax Reform Act have created anxiety on the part of employers regarding their potential liability on this issue and the amount of paperwork that will be required to fulfill the administrative requirements of the federal regulations (once they are promulgated as final rules). In general, employers offering multiple health plans expect that it will be more difficult for them to comply. This factor could have a significant impact on HMOs.

A third issue is retiree medical costs. The Financial Accounting Standards Board (FASB) ruling that liabilities for future retiree medical expenses must be shown on corporate balance sheets is expected to have a major impact on how employers deal with these costs in the future.[15] This issue could have a significant positive or negative effect on HMOs.

A fourth issue concerns "skimming" and allegations that HMOs almost always receive favorable selection in employer offerings with two or more choices of health plans. To avoid a deteriorating relationship with major employers, it is very important for HMOs to confront and respond to this issue. (For a more detailed discussion, see Chapter 8.)

A fifth issue, which is not new but continues to receive heavy emphasis, is the perceived need for "fair HMO premium rates." This concern grew out of allegations concerning (1) HMOs receiving favorable selection, and (2) HMOs employing various competitive pricing methods (i.e., shadow pricing, gouging, charging what the market will bear). (The concerns of employers about these issues are discussed in detail in Chapter 4.)

During the past few years, numerous actions have been taken by major employers to improve their negotiations with HMOs:

1. It has become commonplace for major employers to issue a "request for proposal" (RFP) that specifies the requirements that health plans must meet to be considered by the employer. In addition, the RFP might contain the maximum rates that the employer will pay for the specified health coverage, and other conditions such as the maximum number of plans to be offered, cost-sharing requirements, limitations on services, accessibility or quality requirements, or data reporting requirements.

2. Other employers have decided to simplify their health benefits program either by contracting with a single organization or by

limiting the number of options (one HMO, one PPO, one indemnity option). If a single contractor is used, then there are several possible variations. In some cases, a triple-option plan is offered by the contractor. In other cases, the contractor serves as a vendor for a "managed competition" approach, and enters into arrangements with a limited number of other HMOs and PPOs. In other cases, the contractor operates an open-ended HMO based on a defined network of providers and comprehensive benefits. However, employees may opt out of the provider network and receive service from a nonparticipating provider. In this case, high cost-sharing requirements, in the form of deductibles and coinsurance, usually apply. This exclusive dual or multiple offering usually has a single premium based on the pooled experience of all covered employees and dependents. This pooling of risk for all employees helps to minimize selection bias problems.

3. Some employers have dropped all HMOs from their health benefits program. By offering only one option (health plan), problems from biased selection are eliminated. Some of these employers believe that offering a single self-insured (or indemnity or managed care indemnity) plan allows them to have better control over their health care costs.

4. Some employers have attempted to regulate selection by limiting the frequency of open enrollment periods, by freezing enrollment in selected plans, by having enrollment quotas for various plans, by steering higher-risk persons (such as retirees) into HMOs, or by steering lower-risk persons away from HMOs.

5. Some employers have modified benefits in the non-HMO plan to make it more attractive for lower-risk persons. In addition to limitations on benefits, increased cost-sharing in the form of high deductibles and coinsurance (with appropriately reduced premiums) make an employer's basic plan more attractive to lower-risk persons who do not expect to use health care services.

6. To compensate for differences in health risks among employees, some employers have developed risk-adjusted contributions for the health plans that they offer. In many cases, the employer determines classes (e.g., based on age/sex categories) and sets maximum contribution rates at the level of the indemnity plan's costs for these classes.

7. A recent contract between Allied-Signal and CIGNA has gained wide attention. Under a three-year contract starting 1 March 1988, Allied-Signal's health care costs will not increase more than a stipulated percentage in each plan year. The plan administrator, CIGNA Corporation of Hartford, Connecticut, will absorb any health care costs in excess of the stated increase factor. Under the contract, CIGNA will provide a national managed care network, named "Health Care Connection." This single network replaces a multitude of indemnity plans and contracts with individual HMOs. The "Health Care Connection" will be made available to all of Allied-Signal's 80,000 domestic employees and their families over the next three years. Under the new program, employees will be enrolled in CIGNA Healthplan HMOs nationwide, but employees can also use non-network providers at reduced coverage levels.

8. In a somewhat similar development, First Interstate Bancorp announced their new strategy for managing their health costs, reducing adverse selection, and at the same time maintaining good employee relations. Their plan is called "Health Span," and it is based on a point-of-service HMO/indemnity plan whereby employees can choose to use network or nonnetwork providers at the time they receive health services. Health Span was developed through Metropolitan Life Insurance (Met Life). Starting 1 January 1989, Health Span became available to 29,000 employees and retirees under age 65 in four of the nineteen states where the bank has offices. It is anticipated that most of the remaining 10,000 employees will be phased into Health Span by the end of 1990. Met Life operates the IPA/HMO network portion of the plan and provides claims administration services for the indemnity portion. Employees in California, Colorado, and Oregon can continue to enroll with Kaiser Permanente plans, while Arizona employees can enroll with a CIGNA HMO. All other HMOs previously offered by First Interstate were discontinued.

9. A different approach is being implemented by Xerox Corporation, which has identified their major problems as no cost controls, no quality measurement systems, too many vendors, too much administrative complexity, too little focused purchasing power, and no provider accountability for results. Xerox has

decided to implement the "managed competition" approach recommended by Enthoven and others. Under their model, Xerox will contract with a limited number of vendors who will be responsible for managing nationwide networks of providers. Competitive bidding will be used for procurement of the major vendors using an RFP with detailed specifications.[16]

In general, employers have become increasingly sophisticated purchasers of health services, and they have devoted considerable resources to developing methods to negotiate with HMOs and other health insurers. In return, HMOs need to devote comparable attention to finding successful ways to respond to the concerns of employers.

The potential dangers to established HMOs are real. There have been many cases where HMOs with long-standing contracts have been dropped by major employers. In other cases, HMOs have been forced to swallow bitter medicine, in the form of specified rates or other contractual features, as a condition for continued participation. It is likely that these mechanisms will proliferate in the future and that, in order to survive, individual HMOs will have to find ways to respond successfully.

In an era of high competition among health plans, some of the historical trends in the health insurance industry are likely to recur, with implications for HMOs in highly competitive areas. Examples of these trends include the following:

- A pattern of underwriting cycles where high competition leads to pressure on premiums (possibly with intense price competition in some areas), followed by financial losses and underwriting deficits, followed by inflated premium increases to make up for incurred losses
- A tendency for employers to have the upper hand in negotiations with health plans (including setting conditions for participation and driving hard bargains on prices) due to an excessive supply of alternative health plans and the ability of employers to find at least one plan that will agree to the desired terms and conditions

With respect to the first trend, many HMOs do not have the health insurance underwriting experience to react quickly to changing conditions. Also, many HMOs do not have the substantial reserves that are necessary to withstand the effects of reduced revenues due to price pressures. In the past, many HMOs have been reluctant to raise premiums sufficiently to make up for losses.

In the theory of competitive bidding, the second phenomenon has been termed "the winner's curse" because the winning bidder in these situations has often agreed to terms that guarantee that the health plan will lose money on the contract (expenses will exceed premiums). With an excess of HMOs in many areas, it is likely that astute employee benefit managers will be able to obtain very good bargains by shopping wisely for health coverage.

HMO Cost Savings via Total Replacement Approaches

As described above, employers are using a variety of strategies for dealing with HMOs in order to improve their health benefits programs. The "managed competition" approach is being implemented in different ways to maintain competition while reducing the total number of HMOs offered.

From both the HMO and the employer perspectives, however, perhaps the most effective rebuttal to charges of "skimming" is for an HMO with high penetration in an employer group to offer to assume full responsibility for all eligible employees and dependents (in effect, a 100 percent takeover of the group by the HMO).[17] This option would be particularly attractive to an employer with high HMO penetration and a relatively small residual indemnity plan that is experiencing an adverse selection spiral. In addition to resolving the selection bias issue, this approach allows HMOs to demonstrate their alleged ability to manage care and contain health costs.

The most widely publicized example of this tactic, also referred to as "sole sourcing," was CIGNA's contract with Allied-Signal for a nationwide effort using this approach. In this case, CIGNA assumed financial responsibility for cost savings by guaranteeing multiyear rates.[18]

Traditionally, a key component of HMO philosophy has been "voluntary participation" (i.e., that all persons should be given a choice between enrolling in an HMO or choosing an alternative health plan). In the early days of the prepaid group practice plans, this feature was necessary to avoid charges of restricting "freedom of choice of medical practitioner," a fundamental axiom of American medicine.

With respect to whole group takeovers or "total replacements," it is necessary for the HMO to offer some form of open-ended or multi-option plan to ensure freedom of choice. Although the HMO's cost-control capability will be tested under open-ended plans, an "opt-out" option is critical to maintaining some level of freedom of choice and avoiding employees being "locked in" (i.e., to permit patients to maintain their relationship with their personal primary care physician, or to seek care outside of the HMO panel, if desired). Some plans have found that indemnity-type cost sharing on out-of-plan services (e.g., $200 deductibles per individual and 20 percent coinsurance) provides sufficient financial incentives to keep a very high proportion of patients within the HMO system.

Other factors that HMOs need to consider regarding whole group takeovers (total replacements) include underwriting, rating, and data systems capabilities. An HMO needs defined underwriting procedures to determine which groups should be accepted or denied and the terms and conditions for different underwriting situations. The following rating considerations should be included:

- How should first-year rates be determined for the whole group (a blend of rates for indemnity and HMO enrollees based on past experience, under a prospective experience-rating arrangement)?

- How should rating be handled for retirees and other special categories of eligibles covered under the employer's health benefits program?

- Should residual indemnity eligibles be assumed at rates equal to the indemnity plan's current rates plus projected inflation for the next year (possibly with adjustments for benefit differences)?

- To demonstrate the HMO's confidence in containing costs, should multiyear fixed rates (with inflation adjustments) be offered (possibly with joint risk sharing for losses and division of cost savings in future years)?

Finally, HMOs need to assess whether their data systems are capable of adapting to the requirements of this type of program. In some cases, joint ventures with insurance companies or third-party administrators may be advisable for claims processing or other tasks.

Limited initial experience from some HMOs appears to indicate that whole group takeovers should be considered by HMOs that can offer some form of open-ended plan. A well-designed plan, including appropriate financial incentives for in-plan use, appears to be sufficient to keep a high proportion of in-system services. In addition, this approach presents an excellent opportunity to respond to charges of "skimming" and to demonstrate that the HMO can effectively contain the employer's health care costs. The feasibility of this approach, however, depends on a variety of factors such as the level of indemnity premium rates, prior utilization experience of non-HMO eligibles, benefit differences, retiree coverage, acceptable cost-sharing features, participation rates, and the size and stability of the group. In many cases, though, an HMO will be financially rewarded while at the same time saving money for the employer (assuming that appropriate rating and underwriting procedures have been utilized).

Although this approach has been implemented only in a limited fashion in some areas of the United States, the total replacement approach is defended by some as the type of major restructuring that is needed to control costs. There are certainly potential problems, such as restricted freedom of choice and employee dissatisfaction. It appears that, at a minimum, the following elements are necessary to make this approach work:

1. As many enrollees as possible must be offered as much care as possible within the most efficient HMO or managed care environment, using a combination of financial incentives/disincentives, employer support and recommendations, benefit differentials, employee education on cost and quality of HMO care, and emphasis on the overall goals and objectives of the new (restructured) health benefits program.

2. There also has to be a very good "match" between the HMO and the employer with respect to location, perceived image and reputation, services offered (including mental health, substance abuse), and provider acceptability (including physician panel, hospitals used).

3. The HMO should be well known among the workforce, as evidenced by a current high penetration rate.

4. The employer has to be willing to "pay the price" for the 100 percent conversion. In a well-structured situation, cost savings will be virtually guaranteed, but there will also be a certain level of initial employee dissatisfaction. Good planning for the transition period and a well thought-out communication/educational program for employees are essential. Transition aids such as "hot lines," assistance in starting to use the HMO (new member programs, how to make appointments, how to get urgent care), and thorough explanation of the new program (written materials, employee meetings) are also important to successful total replacement.

5. Non-HMO care has to be kept to a minimum. Unless there are good reasons for the out-of-plan services (e.g., the HMO does not serve some areas where employees live), the program may be in jeopardy if non-HMO care exceeds 10 percent.

6. The HMO must offer experience-rated premiums. If the HMO is truly experience rated, then the number of enrolled HMO members is irrelevant—the only thing that matters is the volume of care that is provided by the HMO versus non-HMO providers. Thus, if the HMO offers experience-rated premiums, then the employer can enroll all employees in the HMO and focus on directing as much care as possible into the HMO setting. In this case, the key issue is the level of non-HMO care. It is important to develop a coordinated approach for minimizing non-HMO care while maintaining employee satisfaction with the overall health benefits program.

7. Interaction effects. Based on a very small sample, it appears that if the employer does a 100 percent conversion to a single HMO (with a well-designed, limited opt-out option), then the level of non-HMO care can be very small (under 5 percent of total expenditures). This might occur because (1) the employer strongly supports the HMO and actively demonstrates this support to employees, (2) the HMO previously had a high penetration in the group, (3) the HMO enrollees were highly satisfied and there was good "word-of-mouth" public relations for the HMO, and (4) the employer might have conducted an effective communication/education program for employees in conjunction with the switch to the new program. In a number of cases where this approach has been implemented (at the urging of the employer), it appears that there have been positive interaction effects, and the level of non-HMO care has been smaller than projected.

8. Primary care must be accessible. In the case of a 100 percent conversion with a closed-panel HMO, it is essential to have outpatient clinics (or a contractual relationship with primary care physicians) in all areas where the firm's employees live and work. If not, then there is a high risk that a significant proportion of the workforce will be "left out in the cold" without access to the HMO's primary care providers.

9. The HMO needs an effective "opt-out" option. Employees

should feel that they have a viable option to use non-HMO services (at the point of service). At the same time, it is essential that the opt-out option be properly structured to provide financial incentives for employees to use the HMO and to minimize the volume of non-HMO services.

10. The reimbursement for non-HMO services can be handled by the HMO, the employer, or a TPA. From the employer's perspective, it is critical to monitor the level of non-HMO payments on an ongoing basis, including estimating incurred-but-not-reported claim expenses.

In summary, the "total replacement" approach certainly eliminates all questions about "biased selection" and "HMO skimming." However, several potential problems need to be considered carefully before an employer or an HMO can successfully implement such a program.

HMOs and Physician Providers

There have been several cycles in the relationship between HMOs and their physician providers. Initially (in the 1970s and earlier), many physicians were reluctant to contract with or participate in HMOs. Over time, their resistance softened and many physicians decided to join HMOs, if only to be assured of a future source of income. Now it appears that the pendulum may be swinging back toward its original position. There have been several examples of confrontations between HMOs and physician groups over matters including capitation reimbursement, return of withholds, fee schedules, methods for utilization review and quality assurance, and changes in risk-sharing arrangements.

Acrimonious negotiations are not uncommon between a group-model HMO and its primary medical group as they debate over the rates to be paid to the group on a capitation basis. In some cases, lawsuits have been filed, and the cases have eventually been settled in court.

Due to the high degree of dependence between IPA-model plans and the group of private practice physicians that participate in the HMO, there are many issues that can cause dissension. For example, one of the hardest tasks for IPAs is to control utilization through a combination of financial incentives, utilization control mechanisms, and risk-sharing arrangements. Some plans pay providers on a capitation basis and place providers at risk for a set of specified services (e.g., primary care, referrals, ancillary services, and inpatient hospital).

Many plans withhold a portion of the physician's reimbursement and use it as a risk pool in case of adverse financial experience (e.g., if the HMO loses money, or budget targets are not met, then physicians share in the adverse experience by forfeiting all or part of the withheld payments in the risk pool). Although the conditions are usually specified in the contracts between the HMO and the participating physicians, many confrontations have occurred when the HMO did not return all or most of the physicians' withhold.

HMOs and the Federal Government

The federal government is another key constituency for HMOs. For federally qualified plans, the Office of Prepaid Health Care in the Health Care Financing Administration exercises substantial influence over the implementation of the federal regulations concerning the federal qualification process. In particular, OPHC is responsible for issuing and implementing the regulations concerning adjusted community rating. In addition, the federal government provides a major source of revenue to many plans through the Federal Employees Health Benefits Program and Medicare.

The FEHBP involves a specialized contracting process in order for HMOs to be able to enroll federal workers and annuitants. With respect to rate setting, the Office of Personnel Management has its own regulations that specify the rules that HMOs must follow. Any plan that is participating in FEHBP and that is considering changing its rate-setting system should give special attention to both the impact of the change on FEHBP enrollees and the restrictions imposed by OPM. For example, health plans are allowed to be experience rated under FEHBP. However, a variety of specific rules apply to experience-rated plans (e.g., limits on types of administrative costs). In addition, OPM will probably have its own interpretation of what is allowed under adjusted community rating.

Medicare risk contracts have become a major source of revenue for many HMOs. However, there is widespread concern among HMOs regarding the adequacy of the HCFA payment rates. In addition, as discussed in previous chapters, there are many HCFA requirements that must be met by participating plans regarding reimbursement and other issues.

In summary, the federal government plays an important role for many HMOs, as both regulator and purchaser of health services. Any plan that is considering changing its rating system should thoroughly evaluate the potential implications from the standpoint of its relationship with the federal government.

9.7   Conclusion

It is impossible, within the scope of this book, to identify all of the issues and factors that can affect the competitive position of an HMO and related competitive strategies. Yet it is difficult to generalize because few, if any, strategies are applicable to every plan. Nonetheless, appropriate competitive strategies for HMOs generally are likely to depend upon the following factors:

- The plan's overall competitive position
- The plan's relationship with its providers
- The financial strength of the plan
- The strategy used by each of the plan's major competitors
- The commitments and capabilities of the plan
- Pressures from employers and other purchasers
- The feasibility of developing and implementing new rating and underwriting methods
- The cost and feasibility of improving data systems and management information
- The desirability of improving the plan's competitive position by major corporate restructuring
- The feasibility of significantly lowering the plan's cost structure through improved internal cost containment and utilization review/quality assurance procedures
- Opportunities for product line diversification
- Opportunities for joint ventures with insurers or providers
- Other opportunities in the plan's marketplace

This section focuses on (1) the need for appropriate and effective risk sharing, (2) the need for a coordinated and multifaceted approach to strategic planning, and (3) the importance of top management in the effective development and implementation of competitive strategy.

Appropriate and Effective Risk Sharing

One of the defining characteristics of an HMO is the development and implementation of appropriate risk-sharing arrangements to encourage the efficient use of resources by providers. In a broader sense, effective control of health care costs requires an appropriate sharing of risk between consumers, providers, payers, and the insuring organization.

Consumers need to be at risk for some of the financial consequences of their decisions so that they are more price-sensitive when making decisions regarding choice of health plans or specific health services. Health plans (HMOs and indemnity carriers) are necessarily at risk in their roles of insuring and delivering health services. Payers (employers, federal and state governments) will not be able to escape being at risk since they are responsible for paying a large portion of health expenditures.

Perhaps the most critical players, however, are the providers (in particular, the participating physicians in a health plan). Unless providers practice cost-effective medicine, health care costs will continue to escalate. Certainly, physicians should have appropriate economic incentives and should be at some economic risk. But it is most important for them to have professional norms that are consistent with the goals and objectives of the HMO-type plans that are trying to control utilization and costs. If they do not (if physicians behave according to fee-for-service practice patterns), it is extremely difficult for HMOs to effectively impose financial incentives and control mechanisms on participating providers. For this reason, closed-panel plans are usually more successful at developing the professional norms and practice patterns that are necessary for cost-conscious health care delivery systems.

The Importance of Top Management

The chief executive officer and the top-tier management team of an HMO may be the most important contributors to the plan's ultimate success or failure. Because most HMOs are local organizations (with relatively small to moderate-sized administrative staffs) and because there are innumerable plan-specific factors that affect the course of development of an HMO, the CEO has the inherent power to exert an enormous influence over both the daily operations and the long-term strategic course of the plan. This characteristic is unlike most insurance companies and Blue Cross plans.

Discussions of HMO competitive strategy must be tempered by consideration of the characteristics of the plan's top management team. For example, it is likely that the competitive strategy of an HMO with a CEO with a strong medical background will differ significantly from the competitive strategy of plans with financially oriented or marketing-oriented CEOs. Competitive strategy ultimately comes down to a finite number of choices, but, in most cases, the preferences and orientation of different CEOs will lead to priorities and perceptions of problems and opportunities that will result in significantly different competitive strategy outcomes.

In the final analysis, a strong CEO with experience and vision is probably the most important asset that an HMO can have in dealing with the current environment. Such persons can get the most out of solid, strong plans by (1) maximizing the financial strength of the plan, (2) resolving problems that could threaten the plan's competitive position, and (3) leading the plan into a secure future under thriving conditions. An excellent CEO can convert a marginal plan into a strong plan and could even save a weak plan that might otherwise fail. The point is not to exaggerate or overemphasize the importance of the CEO. However, the history of the HMO industry has demonstrated the importance of leadership, experience, and vision in this position and the impact of the position on an individual HMO's experience. In large HMOs (e.g., plans with over 100,000 members), the entire top management team plays this crucial role.

A Coordinated and Multifaceted Approach

It is unlikely that a single strategy will be sufficient for an HMO in today's competitive environment. Therefore, it will be necessary to develop broad, coordinated strategies that reflect all facets of the plan's current position and that are based on future goals and objectives with respect to both the overall competitive position of the plan and the major structural elements of the HMO (product lines, providers, customers, financial strength, and the plan's health care delivery system).

To be successful, plans will need to devise and implement a multifaceted approach. Fox and Heinen summarize the current climate:

> [M]anaging an HMO is not easy. Sharper skills are required today than even five years ago because of the veritable revolution taking place in

health care financing and delivery. By the same token, even sharper skills are likely to be needed in the future. Although HMO growth is rapid and shows no signs of abating, individual HMO marketplaces are becoming more crowded, and some of the competitors are not likely to survive. . . .

Employers and insurance carriers are increasingly placing restraints on the fee-for-service system, thereby reducing the utilization differentials that HMOs can achieve. In doing so, they are emulating the approaches that HMOs have originated and refined. . . .

Superior management [for HMOs] will become even more important. The plans that thrive will have leaders who are innovative and capable of rapidly turning threats into opportunities. They will also be able to integrate the various functions of the plan, for example synchronizing the utilization control mechanisms with the financial incentives, assuring that delivery capacity is expanded consistent with enrollment growth, and not losing sight of quality of care in the interests of constraining costs.

Related to the traits of flexibility and creativity is the need to stay abreast of a marketplace that is rapidly changing. This entails both redesigning products and adding to the range of products. . . .

The successful plans will respond to the needs of employers and employees. Employers are increasingly demanding data on performance and greater flexibility in HMOs' premium-setting practices. The HMOs may also have to be more flexible in tailoring benefit packages. . . .

Finally, good relations with physicians, particularly those who deliver primary care, are essential, especially in situations where most participating physicians contract with several plans and can urge patients to shift from one to another.[19]

Summary

The needs for appropriate risk sharing and a multifaceted approach, and the importance of top management, are key factors in the development and implementation of HMO competitive strategy. However, the success of an HMO's strategy during the coming years will depend on (1) accurate assessment of the plan's competitive position and the overall competitive environment in the market area, (2) the adoption of realistic and attainable goals, and (3) the implementation of disciplined measures to accomplish those goals.

Different plans are attempting many different strategies. These strategies range from product line diversification to expansion of provider networks/geographic service areas to joint ventures with insurance companies and provider groups.

To be successful in the coming years, a plan will need astute management with the flexibility and foresight to identify and adapt to rapidly changing competitive conditions. Efforts to improve the competitive position of the plan will require increased attention to marketing approaches, new product development, rating and underwriting practices, provider relations and contract negotiations, cost-containment procedures, data systems and MIS reporting capabilities, utilization review and quality of care protocols, accounting, actuarial and financial-planning methods, and provider reimbursement and risk-sharing arrangements.

Clearly, with the changes that are occurring in health care delivery, organization, and financing, HMOs face a daunting array of competitive pressures, potential barriers, and other obstacles to success. Achieving a high level of success during the next five years will be a demanding and difficult challenge for most HMOs.

The deregulation of the airline industry in the 1970s dramatically increased the level of competition and spawned a host of new entrants and carriers. During the past ten years, however, there were frequent price wars; profitability declined substantially; several major carriers went bankrupt (or were threatened with insolvency); and a series of mergers and acquisitions led to a lesser number of larger, nationwide competitors.

> Today, eight airlines transport 90 percent of all passengers in the U.S. Discount carriers such as People Express, Jet America and New York Air have all closed in recent years. To some, eight airlines might seem like enough to maintain a healthy level of competition. But while many other industries have competitive pricing with fewer than eight participants, . . . it's impossible for all eight airlines to compete against each other in every market across the nation. Instead, most airports are now dominated by just one or two carriers, making the competitive pressures on a local level far less than they might seem nationally.[20]

Thus, major carriers have striven to establish and dominate hubs and to carve out route patterns that are protected from heavy competition. As a result, profitability in the airline industry appears to be recovering as the level of competition recedes.

Whether a similar picture will emerge for HMOs (and the health care industry in general) is still not clear. Although the health care industry has unique characteristics (e.g., the fact that health care is primarily a local business is likely to preclude nationwide HMOs), some similarities are likely to develop. Price competition will drive some plans out of business or into mergers. Many plans will seek secure market niches protected from excessive competition. Large plans will attempt to dominate (one or more) selected local market areas and use their size and economic clout to their financial advantage.

To overcome current obstacles to success, plans with vision will combine top-notch management, effective provider risk-sharing and incentive arrangements, stringent internal cost controls, and a substantially improved relationship with employers. In addition to long-term strategic planning, each plan will have to identify and remedy current deficiencies. Whereas many open-panel plans will be forced to adopt strong cost-control mechanisms, many closed-panel plans will need to make major adjustments in rating and data systems to respond to the increased requirements of a competitive marketplace. As the "sorting out" process continues, the pluralistic nature of the U.S. health system will most likely prevent generic resolutions and lead to a multiplicity of outcomes in different market areas.

Notes

1. Refer to Section 1.4 for a description of the COBRA and Section 89 requirements.
2. The Financial Accounting Standards Board (FASB) has proposed that future liabilities for retiree medical costs be recognized and recorded on the balance sheets of corporations. Retiree medical expenses are now treated as a current expense on a cash basis. Initial estimates indicated that this change in accounting procedures could have a significant impact on the financial results for many corporations. Although final action has not been taken on this issue by FASB, the current proposal calls for these provisions to become effective in 1992. See P. A. Doran et al., *Measuring and Funding Corporate Liabilities for Retiree Health Benefits* (Washington, DC: Employee Benefit Research Institute, 1987).
3. For a broad discussion of current issues affecting employer health benefits programs, see F. B. McArdle, ed., *The Changing Health Care Market* (Washington, DC: Employee Benefit Research Institute, 1987).
4. As of February 1989, there was continuing disagreement over the average increase in the cost of health insurance plans during 1988. A study by the Health Insurance Association of America (HIAA) found that health insurance premiums rose an average of 12 percent between spring 1987 and spring 1988. See J. Gabel et al., "Employer Sponsored Health Insurance in America: Preliminary Results from the 1988 Survey" (Washington, DC: HIAA, January 1989). Other observers believe that the trend increase was 15 to 30 percent. See "Consultants Dispute Survey's Analysis of Group Health Costs," *Business Insurance* 22, no. 52(1988): 1. Some employers would have no increase (or possibly even a decrease) in health premiums, while a substantial number of employers have experienced large increases of 30 percent or more. See "Higher and Higher: 1988 Health Costs Exceed Estimates; No Relief Seen in '89," *Business Insurance* 26, no. 39(1988): 1; "Health Plan Costs Top 10 percent of Pay," *Business Insurance* 23, no.

2(1989): 1; and "Rising Health Costs Dampen Holiday Cheer," *Business Insurance* 22, no. 51(1988): 5.

5. In 1987, approximately two-thirds of existing HMOs experienced financial losses, according to GHAA. This followed the pattern for 1985 and 1986. Many plans had low premium increases in these years (or no increase at all) and attribute the losses primarily to underpricing. Perceived competitive pressure from other HMOs and direct price competition from health insurers also played a role in premium increase decisions by individual HMOs. During this same time period, Blue Cross plans and private health insurance carriers reportedly lost several billion dollars. See H. L. Sutton, "The Future of HMOs in a Chaotic Environment," *Health Section News* (Chicago, IL: Society of Actuaries, January 1989) for an interesting and perceptive assessment of current trends affecting the HMO industry.

6. Some private insurers have consolidated their HMO plans, selling or closing their unprofitable plans and centralizing operations with their strongest plans.

7. The inherent power of physician providers has been demonstrated in several areas in recent years and has led to lawsuits, revised financial arrangements, plan restructurings, and changes in plan management.

8. The other side of this issue is that many corporations now offer numerous HMOs (e.g., national firms may have contracts with 100 HMOs or more). In some cases, selection problems have been severe in highly segmented multiple-option health programs operated by employers. Many companies have hired consultants to assist in reducing the number of HMO offerings to a more manageable number and to develop more effective strategies for dealing with HMOs. Consultants have also provided assistance in determining appropriate factors for risk-adjusted employer contributions to HMOs, which reflect the level of risk represented by the subgroup of employees that enroll with an HMO.

9. See, for example, Jon Christianson, Maureen Shadle, Mary Hunter, Susan Hartwell, and Jeanne McGee, "The New Environment for Rural HMOs," *Health Affairs* 5, no. 1(1986): 105–121; and Jon Christianson, et al., "The Growth of HMOs in Rural Areas," *GHAA Journal* 7, no. 2(1986): 35–42.

10. There are many theories on the topic of the future growth of the HMO industry. Some observers believe that well-managed IPAs have competitive advantages due to their open panels and ease of adapting to open-ended product designs. Other observers favor prepaid group practice models due to their inherent cost advantages and ability to control utilization and practice patterns. Still others believe that strong HMOs, regardless of model type, will benefit from the current environment and experience substantial growth as other HMOs fail (refer to Chapter 2 for a discussion of the record-setting growth experienced by Kaiser Permanente in 1988).

11. In the preceding sections, we have argued that HMOs face serious threats in the current environment and that each plan should rethink its competitive strategy, if it has not already done so. There are a number of other theories on the current situation and the potential effects on HMOs. Some observers

believe that strong HMOs will actually benefit from the current competitive environment and that only weak or marginal plans really have to be concerned about survival (e.g., strong HMOs will be the beneficiaries of the consolidation and restructuring that is taking place). Other observers believe that many HMOs do not have to implement radical changes in order to respond to current competitive pressures. For example, some believe that well-established plans that adhere to traditional prepaid group practice principles will be immune to threats from competition. Others favor well-managed IPAs with effective utilization control mechanisms and physician incentives for long-term success.

12. See Willard G. Manning et al. "Health Insurance and the Demand for Medical Care: Evidence from a Randomized Experiment," *American Economic Review* 77, no. 3(1987): 251–77.

13. The HMO Amendments of 1988 permit federally qualified HMOs to provide up to 10 percent of services through non-HMO physicians. Many HMOs have already developed open-ended HMO products and introduced them into the marketplace.

14. In terms of a baseline for cost comparisons, the total projected cost of the employer's health benefits program for the next year is most important from the employer perspective. HMOs need to redirect their thinking from their own perspective and work jointly with their major employer clients on the larger problem.

15. See note 2 for an explanation of the FASB ruling.

16. Based on remarks by Patricia M. Nazemetz, Xerox Corporation, at 1988 Group Health Institute, Chicago, June 1988.

17. In most cases to date, employers have approached HMOs rather than vice versa. See George C. Halvorson and James R. Hansen, "Developments in the Adverse Selection Debate," paper presented at the 1989 Group Health Institute, Atlanta, GA, June 1989. Halvorson's results indicated that employers using the total replacement approach consistently saved in excess of 10 percent of their total projected health expenditures.

18. A number of other HMOs have employed this strategy with selected employer groups. Although many of these contracts have not been in operation long enough for a thorough assessment of both the HMO's and the employer's experiences, preliminary evidence indicates that many of the arrangements have been profitable from the HMO's perspective and that the employer's overall health care costs have been successfully contained in the process. It is essential, however, for HMOs to pay close attention to carefully underwriting these groups before entering into contractual arrangements. In particular, characteristics of groups that could be associated with adverse selection (e.g., low participation rates) should be thoroughly investigated.

19. P. D. Fox and L. Heinen, *Determinants of HMO Success* (Ann Arbor, MI: Health Administration Press, 1987).

20. J. Koten, "Airlines Pushing Fares Linked to Mileage," *Wall Street Journal,* 13 January 1989, B–1.

Epilogue

In the months since the manuscript for this book was completed, several developments have affected the competitive environment for HMOs and the relationships between HMOs and employers. After a short respite, health care costs increased sharply in 1988. A survey of employers by A. Foster Higgins estimated that the cost of providing group health plans rose 18.6 percent in 1988, more than double the rate of increase for 1986 and 1987.[1] Many employers reported premium increases of 20 to 50 percent or more, and this trend appears to be continuing for 1989 renewals.[2] Other developments have included the following:

1. There has been a general trend toward consolidation and reduction of the number of HMO offerings, especially among larger employers.[3] Although the major goal behind this trend has been to rationalize the number of health plan offerings, the trend has also been related to the need to (1) reduce administrative costs and ease administrative burden, and (2) respond to concerns regarding the potential impact of Section 89 nondiscrimination requirements for health benefit plans.[4]

2. More employers are using Requests for Proposals in HMO contracting. The prevalence of RFPs has increased significantly in recent months. They usually differ in form and content, but the basic thrust has been to negotiate hard on benefits, cost sharing, prices, data, and other contract terms and conditions.[5]

3. There has been increased cost shifting to patients through increased deductibles and co-insurance, and, in some cases, capping and reduction of benefits.[6]

4. There has been a trend from "defined benefit" to "defined contribution" approaches, partly reflecting concerns about the Financial Accounting Standards Board requirements for report-

ing retiree health liabilities that are scheduled to become effective in 1992.[7]

5. With respect to price competition, the trends have been mixed. In some areas, price competition has eased and conditions have stabilized in the marketplace, allowing premiums to rise with improvement in HMO financial results. In other areas, however, heavy price competition continues, with some plans buying market share with below-cost premiums.[8]

6. In several areas, employers are getting directly involved in organizing and delivering health services. For example, employer-sponsored HMOs are being considered in some areas, usually by business coalitions or groups of large employers. In general, it is too early to tell whether these efforts are serious, or if they will be successful.[9]

7. Employers continue to be concerned about pricing, benefit design, quality assurance, biased selection, risk segmentation, and employee satisfaction.[10] But there has been renewed emphasis on *cost containment* and obtaining *value* for the health care dollar.[11]

8. Some employers have initiated major programs using a "managed competition" approach with selective contracting for health plans.[12] Other employers have turned to "sole-sourcing" approaches, in which dual or triple options are offered by a single carrier in an effort to control health care costs.[13] In some cases, employers have restructured their health benefits program and replaced all plans with a single HMO that offers a self-referral option to choose non-HMO providers at the point of service.[14]

9. InterStudy recently reported that HMO enrollment increased by 1.6 million members during the 1988 calendar year, for a total of 31.9 million HMO members as of 31 December 1988.[15] HMOs now constitute 18 percent of enrollment in employer-sponsored health plans.[16] However, the 5.4 percent annual growth rate for the HMO industry in 1988 was substantially below HMO growth rates in previous years. In addition, the number of HMOs had declined to 607 plans as of 1 January 1989, compared to a high of 653 plans as of 1 January 1988.

New HMO development virtually stopped in 1987, and few new plans have begun operations since then. Although enrollment growth rates have varied among individual plans, many established HMOs have experienced high rates of growth as newer plans ceased operation or merged with larger plans. Some plans have continued to suffer serious financial problems. The most notable case is Maxicare, which filed for reorganization under Chapter 11 of the U.S. bankruptcy laws in March 1989 and has undergone major restructuring.[17] The movement toward consolidation in the HMO industry has become quite evident.

10. The Group Health Association of America has reported a significant change in the rate-setting methods used by HMOs. The proportion of plans that used experience rating for some employer groups increased from 13.5 percent in 1985 to 31.2 percent in 1988. In addition, the GHAA survey of the HMO industry found that only 15.8 percent of established HMOs did *not* anticipate using the increased rating flexibility (e.g., adjusted community rating, prospective experience rating) permitted to federally qualified HMOs by the HMO Amendments of 1988 (32.7 percent of plans anticipated a great deal of use, 37.1 percent of plans anticipted limited use, and 14.4 percent of plans were not sure).[18] In addition, several articles have been published concerning experience-rating methods for HMOs.[19] In the Federal Employees Health Benefits Program, approximately 20 plans submitted ACR rates in May 1989 for the 1990 contract year. Detailed instructions concerning permissible adjusted community-rating methods for FEHBP were under development by the U.S. Office of Personnel Management at the time of this writing.

11. After a round of initial enthusiasm for Medicare risk contracts in the mid-1980s, most HMOs have been forced to undertake a more realistic appraisal of the financial viability of this form of contracting. As a result, several plans have recently terminated risk contracts. However, there are currently 133 HMOs with risk contracts serving more than 1 million Medicare members, and a total of almost 2 million Medicare beneficiaries are served by HMOs under either risk or cost contracts.[20] In addi-

tion, various efforts are underway to improve the risk contracts (e.g., Adjusted Average Per Capita Cost [AAPCC] Task Force and diagnostic cost group demonstrations).[21]

12. Perhaps the most interesting development has been the resurgence of the prepaid group practice model plans. From coast to coast, many established staff-model and group-model HMOs have reported record-breaking enrollment growth. Financial results have also been strong for many plans. Some of these plans have found that a more comfortable relationship with health benefit consultants and employer representatives has replaced the adversarial, confrontational relationship that had been common in the last few years. This has been accompanied, to some extent, by acknowledgment of PGP plans that are successful at cost containment.[22]

There are still many difficult issues that need to be resolved. Analysis of HMO selection bias and selection effects in multiple-option health benefits programs is quite complicated, and we still have a lot to learn about that topic.[23] Do HMOs produce cost savings for employers? Although each case involving an HMO and an employer has unique characteristics, HMOs still offer employers one of the few viable options for cost containment. The jury is still out on whether PPOs or indemnity plans with selected managed care features—like preadmission certification and second surgical opinion—are capable of successfully producing long-term cost containment for employers.[24] Some argue that these plans do not sufficiently change the economic incentives, practice patterns, or the methods of health care delivery from the traditional fee-for-service practice of medicine. Although control of health costs will undoubtedly remain a difficult problem for many years, HMO-type plans—especially those that have efficient delivery systems, effective cost-containment procedures, well-defined provider incentives, documented quality assurance methods, and appropriate pricing methods for determining employer premiums—are currently the best hope of employers to control health care costs. It is obviously going to take major efforts by both parties to overcome some of the obstacles in the changing relationship between employers and HMOs. Among other things, each employer will have to determine the best strategy for tackling the health care cost problem and decide if HMOs are part of the overall strategy. For their part, it is incumbent upon HMOs to fully understand and effectively respond to the legitimate concerns of employers, within the framework of a long-term business relationship.

Notes

1. "Double-Digit Inflation Returns to Health Care Plans," *Employee Benefit Plan Review* 43, no. 10(1989): 52.
2. See Jon Gabel et al., "Employer-Sponsored Health Insurance in America," *Health Affairs* 8, no. 2(1989): 116–28; and G. Ruffenach, "Health Insurance Premiums to Soar in '89: Workers Likely to Take on More of Costs," *Wall Street Journal,* 25 October 1988, B–1.
3. A. Peres, J. Mortimer, and C. Shields, "Employers Flex Their Muscles with HMOs," *Business and Health* 6, no. 1(1988): 18–22.
4. H. Stout, "Tax Code's Much-Maligned Section 89 is Likely to Be Amended Before It Can Even Take Effect," *Wall Street Journal,* 2 May 1989, A–20.
5. G. Halvorson, *How to Control Your Company's Health Costs* (Englewood Cliffs, NJ: Prentice-Hall, 1988); "Employers Ask More from HMO Contracts," *Business Insurance* 21, no. 45(1987): 30.
6. See, for example, D. C. Coddington and K. D. Moore, "Employers Looking for More than Health Care Cost Containment," *Health Care Strategic Management* 5, no. 3(1987): 4–9. However, others have argued that there has not been an increase in cost sharing in employer-sponsored health plans, and that, in some cases, coverage and benefits have increased. See, for example, G. Jensen, M. Morrisey, and J. Marcus, "Cost-Sharing and the Changing Pattern of Employer-Sponsored Health Benefits," *Milbank Memorial Fund Quarterly* 65, no. 4(1987): 521–550; J. Gabel et al., "The Changing World of Group Health Insurance," *Health Affairs* 7, no. 3(1988): 48–65.
7. See S. Adler, "Retiree Health Care Accounting Rules to Cut Profits," *Business Insurance* 23, no. 25(1989): 1; R. Ostuw, "How to Control Retiree Health Plan Costs," *Business and Health* 7, no. 3(1989): 12–15.
8. "Double-Digit Inflation Returns to Health Care Plans," *Employee Benefit Plan Review* 43, no. 10(1989): 52–54.
9. D. DiBlase, "Direct Ties with Providers Can Cut Health Care Costs," *Business Insurance* 23, no. 26(1989): 121.
10. P. D. Fox, "The Future of HMOs," *Compensation & Benefits Management* 5, no. 2(1989): 101–106.
11. See R. W. Sorrenti, "How to Assess Managed Care Plans," *Business and Health* 5, no. 11(1988): 14–16; "Active Role in Benefits Mandatory," *Business Insurance* 23, no. 26(1989): 123; B. Dowd, R. Feldman, and J. Klein, "What Do Employers Really Want in a Health Plan?" *Business and Health* 4, no. 3(1987): 44–48.
12. A. C. Enthoven, "Managed Competition: An Agenda for Action," *Health Affairs* 7, no. 3(1988): 25–47.
13. "HMOs Must Meet Employer Demands: Expert," *Business Insurance* 23, no. 26(1989): 121.
14. G. C. Halvorson and J. R. Hansen, "Developments in the Adverse Selection Debate," Paper presented at the 1989 Group Health Institute, Atlanta, Georgia, June 1989.

15. "HMO Enrollment Growth in 1988 Near Record Low," *Business Insurance* 23, no. 22(1989): 1.

16. Jon Gabel et al., "Employer-Sponsored Health Insurance in America," *Health Affairs* 8, no. 2(1989): 117.

17. "Court Blocks States' Attempt to Rehabilitate Maxicare Units," *Business Insurance* 23, no. 25(1989): 2.

18. Group Health Association of America, *HMO Industry Profile,* vol. 1; *Benefits, Premiums, and Market Structure in 1988* (Washington, DC: Group Health Association of America, 1989), 35 and 74.

19. See, for example, Randall P. Herman and Daniel E. Freier, "Experience Rating and Administrative Services Only Arrangements for HMOs," *GHAA Journal* 9, no. 1(1988): 69–79; David V. Axene, "Alternate Premium Financing Methods for the Managed Care Plan," in *Proceedings of 1989 Group Health Institute* (Washington, DC: Group Health Association of America, 1989); Karen R. Bauder, "Minimum Premium Arrangements in Health Maintenance Organizations," in *Proceedings of 1988 Group Health Institute* (Washington, DC: Group Health Association of America, 1989); Douglas G. Cave, Stuart O. Schweitzer, and Peter A. Lachenbruch, "Community Rating by Class as a Method of Adjusting Community Rated Employer Group Capitation Payments," *GHAA Journal* 9, no. 1(1988): 80–96; Gordon R. Trapnell and Charles W. Wrightson, "HMO Pricing Issues from an Actuarial Perspective," in *Proceedings of 1988 Group Health Institute* (Washington, DC: Group Health Association of America, 1989).

20. U.S. Department of Health and Human Services, Office of Prepaid Health Care, "TEFRA HMO/CMP Contracts: Monthly Report" (Washington, DC: Health Care Financing Administration, 1 April 1989).

21. C. Carter, Presentation on Medicare risk contracts from the Office of Prepaid Health Care (HCFA) at the 1989 Group Health Institute, Atlanta, Georgia, June 1989.

22. The discussion of this development is based on (1) review of recent HMO enrollment statistics, and (2) conversations with numerous HMO officials during the spring of 1989. It should be noted that, although many staff-model and group-model HMOs have participated in this resurgence, other prepaid group practice plans have experienced flat enrollments or have suffered adverse financial results.

23. For excellent overviews and discussions of current issues related to this topic, see David Mechanic, "Consumer Choice among Health Insurance Options," *Health Affairs* 8, no. 1(1989): 138–48; and Harold S. Luft and Robert H. Miller, "Patient Selection in a Competitive Health Care System," *Health Affairs* 7, no. 3(1988): 53. Some experts continue to believe that HMOs consistently receive favorable selection: "It is no secret that healthy young adults dominate the rosters of HMOs." (Regina E. Herzlinger, "The Failed Revolution in Health Care—The Role of Management," *Harvard Business Review* 67, no. 2(1989): 95–103.) For HMO disenroll-

ment, see William Wrightson, James Genuardi, and Sharman Stephens, "Demographic and Utilization Characteristics of HMO Disenrollees," *GHAA Journal* 8, no. 1(1987): 22; and Stephen H. Long, Russell F. Settle, and Charles W. Wrightson, "Employee Premiums, Availability of Alternative Plans, and HMO Disenrollment," *Medical Care* 26, no. 10(1988): 927–38.

24. See, for example, Thomas Rice, Jon Gabel, and Gregory de Lissovoy, "PPOs: The Employer Perspective," *Journal of Health Politics, Policy and Law* 14, no. 2(1989): 367–82; T. M. Wickizer, J. R. C. Wheeler, and P. J. Feldstein, "Does Utilization Review Reduce Unnecessary Hospital Care and Contain Costs?" *Medical Care* 27, no. 6(1989): 632–47; J. R. Schiffman, "Revising Second-Opinion Health Plans: Companies Find Such Programs Fail to Cut Costs," *Wall Street Journal,* 24 May 1989, B–1; Howard Larkin, "PPOs Join Forces for Economy, Market Leverage," *Hospitals* 63, no. 3(1989): 66; P. J. Feldstein et al., "Private Cost Containment: The Effects of Utilization Review Programs on Health Care Use and Expenditures," *New England Journal of Medicine* 318(20):1310, 1988; *Issues in Managed Health Care* (Brookfield, WI: International Foundation of Employee Benefit Plans, 1989).

Glossary of HMO Actuarial Terminology

Access. An individual's ability to obtain medical services on a timely and financially acceptable basis.

Actuary. A professional trained in the science of loss contingencies, investments, accounting, statistics, and subjects relating to insurance programs and systems.

Administrative Loading. Or retention, as in insurance. The amount added to the prospective actuarial cost of health care services (pure premium) for expenses of administration, marketing, and profit.

Adverse Selection. Disproportionate enrollment of adverse risks, like an impaired or older population, with a potential for higher health care utilization than budgeted for an average population.

Capitation. A method of payment for and charging for health services in which an HMO, medical group, or institution is paid a fixed amount for each person served, usually monthly. The amount of money paid covers services provided regardless of the actual value of those services. Specific service costs are often expressed as dollars per member per month in development of capitation rates and premiums.

Community Rating. A general method of establishing premiums for financing health care in which the individual's premium or capitation rate is based on the actual or anticipated average cost of health services used by all HMO members in a specific service area. Acceptable methods are defined in federal statutes.

Source: Sutton, Harry J., Jr., FSA, and Allen J. Sorbo, FSA, *Actuarial Issues in the Fee-for-Service/Prepaid Medical Group,* one in a series of seven monographs, the "Going Prepaid" series (Denver, CO: Center for Research in Ambulatory Health Care Administration, research arm of the Medical Group Management Association, 1987), 74–77. Reprinted by permission of the publisher.

341

Community Rating by Class. A modification of established community rating principles, whereby individual groups can have different rates depending on the composition by age, sex, marital status, and industry. The changes were included in the 1981 amendments to the Federal HMO Act affecting qualified plans.

Completion Method. A method of determining outstanding claim liabilities whereby the claims already paid are divided by a factor indicating the percentage of estimated claims paid to date.

Compositing. A term used for combining a multiple tiered rate structure into a tier structure with fewer tiers. For example, combining a rating system using two-person contracts and three or more person contracts into a premium structure which includes all families of two or more.

Contract Type. Classification of employees into categories usually based on enrolled dependent status. Typical would be a single employee, an employee with one dependent, or an employee with two or more dependents.

Conversion Factor. An arithmetic number which is multiplied by the HMO capitation rate to produce a rate for single employees.

Coordination of Benefits (COB). A typical insurance provision whereby responsibility for primary payment for medical services is allocated between carriers where a person is covered by more than one employer-sponsored health benefit program. This coordination avoids a person's being reimbursed twice for the same medical services.

Copayments. Any extra charges specified in the contract for certain services not fully covered through prepayment. Payments must be made by user of services.

Dual Choice. An option offered individuals in an employer group to choose between two or more different health care benefit programs, i.e., between the employer's health benefit plan and an HMO.

Experience Rating. A rating system in which the premium rates reflect the cost experience of the particular group enrolled.

Feasibility Analysis. A study to gather and analyze information and financial data or forecasts to assess criteria and to enumerate influences, deterrents, advantages, and disadvantages of a task, project, program, or action. The feasibility study presents conclusions and strategies or recommendations accordingly.

Health Maintenance Organization (HMO). An organized system of health care that provides directly or arranges for a comprehensive range of basic and supplemental health care services to a voluntarily enrolled group of persons in a geographic area under a prepayment plan. The term HMO is specifically defined in the Federal HMO Act (P.L. 93–222) of 1973 and its amendments.

Incentives. As related to medical care delivery, this term refers to economic incentives for providers to motivate efficiency in patient care management.

Indemnity Insurance. Indemnity insurance typically means coverage offered by insurance companies and Blue Cross plans, whereby individual persons insured are indemnified through reimbursement by the carriers for their medical expenses. Payments may be made to the individual incurring the expense, or, in many cases, directly to providers. The important point is that the indemnity relates only to a specific loss incurred by the insured person after the fact.

Intensity Factor. A multiplier or weighting element used in computations to allow for the quantitative influence of a specific variable.

Lag Factor. Lag factor is a general term indicating a percentage of claims incurred in a given accounting period but received, processed, and paid by specific months following the close of the accounting period.

Loading Factor. See **Administrative Loading.**

Loss Ratio. The ratio between costs incurred for health care services and premiums received.

Member. An individual who has entered into a contractual agreement or on whose behalf a contractual agreement has been entered into with an HMO for the provision of health care services.

Out-of-Area Benefits. Those benefits that the plan supplies to its members when they are outside the geographical limits of the HMO. These benefits always include emergency services.

Penetration. In marketing HMOs, the percentage of possible subscribers within an employment group that enrolls in the HMO. **Participation** or **saturation** is sometimes used.

Premium Rate. A monetary amount charged employers or individuals to prepay the cost of health care services. The premium rates may vary by contract type. The premium is a specific contractual amount agreed on by the HMO (or an insurer) and an employer to fix a cost for medical services for employees over an agreed-on period of time.

Proprietary. Operated for the purpose of gaining a profit.

Qualified. Meeting HMO program standards defined by the federal HMO law.

Reinsurance. Insurance by the HMO with a third party against risks which the plan cannot easily financially manage. For example, insuring for 80 percent of hospital charges in excess of $20,000 for one patient in a year (catastrophic), or total HMO costs in excess of 115 percent of revenue (aggregate).

Risk. The uncertainty of loss or expense levels due to the inability to project with complete confidence the exact health care needs of the HMO population.

Risk Retention.   A description of the limitations of financial liability remaining with a major entity to the HMO program. For example, the HMO may accept all risk to guarantee provision of services to its enrolled population. This risk may be limited by arrangements with reinsurers. Also, the fee-for-service/prepaid medical group may take full risk or limit its risk by contractual arrangements with the HMO corporation.

Service Area.   The geographic area covered by the HMO, within which it provides direct services.

Shared Risk.   In the context of an HMO, an arrangement in which financial liabilities are apportioned between two or more entities. For example, the HMO and the medical group may each agree to share the risk of excessive hospital cost over budgeted amounts on a 50–50 basis.

Stop-Loss.   An arrangement between an HMO (including the FFS/PPD medical group) and a reinsurer whereby absorption of prepaid patient expenses is limited, either in terms of overall expenditures and deficits, or by limiting losses on an individual expensive hospital and/or professional services claim.

Subrogation.   Seeking, by legal or administrative means, reimbursement from others responsible for certain categories of medical expenses such as workers' compensation, third party negligence liability, or no-fault auto medical coverage.

Subscriber.   An employment group or an unaffiliated individual that contracts with an HMO.

Utilization.   The extent to which a given group uses specific services in a specific period of time, usually expressed as the number of services used per year per 1,000 persons eligible for the services; utilization rates may be expressed in other types of ratios, i.e., per eligible person covered.

Venture Capital.   Private capital offered in return for a large share of ownership in a new business venture where the chance of failure may be high but success will produce extreme financial gain.

Index

A

AAPCC. *See* Adjusted average per capita cost

Accreditation Association for Ambulatory Health Care, 75

ACR. *See* Adjusted community rating

Actuarial/fee-for-services method. *See* Capitation rate

Actuaries, 248, 307, 328; capitation and, 150, 153, 155, 158–64; rating and, 114, 119, 126, 205; tasks of, 140, 221, 267, 270–71, 273

Adams, Brock, 101

Administrative services only (ASO), 30, 80, 118, 152, 311

Adjusted average per capita cost (AAPCC), 7, 10, 264, 270–71, 336

Adjusted community rating (ACR), 10, 214, 312, 335; adjustment factors, 170, 200–203; group-specific. *See* Group-specific rating; HMO legislation and, 6, 78, 89–90, 101–3, 147, 199–206, 237, 242n7, 323; relative experience ratio and, 227–28

Adverse selection, 82, 87, 104n8, 219, 256, antiselection, 127, 136, 249, 297; causes of, 261–64; defined, 127; selection bias and, 246–48, 250; spiral, 74, 102, 265; underwriting and, 250–51

AETNA Life & Casualty, 13, 299

AHA. *See* American Hospital Association

AHCCCS. *See* Arizona Health Care Cost Containment Study

Allied-Signal Technologies Inc., 316, 318

AMA. *See* American Medical Association

AMCRA. *See* American Medical Care and Review Association

American Hospital Association (AHA), 27

American Medical Association (AMA), 26–27

American Medical Care and Review Association (AMCRA), 98

Antiselection. *See* Adverse selection

Arizona, HMOs in, 37, 40, 316

Arizona Health Care Cost Containment Study (AHCCCS), 305

ASO. *See* Administrative services only

B

Benefits programs, xiv, 248, 264, 271, 304, 315, 320. *See also* Employers; design options of, 86, 152, 197, 219, 241n1, 307–8, 319, 327, 333; multiple-option, 33, 70, 84, 87, 102–3, 246–47, 256, 261, 265, 267–68, 311, 314, 316, 336; service and, 50–51; triple-option, 30,

33, 197, 296, 311, 315

Birnbaum, Roger, 96, 98, 143

Blue Cross, 13, 120–21, 143–44, 213; HMOs vs., 34, 49–51, 81, 84, 104n9, 114, 117, 138, 239, 250, 326

Blue Cross/Blue Shield Association, 12–13, 98, 144

Bureau of Labor Statistics, U.S., 161

Byrd, Robert C., 101

C

California, HMO enrollment in, 28, 32, 33, 37, 39–40, 143, 316

Capitation rate, 30, 150, 153, 158–59, 179, 306; actuarial/fee-for-service method, 155, 158–64; development for HMOs, 162–63; fixed, 59; historical data projection, 160–61; reimbursement and, 55, 230, 322; risk-adjusted, 190

CIBNR. *See* Claims incurred but not reported

CIGNA Health Plans, 13, 37, 316, 318

Claims incurred but not reported (CIBNR), 54, 160–62, 193n21, 226, 322

Class rates. *See* Manual rating

Closed-panel plans. *See* Group-model plans; Staff-model plans

CMPs. *See* Competitive medical plans

COBRA. *See* Consolidated Omnibus Budget Reconciliation Act

Colorado, HMO enrollment in, 29, 33, 37, 38, 40, 316

Committee on the Costs of Medical Care, xvii, 26

Community rating, 106, 119–21, 201, 204, 213, 220–21, 264. *See also* Adjusted community rating, Capitation rate; advantages/limitations, 83–87, 103–5nn8–12, 115, 241n2;

conversion factor, 167–68, 181–82; design and implemention, 103n7, 150–53, 174–75, 253, 255; equity in, 118, 120, 148; HMOs, xviii, 29, 71–73, 76–78, 81, 88–89, 139, 144–47, 165, 173–74, 178, 196; flexibility in, 87, 164–69, 171–73; increases in, 153–55, 158, 175; other rating methods vs., 84–85, 104n10, 143–44, 153, 175–76, 185–87, 190, 239; recompositing of, 148, 169, 171, 257; size of group and, 208, 251

Community rating by class, 87, 180–81, 218, 234–36; factors of, 175–77, 182–84, 186–88; HMO legislation and, 72, 88–90, 145–46, 174–78, 187, 189; manual rating and, 121; risks and, 175, 177–81, 190; standard community rating vs., 175–76, 185–87, 190

Competition, 98, 220, 317; health care market and, 11–15, 33, 75–76, 114, 136–37, 153, 263, 306, 316:—changes in, 70, 81–83, 144, 174, 196–97, 205, 237, 301; —cost-containment efforts, 4, 245; —group insurance and, 117–18, 218–20; HMOS and, 81–86, 103–4n8, 114, 264, 296–99, 305–6; managed, 318, 334; selection bias and, 344

Competitive medical plans (CMPS), 7, 10, 95

Competitive strategies. *See also* Cost containment, Cost sharing, Risk sharing; coordination of, 299, 305, 318, 325–37; cost-containment measures, 300, 302–4, 318–22; employers and, 304–5, 313–18; financial strength, 301–2, 305–7, 325–29; government and, 323–34; HMO growth and, 297–99, 305–6; physician providers and, 322–24

Compositing. *See* Premium rate, composite

Consolidated Omnibus Budget Reconciliation Act (COBRA) of 1985, 9, 295

Copayments. *See* Cost sharing

Cost containment, 49–50, 56, 70, 84, 150, 153, 230, 295; as competitive strategy, 300, 306, 311–12, 324, 328; direct measures for, 51–58; need for, 4–5, 88, 334, 336; risk sharing and, 58–64

Cost sharing, 80, 162, 256, 263, 272; as competitive strategy, 11–12, 308–12, 314–15; requirements of, 29, 71, 94, 152, 253, 266

Costs: actual-to-expected, 130–35, 222–30, 235–36; adjusted average per capita, 7, 10, 264, 270–71, 311

Crane, Robert, 96

Cross subsidies, 72, 80, 86, 101, 119, 121, 218, 235–37

D

Data: analysis strategies, 232–41, 312; and community rating, 150–53; dissemination of, HMO use and cost, 75, 80; historical, projection of, 160–62; and rating capabilities, 52, 56, 233–34, 312; systems, 57, 85, 185, 196, 239, 306, 319, 328

Densen, P. M., 258

Department of Health and Human Services, U.S., 61, 79, 93, 95–96, 146, 176–77, 185

Diagnosis-related groups (DRGs), 8, 159, 210–11

Dingell, John D., 101

Donabedian, Avedis, 258

DRGs. *See* Diagnosis-related groups

Dual-choice mandate, 27, 71, 76–77, 92, 93, 99–100

E

Eggers, P., 259, 264

Ellwood, Paul, 25

Employees: coverage options, 5, 11, 48, 77, 263, 266, 309–10, 318–322, 325; satisfaction levels, 70, 79, 320–21

Employers, 196–97, 259, 263, 268, 279n56, 325, 334. *See also* Dual-choice mandate; benefits offered, 72, 80, 158, 197, 219, 248, 271–72, 304, 309, 314, 327; contribution to costs, 4, 11, 70–71, 73, 75–78, 87–88, 89, 91–93, 103n8, 248, 256–57, 300, 312–13; cost savings to, 5, 102–3, 304, 313; HMOs and, 5, 33, 70–81, 88–89, 114, 118, 254, 299–300, 304–5, 313–18, 320–22, 329, 335; legislation and, 7–11, 88–93, 314; preference for experience rating, 199–200; request for proposal (RFP) and, 314, 317, 333

Enrollment, 31, 33, 35–38, 42, 49, 175–76, 334–35. *See also* Health maintenance organizations; composition of, 48, 92, 121, 183, 205, 252, 263–64; freezing of, 315; group, 120–21, 129–30, 138, 228–30, 250, 300, 306, 315; health status of. *See* Skimming; largest U.S. plans, 37–38, 40–41; open, xviii, 230, 302, 315; patterns, 190, 235–36, 246, 249–50, 271; rate setting and, 86, 169–70; selective, 250, 253, 266, 271–72, 303, 334. *See also* Skimmming

Enthoven, Alain, 14–15, 260, 317

Experience rating, 6, 72, 97, 101–2, 118, 145, 151, 217–18, 237, 249, 321; implementation of, 214–15; increases in, 335; large employers and, 78, 215; other rating methods vs., 84–86, 104n10, 121–22, 143, 153, 178, 206; prospective, 90, 122, 196, 199, 201, 214–18. *See also* Group-specific rating; requirements, 114–15, 174, 323; retrospective, 79, 90, 122, 212, 214–18; underwriting and, 137

F

FASB. *See* Financial Accounting Standards Board
Favorable selection. *See* Skimming
Federal Employees Benefits Program (FEHBP), 12, 176, 187, 192n16, 242n7, 259, 278n47, 323, 335
Federal qualification, 27, 36, 172, 323. *See also* HMO Act of 1973, HMO Amendments; rating and, 174, 215; underwriting and, 138–39, 250
Fee-for-service plans, 245, 269–70; HMOs vs., 5, 61, 73–74, 94, 102, 259, 264, 266, 327, 336; prepaid groups vs., 27, 56
FEHBP. *See* Federal Employees Health Benefits Program
Financial Accounting Standards Board (FASB), 295, 314, 329, 333
First Interstate Bancorp Health Span, 316
Florida, HMO enrollment in, 38, 39–40

G

General Accounting Office (GAO), U.S., 63–65
Generic rating method. *See* Experience rating
GHAA. *See* Group Health Association of America
Group Health Association of America (GHAA), 27–28, 33, 75, 97, 100–

101, 147, 335; "1987 Survey of HMO Industry Trends," 145, 335
Group Health, Inc., 38, 262, 269
Group-model plans, 29–30, 32, 36, 38, 42, 103n5, 145, 310; as closed-panel plan, 56, 220, 310, 323, 325; cost-budget method and, 152, 155–57; favorable selection and, 254–55, 261–62, 264; prepaid group plans and, 48, 81, 336
Group-specific rating, 103–4n8, 122, 153, 185, 195, 256; adjusted community rating and, 78, 91, 199–203, 207–13, 230–32, 237, 239, 312; community rating by class and, 174–82, 184–85, 187, 189–91, 218–19; employers' preference for, 79–80; enrollees and, 220–22, 228–30; factors in, 175–78, 221–30; legislation for, 6, 100; premiums of, 177, 198, 214, 239; standard community rating vs., 220–21
"Guidance for Community Rating by Class," 178

H

Hackbarth, Glenn, 96–97
Hancock Insurance, 299
Hatch, Orrin, 101
Hawaii, HMOs in, 33
HCFA. *See* Health Care Financing Administration
Health care, 15, 36, 329; competition in market. *See* Competition; costs of, 5–7, 26, 58, 81, 119, 128–33, 158–59, 247, 249; market, changes in, 3, 13–15, 33, 76–79, 97, 102, 262, 295, 309–10; rationing of, 15, 18n16
Health Care Connection, 316
Health Care Financing Administration (HCFA), 6, 39, 90, 97, 120, 228–29, 231, 264; Office of the Actu-

ary, 270, 273; Office in Department of Health and Human Services, 177; Office of Prepaid Health Care, 101, 323; payment rates of, 270–72, 323

Health insurance, 124–25, 138; group, 114–27, 136–37, 148, 218–19, 221–22; hybrid plans, 30, 34, 51; market, xviii, 12–13, 31–34, 114, 116–18, 174, 246–47; self-insured, 13, 50–51, 80, 95, 102, 120, 197, 315; uninsured, 15

Health Insurance Association of America, 329

Health Maintenance Organization Act of 1973, 3, 14, 28, 36, 48, 76, 94, 144, 251; background, 27–31; equal-dollar contributions and, 77–78, 91; limitations of, 75–76; premium rate setting under, 175–77, 199; requirements of, 27, 29–30, 71–72, 212

Health Maintenance Organization Act Amendments, 29, 146, 214, 255; 1981, 72, 146, 174. *See also* Community rating by class; 1986, 94; 1988, 70, 79, 103n7, 256; adjusted community rating under, 78, 89–90, 196, 199–206, 219; congressional testimony and action for, 89–92, 94–101; deductibles and physician services, 93–94; employer contributions, 91–93; flexibility of, xviii, 6, 147, 335; provisions of, 94–96; rating methods of, 90–91

Health Maintenance Organization Advisory Group. *See* Washington Business Group on Health (WBGH)

Health Maintenance Organization Assistance Act, 100

Health maintenance organizations (HMOs), xiv, 46–49. *See also* Fee-for-service plans; Blue Cross vs., 34, 49–51, 81, 84, 104n9, 114, 117, 138, 239, 250, 326; geographic markets, 32, 34, 72–73, 81, 148–49, 174, 257, 296, 327. *See also* Individual states; goals of, 49, 79, 266, 321; growth of, 13–15, 31–39, 54, 76–77, 79, 82, 255, 256, 296–307, 327, 330, 334–36; health insurance options vs., 49–51; history of, 25–44, 326. *See also* Prepaid group plans; hybrid plans, 30, 34, 51; management of, 94–95, 116, 150–53, 325–29; open-ended, 30, 33, 98, 209–13; PPOs vs., 5, 49–50, 81–82, 95, 102, 255; premium rate setting and, 5, 6, 71–75, 81–89, 101–3; selection bias and, 263–69, 315

Health Subcommittee on the House Ways and Means Committee, 62

Herbert, Michael, 96

Higgins, A. Foster, 333

Hospital Cost Containment Act of 1977, 17n5

House Committee on Energy and Commerce, 92, 96; Health and Environment Subcommittee, 96

Humphrey, Gordon, 101

Hybrid plans, 30, 34, 51

I

ICF study, 62, 63

Illinois, HMO enrollment in, 37, 39–40

Indemnity insurance plans, 50, 81, 95, 103, 114, 291, 299; HMOs vs., 80, 92, 103n4, 309, 313; managed care and, 14, 33, 197, 255, 336; premiums of, xix, 32, 72–74, 102, 104–5nn8–9, 319; rating and, 132, 169, 265–66, 297, 299

Individual practice associations

(IPAs), 27, 32, 48, 82, 152, 227, 272, 311

Individual practice association— model plans, 29, 36, 39, 42, 59– 60, 103n5, 310, 322; adverse selection and, 261–62; capitation and, 150; community rating and, 145; cost-budget method and, 153; as open-panel plan, 297–99, 302, 330n10

Internal Revenue Service Code, 9, 241n1

InterStudy reports, 34, 334–35

IPAs. *See* Individual practice associations

J-L

Jackson-Beeck phenomenon, 255, 259, 261–63, 269, 275n17

JCAHO. *See* Joint Commission on the Accreditation of Healthcare Organizations

Joint Commission on the Accreditation of Healthcare Organizations (JCAHO), 75

Kaiser Permanente: adjusted community rating system, 41, 43, 206–13, 242n6; Foundation Health Plan, 28, 33, 37, 206; prepaid group practice program, 46–48

Kennedy, Edward, 11, 101, 195

Legislation. *See* National health policy; individual acts

Lent, Norman F., 101

Lincoln National, 299

Luft, Harold, 14, 48, 258, 260

M

Madigan, Edward R., 101

Managed health care. *See* Indemnity insurance plans

Management information systems (MIS), 52, 197, 239, 241, 302, 306, 328

Manual rating, 121, 179. *See also* Community rating by class

Maryland, HMO enrollment in, 29

Massachusetts, HMO enrollment in, 29, 32, 33, 37, 39–40

Mathematica Policy Research, 259, 262

Matsunaga, Spark M., 101

Maxicare, 3, 34, 37, 38, 335

Medicaid, 4, 7, 10, 57, 61, 118, 173, 178, 264–65; Capitation Demonstration Evaluation, 260

Medicare, 57, 120, 178, 231; capitation and, 7; coverage selection, 11, 261–62; eligibility, 174, 259, 264– 65; risk contracts, 4, 7–8, 10, 39, 61, 90, 118, 199–200, 213, 227, 267, 269–73, 323, 335–36; underwriting and, 138; voucher proposal, 11

Medicare Catastrophic Act, 8–9

Metropolitan Life Insurance, 13

Michigan, HMO enrollment in, 28, 33, 37, 39–40

Minnesota, HMO enrollment in, 28, 32, 33, 37, 38, 40

MIS. *See* Management information systems

Missouri, HMOs in, 28

N

National Advisory Commission of Health Manpower, 26–27

National Committee for Quality Assurance, 75

National Evaluation of the Medicare Competition Demonstrations, 259, 262

National health policy, 3–4, 6–7, 15,

31; congressional proposals, 10–11, 27, 60–61; federal initiatives, 7–10

Network models, 38, 40, 42, 44, 60, 150, 153, 220, 310; as open-panel plan, 299, 305

New Jersey, HMOs in, 37

New York, HMOs in, 32, 33, 37, 39–40

Nixon administration, 25, 27

O

Office of the Actuary. *See* Health Care Financing Administration

Office of Health Maintenance Organizations (OHMO), 146

Office of Personnel Management (OPM), U.S., 120, 187, 242n7, 323, 335

Office of Prepaid Health Care. *See* Health Care Financing Administration

Ohio, HMOs in, 28, 33, 38, 39–40

Oklahoma, HMOs in, 28

Omnibus Budget Reconciliation Act of 1986, 60–61

Open-panel models. *See* Network models; Individual practice associations

OPM. *See* Office of Personnel Management

Opt-out (wrap around) plans, 310–11, 315, 318, 321–22

Oregon, HMOs in, 28, 32, 33, 37, 40, 316

P

Pennsylvania, HMO enrollment in, 28, 37, 39–40

Peres, Alan, 97, 99–100

PGPs. *See* Prepaid group practices

Physicians, 32, 51–52, 150; incentive payments of, 10, 61–65, 325; out-of-plan, 89, 94, 98, 311; practice patterns of, 60, 73, 152, 325; relationship with HMOs, 303–4, 306, 322–23, 327; risk sharing. *See* Risk sharing, with providers; services, 93–94

Point-of-service plans. *See* Benefit programs, multiple-option

Preferred provider organizations (PPOs), 261, 297–98, 301, 336; competition and, 12, 30, 33, 117, 197; development of, 296, 299, 311; HMOs vs., 5, 49–50, 81–82, 95, 102, 255

Premium rate setting, 151, 196–98. *See also* Adjusted community rating, Community rating, Experience rating, Group-specific rating; community rating by class and, 174–78; employers' perspective, xviii, 5, 69–71, 101–2, 327; flexibility in, 89; HMOs and, 5, 6, 71–75, 81–89, 101–3; selection bias and, 249–50, 268

Premium rates, 32, 145, 175, 182, 263, 313, 317; community rating and, 73–74, 83–87, 89; composite, 176, 189; cost per member and, 164–69; defined, 115; development of, 150, 152–53, 164, 179–82; employers and, 88, 249, 300; fairness in, 118–19, 205, 256–57, 314; group health and, 118; increases in, 102, 312–13, 330n5, 333; requirements of, xviii, 101–2, 122; risk adjusted, 260–61; schedules, 148, 154, 165; self-supporting, 119; structures, 148–49, 151, 165, 173, 189

Prepaid group practice (PGP) plans, 26–27, 144–45, 148, 336; as basis for HMOs, 28–32, 45–48, 196, 239, 318

Primary care swing plans, 310
Prospective payment system (PPS), 8
Provider reimbursement, 54–55, 152–53, 307, 323, 328
Public Health Service Act (Title XIII), 96–98, 99

R

Rating, 74, 217. *See also* Adjusted community rating, Community rating, Community rating by class, Underwriting, community; data analysis and, 232–41, 312; equity in, 17, 118, 120, 205–6, 238; experience. *See* Experience rating; fixed structures, 87, 115, 118, 146, 148, 153–54, 164–65, 238; group-specific. *See* Group-specific rating; HMOs and, 87–88; implementation of, 122, 198; increases in, 232–33; manual. *See* Manual rating; objectives/requirements of, 116–20, 197–98, 238–41; prospective. *See* Adjusted community rating; strategies for, 119–20, 135–37, 205, 232–41, 306–7, 312–13, 325–29; systems, 115, 116–23, 189–90, 198
Reagan administration, xviii, 6–7, 88, 101
Recompositing, 146, 148, 169, 170–71, 184, 257
Regression to the mean, 103, 252, 259, 262–64, 267, 271
Relative experience ratio (RER), 224–28
Request for proposal (RFP). *See* Employers
RER. *See* Relative experience ratio
Retirees, coverage, 314, 319, 333–34
Risk classes, 165, 178–79, 190, 249
Risk contracts, 4, 39, 49, 58–63, 162, 170, 174, 269–73

Risk sharing, 56, 220, 313, 327; employer preferences, 80; models of, 58–64; with providers, 61–64, 150–52, 159, 230, 307, 325
Ross-Loos Medical Foundation, 28, 143

S

Selection bias, 247–51, 318, 322, 336. *See also* Adverse selection, Skimming; analysis of, 251–52; causes of, 261–63; measurement, 102, 263, 268; Medicare risk contracts and, 269–73; overview, 258–73; premium rate setting and, 249–50; and relationship to HMOs, 263–69, 315; results of, 245–46
Senate Committee on Labor and Human Resources, 100–101
Shadow pricing, 72–73, 80, 91, 102
Simon, Paul, 101
Sixth Omnibus Budget Reconciliation Act (SOBRA), 10
Skimming, 221, 246, 264, 266; allegations of, 72–73, 80, 87, 253–54, 313–14, 318–19, 322; favorable selection, 254–57, 261, 265–66, 269
SOBRA. *See* Sixth Omnibus Budget Reconciliation Act
Social Security Act, 95
Sole-sourcing, 197, 318, 334
Staff-model plans: closed-panel plan as, 310, 321, 325; competition and, 36, 82; cost-budget method and, 153–55, 156–57; costs per case and, 227–28; favorable selection and, 261–62, 264; prepaid group plans and, 48, 336
Stark, Fortney, 62
Stop-loss adjustments, 60, 209–10, 213
Strategic planning, 313, 329. *See also* Competitive strategies